Communication within Animal Cells

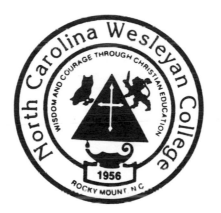

Communication within Animal Cells

Greg J. Barritt

Reader in Medical Biochemistry,
School of Medicine, Flinders University

OXFORD   NEW YORK   MELBOURNE   TOKYO
OXFORD UNIVERSITY PRESS

Oxford University Press, Walton Street, Oxford OX2 6DP

Oxford New York Toronto
Delhi Bombay Calcutta Madras Karachi
Kuala Lumpur Singapore Hong Kong Tokyo
Nairobi Dar es Salaam Cape Town
Melbourne Auckland Madrid
and associated companies in
Berlin Ibadan

Oxford is a trade mark of Oxford University Press

Published in the United States by
Oxford University Press Inc., New York

© Greg J. Barritt 1992

First published 1992
Reprinted 1994

A catalogue record for this book is
available from the British Library

Library of Congress Cataloging in Publication Data
(Data available)

ISBN 0 19 854727 7 (Hbk)
ISBN 0 19 854726 9 (Pbk)

Printed by Butler & Tanner Ltd, Frome, Somerset

Preface

The idea of writing this book occurred several years ago at a time when there were very rapid developments in knowledge of the intracellular functions of the inositol polyphosphates and Ca^{2+} and of the structures of the plasma-membrane receptors. Although many excellent reviews have been published on specific elements of the intracellular signalling systems, such as the inositol polyphosphates and subgroups of protein kinases, there are few works which deal with the concept of intracellular communication as a whole. A major objective of this book is to attempt to provide an overall framework in which to view the present knowledge of the pathways of intracellular communication and future advances in this knowledge. Another major objective is to attempt to place in perspective the detailed knowledge of the different components comprising the network of signals which transfer information from one part of a cell to another.

This book is a description of just one of a number of important areas of knowledge which are encompassed in the discipline known as cell biology. The information presented builds on a basic knowledge of biochemistry and cell biology. It is intended that the book will be used by final year undergraduate science students, medical and pharmacology students in the early or middle years of their courses, students undertaking an honours science degree, and by postgraduate students and more senior scientists who are studying topics in intracellular communication or who wish to obtain a broad perspective of the field.

It has sometimes been difficult to define what is meant by the term 'intracellular communication'. There are many well established pathways of communication such as the mobile intracellular messengers and protein kinases. However, there are other intracellular processes which might also be considered to transfer information within the cell, but which primarily function to maintain the structure and metabolic functions of the cell. These processes include the metabolic pathways themselves and the movement of proteins and membrane vesicles within the cell. The limitations inherent in the conventional treatment of the pathways of intracellular communication presented here are realized. However, it is hoped that the present work will provide a framework for a more imaginative treatment in the future.

The first chapter presents a view of the nature of the processes of intracellular communication and describes the major pathways by which information is transmitted from one part of a cell to another. In the second chapter an attempt has been made to emphasize the importance of the knowledge of cell structure in considering the pathways and processes of intracellular communication, constraints on the spatial distribution of components of these pathways, and the roles of the movement of proteins, membrane vesicles, and organelles in transferring information within cells. This chapter was particularly difficult to write because knowledge of the spatial aspects of pathways of intracellular communication has only recently begun to evolve.

The properties of the various components of the pathways of intracellular communication are examined in Chapters 3 to 10 beginning with the plasma-membrane receptors and the oligomeric GTP-binding regulatory proteins (Chapter 3) and concluding with the sequence-specific DNA-binding proteins of the nucleus (Chapter 10). Pathways present in the cytoplasmic space are divided into the protein kinases (Chapter 4), cyclic nucleotides (Chapter 5), inositol polyphosphates and diacylglycerols (Chapter 6), calcium (Chapter 7), and other metabolites, including those involved in metabolic regulation (Chapter 8). In Chapter 9 the arachidonic acid metabolites are considered. Although these act principally as extracellular messengers, they can readily move between extra- and intracellular spaces and some may act as true intracellular messengers.

Chapter 11 describes the known oncogenes, the importance of the proteins encoded by the normal counterparts of oncogenes, how oncogenic proteins differ in structure and function from their normal counterparts, and the information that knowledge of the actions of the oncogenic proteins has provided about pathways of intracellular communication. Recent advances in knowledge of the functions of the normal forms of oncogenic proteins have meant that many of these proteins can now be discussed in terms of their role in the normal processes of intracellular communication. In Chapter 12 some of the interactions between pathways of intracellular communication are described and an attempt is made to consider pathways in their entirety, using the stimulation of cell growth as an example.

Within each chapter, some key references have been cited. These have been chosen in order to identify important experiments which have contributed to the body of knowledge on intracellular communication. However, it has been necessary to be selective in the choice of references since this area of knowledge is large and the length of the book finite.

Our present knowledge of some aspects of the systems of intracellular communication, for example the protein–tyrosine kinases, sequence-specific DNA-binding proteins, the network of proteins which control the transcription of DNA, and spatial aspects of pathways of intracellular communication is only a partial view of the true picture. An attempt has been made to describe the principles of the pathways of intracellular communication and the actions of their component parts while giving some indication of the interesting questions still to be answered. The line between established knowledge and speculation has not always been easy to draw, especially where close inspection of present knowledge, for example of the mechanism of activation of protein kinase C, reveals many uncertainties. It has been difficult to reach a good balance between a clear statement of the overall theme and the need to present the processes under consideration in a sufficiently challenging manner. These problems are compounded by the very rapid rate of expansion of knowledge that is occurring at present.

Adelaide   G.J.B.
August 1991

Acknowledgements

I would like to thank the following scientists for their written comments and advice used in the preparation of this book.

Chapter 1   Dr Peter R. Dunkley, The University of Newcastle, New South Wales
Dr Greg B. Ralston, The University of Sydney, New South Wales

Chapter 2   Dr Greg B. Ralston, The University of Sydney, New South Wales
Professor Colin J. Masters, Griffith University, Queensland
Professor George E. Rogers, The University of Adelaide, South Australia
Dr Brian K. May, The University of Adelaide, South Australia

Chapter 3   Professor Jim W. Goding, Monash University, Victoria

Chapter 4   Dr Peter R. Dunkley, The University of Newcastle, New South Wales
Dr Bruce E. Kemp, St. Vincent's Institute of Medical Research, Victoria

Chapter 5   Professor Michael G. Clark, University of Tasmania, Tasmania

Chapter 6   Dr Majorie E. Dunlop, The University of Melbourne, Victoria

Chapter 7   Dr Fyfe L. Bygrave, The Australian National University, Australian Capital Territory

Chapter 8   Dr Dallas G. Clark, CSIRO Division of Human Nutrition, South Australia
Dr Majorie E. Dunlop, The University of Melbourne, Victoria
Dr Lance Macaulay, The University of Melbourne, Victoria
Dr Anthony M. Edwards, Flinders Medical Centre, South Australia

Chapter 9   Professor Nick H. Hunt, The University of Sydney, New South Wales

Chapter 10   Dr Peter J. MacKinnon, The University of Adelaide, South Australia
Dr Michael J. Bawden, The University of Adelaide, South Australia

Chapter 11   Professor Anthony W. Burgess, Ludwig Institute for Cancer Research, Royal Melbourne Hospital, Victoria
Dr David R. Turner, Flinders University, South Australia

Chapter 12   Dr Bernard P. Hughes, Flinders University, South Australia

My thanks are also due to Professor Michael A. Denborough, The Australian National University, Australian Capital Territory, for reading the complete manuscript; to Ms Diana Tanevski for typing the manuscript; to Ms Margaret Menadue, Ms Heather Halls; Ms Kathie M. Hurst and Ms Annabel E. Barritt for background research; to Professor Michael N. Berry for providing a stimulating environment for research and teaching; and to Lenore, Annabel, and Joe Barritt for their constant support without which the preparation of this book would not have been possible.

Credits

Permission granted by authors and publishers to adapt material for the preparation of figures is gratefully acknowledged; sources are accredited in the appropriate figure legends. Material published by the following publishers was used with permission in preparation of the following figures: **Fig. 1.2,** Lea & Febiger, Philadelphia, U.S.A. © 1987; **Fig. 1.3,** Raven Press, New York, U.S.A. © 1984; **Fig. 1.4,** Macmillan Magazines Ltd., Basingstoke, United Kingdom © 1987; **Fig. 1.10,** IRL Press Ltd., Eynsham, United Kingdom © 1986; **Fig. 2.1,** W.B. Saunders Company, Philadelphia, U.S.A. © 1970; **Fig. 2.4,** Springer-Verlag, Heidelberg, Germany © 1979; **Fig. 2.5,** Springer-Verlag, Heidelberg, Germany © 1986; **Fig. 2.10,** Elsevier Science Publishers B.V. (Biomedical Division), Amsterdam, The Netherlands © 1989; **Fig. 2.11,** Scientific American Inc., New York, U.S.A © 1981; **Fig. 2.14,** Academic Press Inc., London, United Kingdom © 1983; **Fig. 3.3,** Elsevier Science Publishers B.V. (Biomedical Division), Amsterdam, The Netherlands © 1985; **Fig. 3.4,** Cambridge University Press, Cambridge, United Kingdom © 1985; **Fig. 3.5,** Macmillan Magazines Ltd., Basingstoke, United Kingdom © 1985; **Figs 3.6 and 3.7,** Elsevier Science Publishers B.V. (Biomedical Division), Amsterdam, The Netherlands © 1985; **Fig. 3.12,** The American Society of Clinical Investigation, New York, U.S.A. © 1979; **Fig. 3.22,** Macmillan Magazines Ltd., Basingstoke, United Kingdom © 1987; **Fig. 3.23,** American Association for the Advancement of Science, Washington DC, U.S.A. © 1988; **Fig. 4.3,** Springer-Verlag, Heidelberg, Germany © 1980; **Fig. 4.9,** Macmillan Magazines Ltd., Basingstoke, United Kingdom © 1982; **Figs 4.10 and 4.11,** American Society of Biological Chemists Inc., Bethesda, U.S.A. © 1975 and 1989, respectively; **Fig. 4.12,** Springer-Verlag, Heidelberg, Germany © 1980; **Figs 4.18, 5.3, 5.8 and 5.10,** American Society of Biological Chemists Inc., Bethesda, U.S.A. © 1987, 1971, 1957 and 1987, respectively; **Figs 5.14, 5.15 and 5.18,** The Biochemical Journal, London, United Kingdom © 1987; **Fig. 5.20,** Raven Press, New York, U.S.A. © 1984; **Fig. 5.23,** Academic Press Inc., London, United Kingdom © 1980; **Fig. 5.26,** Elsevier Science Publishers B.V. (Biomedical Division), Amsterdam, The Netherlands © 1985; **Figs 5.30, 6.4 and 6.6,** American Society of Biological Chemists Inc., Bethesda, U.S.A. © 1986, 1953 and 1987, respectively; **Fig. 6.7,** The Biochemical Journal, London, United Kingdom © 1983; **Fig. 6.11,** The Rockefeller University Press, New York, U.S.A. © 1978; **Fig. 6.14,** American Society of Biological Chemists Inc., Bethesda, U.S.A. © 1984; **Fig. 6.15,** Cell Press, Cambridge, U.S.A. © 1986; **Fig. 6.20,** The Biochemical Journal, London, United Kingdom © 1979; **Fig. 6.21,** American Society of Biological Chemists Inc., Bethesda, U.S.A. © 1985; **Fig. 6.23,** Macmillan Magazines Ltd., Basingstoke, United Kingdom © 1987; **Fig. 6.25,** The American Society of Clinical Investigation, New York, U.S.A. © 1979; and American Society of Biological Chemists Inc., Bethesda, U.S.A. © 1985; **Fig. 6.28,** American Society of Biological Chemists Inc., Bethesda, U.S.A. © 1986; **Fig. 6.29,** Macmillan Magazines Ltd., Basingstoke, United Kingdom © 1983; **Figs 6.30 and 6.31,**

Contents

Abbreviations

ANP	atrial natriuretic peptide
$[Ca^{2+}]_i$	intracellular free Ca^{2+} concentration
CSF	colony-stimulating factor
DNA-binding protein	sequence-specific DNA-binding protein
EDRF	endothelium-derived relaxing factor
EGF	epidermal growth factor
G protein	oligomeric GTP-binding regulatory protein
G_s	G protein which activates adenylate cyclase
G_i	G protein which inhibits adenylate cyclase
G_t	transducin
G_o	'other' G protein
HLH	helix–loop–helix
Ins 1,4,5 P_3	inositol 1,4,5-trisphosphate
LTD_4	leukotriene D_4
NGF	nerve growth factor
PDGF	platelet-derived growth factor
PGE_1	prostaglandin E_1
PGE_2	prostaglandin E_2
PGI_2	prostaglandin I_2 (prostacyclin)
PtdIns	phosphatidylinositol
PtdIns 4 P	phosphatidylinositol 4-phosphate
PtdIns 4,5 P_2	phosphatidylinositol 4,5-bisphosphate
TXA_2	thromboxane A_2

1 Networks of extracellular and intracellular signals

1.1 The functions of animal cells and the need for intracellular communication

One view of the function of an animal cell is that each type of cell within a multicellular organism makes a small but essential contribution to the existence of the whole organism. This contribution is not only important to the function of the organism as it exists in the present but, together with the DNA and structural components of the cell, also provides the framework which permits evolution of the organism. Some examples of the types of contribution made by individual animal cells to multicellular organisms are listed in Table 1.1. Most cells in a multi

cellular organism perform only a limited range of functions.

An animal cell might further be viewed as being inserted into a network of extracellular signals which direct the function of the cell. This idea is represented in Fig. 1.1. In this model, the cell is shown as a vehicle by which the information contained in the set of extracellular signals is translated into a set of specific responses. In single animal cells, such as the amoeba, the multiple extracellular signals are derived solely from the external environment. The multiple responses of the cell contribute to the existence of the individual cell and to the animal of which it is a part.

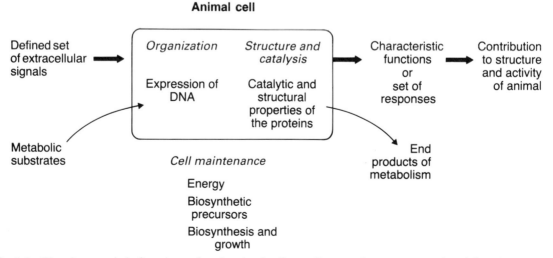

Fig. 1.1 The characteristic functions of each animal cell contribute to the structure and activity of the whole animal. These functions are usually under the control of a defined set of extracellular signals. Together with the reactions required to maintain the structure and chemical components of the cell, expression of the characteristic cell functions requires metabolic substrates.

A number of properties define each type of animal cell. These are the macromolecular structure (Fig. 1.2) which includes intracellular membranes and the cytoskeleton, the chemical pathways of metabolism, and the spatial arrangement of these pathways. The chemical pathways include those involved in the provision of energy and biosynthetic precursors, in growth and cell division, in movement of the cytoskeleton, and in the activities of specialized metabolic pathways. This basic framework of physical and chemical structures allows the cell to perform a specific set of functions. Much of the energy utilized by each cell is required for maintenance of this basic framework.

The specific set of functions performed by each animal cell and the maintenance of basic cell structure require co-ordination of the structures and chemical reactions. This co-ordination is achieved by a variety of lines of intracellular communication which respond to a network of extracellular signals.

1.2   The nature of the network of extracellular signals

There is a large number of different types of external signal to which an animal cell can be exposed. These signals include hormones,

Table 1.1   *Examples of the activities of animal cells which contribute to the survival of the animal, and some of the extracellular signals which direct these activities*

Activity	Cell	Extracellular signals
Structure		
Mineralization of bone	Osteoblast	Calcitonin, parathyroid hormone
Formation of collagen		
Movement		
Transport of blood	Heart muscle	Hormones
Digestion	Smooth muscle	Neurotransmitters, peptides
Mobility of animal	Skeletal muscle	Neurotransmitters
Supply of metabolites		
Blood glucose	Liver cells	Glucagon, insulin, glucocorticoids
Fatty acids	White adipocytes	Glucagon
O_2	Alveola cells (lung)	O_2 concentration
Perception of environment		
Nerve impulse to brain	Rod cells	Light
Defence		
Synthesis of antibodies	Lymphocytes	Cytokines
Formation of blood clot	Platelets	Thrombin, collagen
Synthesis of acute phase proteins	Liver	Cytokines
Growth		
Fertilization	Egg	Spermatozoa
Mitosis	Most cells	Growth factors, hormones
Synthesis of growth factors	Most cells	Growth factors, hormones
Communication		
Nerve transmission	Nerve cells	Neurotransmitters
Secretion of neurotransmitters	Nerve cells	Depolarization
Secretion of hormones	Endocrine cells	Hormones, neurotransmitters
Fluid balance		
Secretion of fluid and ions	Secretory cells	Hormones, neurotransmitters

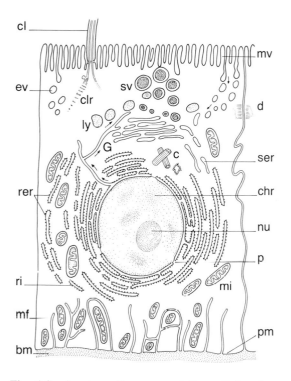

Fig. 1.2 A schematic representation of the ultra-structure of an animal cell. The structures shown are the rough (granular) endoplasmic reticulum (rer), the smooth (agranular) endoplasmic reticulum (ser), the basal membrane (bm), the centriole (c), the chromosomes (chr), a cilium (cl), a cilial root (clr), a desmosome (d), the Golgi complex (G), the lysosomes (ly), membrane folds (mf), mitochondria (mi), microvilli (mv), the nucleolus (nu), a pore in the nuclear membrane (p), plasma membrane (pm), endocytotic vesicles (ev), ribosomes (ri), and secretory vesicles (sv). From De Robertis and De Robertis (1987).

Table 1.2 *The major types of extracellular signals which regulate the activity of animal cells*

Hormones (endocrine system)
    Steroid hormones
    Thyroid hormones
    Proteins (e.g. insulin)
    Polypeptides
    Small organic molecules (e.g. adrenalin)

Neurotransmitters (synaptic space)
    Acetylcholine
    Amines
    Peptides
    Amino acids

Local hormones (intercellular space or restricted region of blood)
    Peptide growth factors
    Metabolites of arachidonic acid
    Cytokines

Morphogens
    Retinoic acid

Metabolites
    Glucose
    Amino acids
    Fatty acids

Environmental elements
    Light
    Odour
    Toxins
    Drugs

Extracellular structures
    Extracellular matrix
    Surfaces of neighbouring cells

Foreign proteins and cells
    Antigens
    Bacteria
    Viruses

Metabolic and electrical signals which move through gap junctions

---

neurotransmitters, local hormones, morphogens, metabolites, extracellular structures such as the extracellular matrix, other natural chemicals in the cell environment, foreign chemicals, and light (Table 1.2). The major types of external signals are hormones, local hormones, neurotransmitters, and metabolites. The local hormones include growth factors, cytokines, metabolites of arachidonic acid, and may also include phospholipids released from cells.

Almost all the extracellular signals consist of a change in the concentration of a given type of molecule in the environment of the cell. Each cell is exposed to a variety of extracellular signals. Only some of these are likely to be active at any given time. For example, a liver cell is exposed constantly to hormones which control intermediary metabolism but will be exposed to growth factors chiefly during the early development of the animal, or if the liver is damaged.

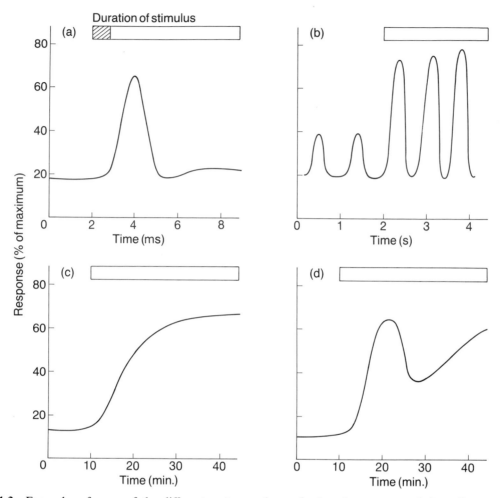

Fig. 1.3 Examples of some of the different patterns observed when the response of the cell to an agonist is measured as a function of time. The duration of the stimulus is indicated by the bar above each part. (a) A transient response to either a brief (shaded bar) or a prolonged (open bar) stimulus. An example of a response to a brief stimulus is the release of neurotransmitter or the contraction of muscle fibres stimulated by membrane depolarization. An example of a response to a prolonged stimulus is the release of histamine from mast cells. (b) An increase in the amplitude of a pre-existing periodic response during a sustained stimulus (open bar). For example, the response of heart muscle cells to adrenalin. (c) A sustained response to a sustained extracellular signal (open bar). For example, the production of aldosterone from adrenal glomerulosa cells stimulated by angiotensin II. (d) A biphasic response to a sustained extracellular signal (open bar). For example, the secretion of insulin from beta cells of the pancreas stimulated by glucose. From Rasmussen et al. (1984).

There are considerable differences in the time during which an extracellular signal is maintained, in the rate at which cells respond to an extracellular signal, and in the length of time that the response is maintained. Some examples of differences in the time of onset and time-courses for responses are shown in Fig. 1.3. Nerve cells respond very rapidly to a brief increase in the concentration of a neurotransmitter at the pre-synaptic terminus with depolarization of the plasma membrane and the release of neurotransmitter at the post-synaptic termi-

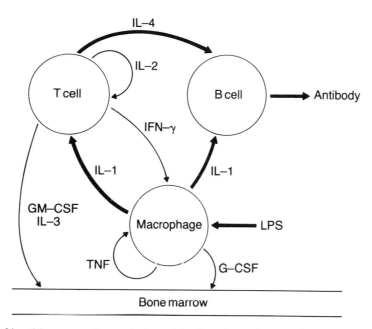

Fig. 1.4 The role of local hormones in regulation of the functions of macrophages and T and B lymphocytes (T and B cells). Lipopolysaccharide (LPS) derived from bacteria stimulates the release of interleukin-1 (IL-1), tumour necrosis factor (TNF) and granulocyte colony-stimulating factor (G-CSF) from macrophages. IL-1 together with interleukin-4 (IL-4) stimulates the production of antibody by B cells (bold arrows) with the help of T cells. TNF and IL-2 act in an autocrine manner on macrophages and T cells, respectively. The interleukins (IL-1, Il-2, Il-3, and Il-4), G-CSF, granulocyte macrophage CSF (GM-CSF), TNF and interferon-γ (IFN-γ) are all polypeptides. From Old (1987).

nus. On the other hand, the prolonged exposure of skin fibroblasts to an increased concentration of growth factor causes a stimulation of growth and cell division which is slow in onset and is maintained for a long period of time. In contrast to stimulation of the nerve cell, which involves the activation of pre-existing enzymes, the stimulation of cell growth involves the synthesis of new enzymes and proteins.

Hormones generally travel long distances, in the blood stream of an animal, between the organ of secretion and the target organ. By contrast, the distances travelled by neurotransmitters and local hormones are much shorter. For example, the cytokines and other local hormones which regulate the function of T and B lymphocytes (Fig. 1.4) are confined to the intercellular space or to a restricted region of a tissue.

Some local hormones, for example the inter-

leukins and metabolites of arachidonic acid, act on the same cell from which the local hormone is secreted as well as acting on neighbouring cells. The action of a local hormone on the cell in which it is produced is called an autocoid action. An example is the role of thromboxane A_2 in the regulation of platelet aggregation. The release of thromboxane A_2 by a given platelet increases the aggregation potential of that platelet as well as that of neighbouring platelets.

1.3 Reception of extracellular signals

There are three main mechanisms by which external signals are received by animal cells. These are: receptors located on the external surface of the plasma membrane, sequence-specific DNA-binding receptor proteins located in the cytoplasmic space, and certain enzymes in path-

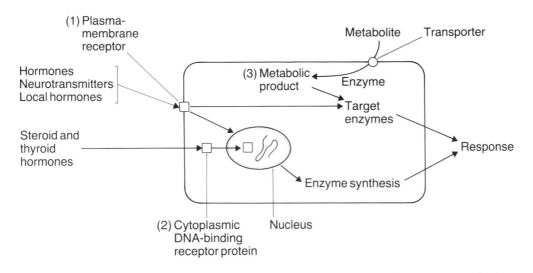

Fig. 1.5 Animal cells recognize extracellular signals through (1) plasma-membrane receptors for hormones, neurotransmitters, and local hormones, such as cytokines, (2) sequence-specific DNA-binding receptor proteins for hormones or morphogens which are located in the cytoplasmic space, and (3) certain enzymes in the cytoplasmic space which metabolize extracellular metabolites.

ways of intermediary metabolism (Fig. 1.5). The majority of extracellular signals are received by plasma membrane receptors.

In some cells extracellular signals are also received through gap junctions. The anatomical structure of such a junction is shown in Fig. 1.6. An example of this type of extracellular signal are the electrical signals which are transmitted from the sarcolemma of one myocardial muscle cell to the sarcolemma of adjacent cells through the gap junctions. These junctions also permit the controlled movement of metabolites and ions from one cell to another.

Although most extracellular metabolites which reach cells are substrates for the reactions of intermediary metabolism, there are some instances in which a metabolite present in the extracelluar medium acts as an external signal in a manner similar to a hormone. These extra-cellular signals are initially received by an enzyme in the cytoplasmic space (Fig. 1.5). One or more intracellular metabolic products of the reaction catalysed by this enzyme initiates a set of specific cell responses by altering the concen-

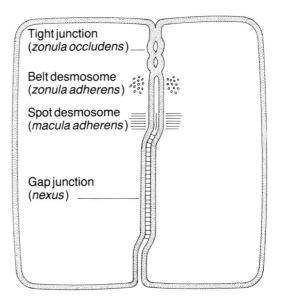

Fig. 1.6 In cells which are part of the network of cells in a tissue, signals from neighbouring cells can be received through the gap junctions. These are composed of junctional channels which allow the passage of metabolites and ions. The belt desmosomes (*zonula adherens*) and spot desmosomes (*macula adherens*) are responsible for mechanical adhesion between cells. In heart muscle and in a number of other cells, the gap junctions permit electrical coupling between cells.

trations of mobile intracellular messengers. An example of this type of signal is the stimulation, by glucose and other metabolites, of insulin secretion from β-cells of the pancreas. Although the mechanism is not yet fully understood, it seems that the initial signal for insulin release is the metabolism of glucose by the β-cell. In this case the metabolic pathway acts as a sensor and the metabolic flux amplifies the initial signal.

1.4 The major pathways of intracellular communication

The major pathways by which information is transferred within cells are summarized in Table 1.3. These have been divided into pathways which primarily co-ordinate maintenance functions of the cell and pathways which primarily

Table 1.3 *Major pathways of communication within animal cells*

Co-ordination of maintenance functions of the cell
   Regulation of transcription of selected genes
   Transport of metabolites and ions across
     intracellular membranes
   Regulation of metabolic pathways by effector
     metabolites
   Movement of proteins within directed pathways

Transfer of information contained in extracellular signals which induce cellular responses
   Interaction of receptors with GTP-binding
     regulatory proteins at the plasma membrane
   Movement of intracellular messengers within the
     lipid bilayer
   Movement of intracellular messengers and
     metabolites within the cytoplasmic and
     organelle spaces
   Movement of lipid-soluble hormones and
     morphogens from the extracellular space to the
     nucleus
   Movement of DNA-binding receptor proteins
     from the cytoplasmic space to the nucleus
   Interaction and movement between protein
     kinases and phosphoprotein phosphatases
   Synthesis and movement of specific enzymes and
     proteins, and the reactions catalysed by these
     proteins

---

transfer information contained in extracellular signals.

The pathways of intracellular communication used when a cell responds to extracellular signals might be considered as being superimposed on those pathways of communication involved in the control of maintenance functions of the cell. Although each of the mechanisms listed in Table 1.3 is essential to the function of a given cell, it is likely that most information flows through diffusible intracellular messengers in the cytoplasmic space, through the protein kinase network, and through the actions of newly synthesized proteins. Before describing in more detail each of the major pathways of intracellular communication listed in Table 1.3, some stepping-stones in the processes by which these pathways were discovered will be considered.

1.5 Some landmarks in the discovery of the pathways of intracellular communication

Knowledge of the pathways of intracellular communication has evolved during a period of more than a century. The first major development was the accumulation of a large body of information on the nature and physical structure of cells. This began with the first microscopic examination of the external forms of cells by Robert Hooke in 1655 and culminated in the deductions about cell structure which were made in the late 19th century and in the first half of the 20th century. From about 1930 onwards, these observations of the physical structure of cells were accompanied by elucidation of the chemical structures of metabolites such as glucose and ATP, and of the nature of the different metabolic pathways and some of the intermediates in these pathways.

Two important areas of further knowledge developed between 1940 and 1970. One was the elucidation of the chemical structures of biological macromolecules, including DNA, RNA, proteins, phospholipids, and complex carbo-hydrates, and the development of knowledge of the pathways for the synthesis of these macro-molecules. An important component of this knowledge was the elucidation of the genetic code. The second area was knowledge of the mechanisms by which enzymes catalyse chemical reactions, and development of the concept that flux through metabolic pathways is closely regu-lated. This area included the discoveries of feedback-control systems in metabolic path-ways, and of allosteric enzymes and allosteric effectors.

The growth of knowledge of the structure and function of individual cells was accompanied by discovery of the extracellular pathways by which information is transmitted between different cells and different tissues. Two fundamental steps in the development of the knowledge of the processes by which cells communicate with each other were the elucidation of the nature and function of the nervous system and the dis-covery of hormones. The discovery of insulin in 1921 laid the foundation for the concept that hormones are specific chemicals which are sec-reted by one type of cell in an animal and act on various target cells (Banting and Best 1922). Investigation of the mechanisms of action of hormones, neurotransmitters, and drugs led to the pharmacological concept that it is receptors located on or within a cell which receive extracel-lular chemical signals. It was considered that these receptors may be present either on the cell surface or within the cytoplasmic space.

In about 1955 investigations of the regulation of cellular metabolism and of the mechanism of action of hormones on target cells converged. At that time, Sutherland and his colleagues were studying the mechanisms by which adrenalin and glucagon stimulate glycogenolysis in liver cells. Their experiments led to the discovery of cyclic AMP (Rall *et al.* 1957). This cyclic nucleo-tide was viewed as a molecule which conveys information through the cytoplasmic space from a hormone receptor to a given target enzyme in a metabolic pathway. Since the hormones, which are responsible for carrying information to cells through the bloodstream, had been con-sidered as first messengers, cyclic AMP was de-scribed as a second messenger. Later the concept of second messengers was found to apply to other diffusible molecules.

The principle behind second-messenger func-tion had been observed much earlier than the discovery of cyclic AMP in a slightly different form—that is, the function of intracellular Ca^{2+} in the stimulation of contraction in skeletal muscle cells. The experiments of Heilbrunn (1940) and Heilbrunn and Wiercinski (1947) pro-vided the first direct indication that Ca^{2+} stimu-lates contraction of myofibrils. These and many other experiments led to the proposal that in muscle cells, Ca^{2+} acts as a coupling factor which links depolarization of the sarcolemma to the contraction of myofibrils. Transient changes in the concentration of free Ca^{2+} in the myoplasm were first observed experimentally by Jobsis and O'Connor (1966) and by Ridgway and Ashley (1967).

The next stage in the elucidation of the intra-cellular functions of cyclic AMP and Ca^{2+} was the discovery of the mechanisms by which these molecules exert their effects on target enzymes or proteins. The protein complex troponin was discovered in 1965 by Ebashi and Kodama. The troponin complex contains troponin C which binds Ca^{2+} and, through its interaction with actin and myosin, allows Ca^{2+} to activate con-traction of the myofibrils in muscle cells. Twenty years later, calmodulin, a Ca^{2+}-binding protein which mediates many of the actions of Ca^{2+} in the cytoplasmic space, was identified (Cheung 1970).

Cyclic AMP-dependent protein kinase, the enzyme which mediates the effects of cyclic AMP on target enzymes, was described in 1968 (Walsh *et al.* 1968) soon after the discovery of cyclic AMP. Not only did the discovery of this enzyme establish the mechanism of action of cyclic AMP but it also laid the foundation for future elucidation of the nature of the extensive network of protein kinases in animal cells.

At about the same time as the mechanism of action of cyclic AMP was elucidated, an important observation was made on the nature of the process by which agonists stimulate the synthesis of this cyclic nucleotide. This was the discovery of the GTP-binding regulatory protein which couples agonist–receptor complexes to adenylate cyclases (Rodbell *et al.* 1971).

Investigations conducted during the past 15 years have built on the general principles provided by the discovery of the intracellular messenger functions of cyclic AMP and the role of Ca^{2+} as a coupling factor in muscle cells. These have revealed more details of the molecular events involved in the processes by which cyclic AMP acts as an intracellular messenger.

Knowledge of the role of Ca^{2+} in muscle contraction contributed to the discovery that Ca^{2+} acts as an intracellular messenger in many other cells, in addition to its function in muscle and nerve cells. Although this point was established in the late 1970s, it was not clear then how extracellular agonists induce the release of Ca^{2+} from intracellular stores in non-excitable cells. A pointer to the answer to this question was provided by a much earlier observation by Hokin and Hokin in 1953. They showed that agonists stimulate phosphatidylinositol hydrolysis. Investigation of the link between phosphoinositide hydrolysis and Ca^{2+} movement (Michell 1975) led to the elucidation of the role of inositol 1,4,5-trisphosphate (Ins 1,4,5 P_3) in releasing Ca^{2+} from an intracellular store, probably the endoplasmic reticulum (Streb *et al.* 1983).

The earlier deductions that cyclic AMP and Ca^{2+} act as intracellular messengers paved the way for the discovery of the roles of cyclic GMP, diacylglycerol, Na^+, and H^+ as intracellular messengers. Likewise, knowledge of cyclic AMP-dependent protein kinase encouraged the search for a number of other protein kinases, including (Ca^{2+} + calmodulin)-dependent protein kinase (De Lorenzo 1976), protein kinase C (Inoue *et al.* 1977) and the protein–tyrosine kinases (Eckhart *et al.* 1979).

During the period in which knowledge of plasma-membrane receptors, intracellular messengers, and protein kinases developed, steroid and thyroid hormones were discovered and their interactions with cells described. Experiments conducted between about 1945 and 1970 showed that steroid and thyroid hormones act by mechanisms which are quite different from the processes which involve plasma-membrane receptors, mobile intracellular messengers, and the network of protein kinases. The major steps in the elucidation of these mechanisms were the observation that steroid and thyroid hormones stimulate the synthesis of one or more specific proteins (Tipton and Nixon 1946; Thompson *et al.* 1966; Notides and Gorski 1966), the discovery of nuclear receptors for these hormones (Talwar *et al.* 1964; Toft and Gorski 1966), and elucidation of the process by which the hormone–receptor complex interacts with specific regions of the chromosome (Payvar *et al.* 1981).

During the past six years, the techniques of molecular biology have increasingly provided knowledge of the structures of the key proteins involved in intracellular communication (Ullrich *et al.* 1984). These proteins include plasma-membrane receptors, DNA-binding hormone receptors, ion channels, GTP-binding proteins, and protein kinases. Knowledge of the structure of these proteins has, in turn, led to knowledge of the molecular mechanisms through which interaction between these proteins occurs.

The nature and function of the receptors for extracellular signals and of the components of the major pathways by which information is transferred through the cytoplasmic space is now reasonably well understood. Rapid advances are currently being made in the elucidation of the mechanisms by which receptors couple with intracellular pathways. Less is known about the interactions between the various intracellular messengers and about the nature of the target enzymes and proteins affected by the mobile intracellular messengers and by plasma-membrane receptor protein–tyrosine kinases.

1.6 Terms used to describe the mobile intracellular messengers

The pathways of intracellular communication are more complex than envisaged when it was first proposed that cyclic AMP functions as a second messenger. Two examples of this complexity are Ins 1,4,5 P_3 and fructose 2,6-bisphosphate. These two intracellular messengers are required to transfer information carried by an extracellular signal to intracellular target enzymes. In many cells an increase in Ins 1,4,5 P_3 precedes an increase in the cytoplasmic free Ca^{2+} concentration. Changes in the concentration of fructose 2,6-bisphosphate mediate some of the effects of glucagon on glycolysis in a number of cells, including liver. In conjunction with cyclic AMP and cyclic-AMP-dependent protein kinase, this metabolite functions as a second messenger with a restricted sphere of action.

Three terms have been used to describe the actions of cyclic AMP, Ca^{2+}, Ins 1,4,5 P_3, fructose 2,6-bisphosphate, and other molecules and ions which transfer information within cells. These are 'second messenger', 'coupling factor', and 'intracellular messenger'. In keeping with the original definition, the term 'second messenger' might best be used to describe a readily diffusible molecule involved at some stage in

conveying information, which reaches a cell from an external source, to the principle target enzymes within the cell. The extracellular signal concerned may be an agonist which combines with a plasma-membrane receptor, depolarization of the plasma membrane (initially induced by a neurotransmitter), or a metabolite. The term 'intracellular messenger' might be considered as a broader term which encompasses both the 'second messengers' as just defined and other diffusible molecules such as fructose 2,6-bisphosphate, free fatty acids, allosteric effectors, and other metabolites which convey information from one part of the cell to another.

1.7 The links between extracellular signals and intracellular messengers

Extracellular signals regulate the concentrations of mobile intracellular messengers in one of three ways: through the direct coupling of plasma membrane receptors to enzymes or ion channels; through the indirect coupling of plasma-membrane receptors to ion channels by depolarization of the plasma membrane; or through the metabolism of an extracellular metabolite by an intracellular enzyme. The direct coupling of receptors to the generation of intracellular messengers or to the movement of ions is achieved by GTP-binding regulatory proteins.

One of the best examples of the function of membrane depolarization as the link between receptors and a change in the concentration of a mobile intracellular messenger is the release of neurotransmitter from the pre-synaptic nerve terminal (Fig. 1.7). Depolarization of the nerve is induced by the binding of a neurotransmitter, for example acetylcholine, at the post-synaptic terminal. The resulting wave of depolarization causes an increase in the concentration of free Ca^{2+} in the cytoplasmic space, the movement of secretory granules which contain neurotrans-

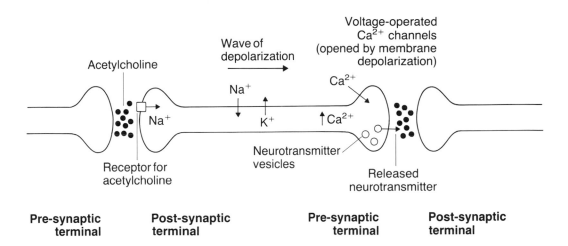

Fig. 1.7 The roles of Na^+, K^+, and Ca^{2+} in the transfer of information along the nerve axon. In the example shown, the binding of acetylcholine to nicotinic acetylcholine receptors on the post-synaptic membrane opens Na^+ channels and initiates depolarization of the plasma membrane. The wave of depolarization, which is propagated by the opening of voltage-operated Na^+ and K^+ channels, moves from the post-synaptic to the pre-synaptic terminal. At the pre-synaptic terminal depolarization of the plasma membrane opens voltage-operated Ca^{2+} channels. This leads to an increase in the concentration of free Ca^{2+} in the cytoplasmic space and to the secretion of neurotransmitters.

mitter to the plasma membrane, and release of the neurotransmitter by exocytosis at the pre-synaptic terminal.

1.8 The mobile intracellular messengers, metabolites, and proteins in the cytoplasmic space

The diffusible ions and metabolites that have a defined intracellular messenger function are summarized in Table 1.4. Most of the metabolites and ions listed in Table 1.4 have widespread roles and are present in almost all animal cells. However, others such as fructose 2,6-bisphosphate, free fatty acids, and metabolites of arachidonic acid probably play a restricted role in intracellular communication.

The majority of mobile intracellular messengers are water-soluble molecules that can diffuse through aqueous regions of the cytoplasmic space (Table 1.4). The functions of the cyclic nucleotides, Ins 1,4,5 P_3, Ca^{2+}, and fructose 2,6-

bisphosphate are now reasonably well defined. In addition to these compounds, it has also been proposed by some workers that polyamines act as water-soluble intracellular messengers. Although it has been suggested that polyamines may regulate the rate of synthesis of DNA, RNA, and protein, the activities of enzymes required for maintenance of cytoskeletal function, and the activities of certain regulatory enzymes in pathways of intermediary metabolism, these putative actions of polyamines have not yet been clearly established.

The movement of the lipid-soluble, mobile intracellular messenger, diacylglycerol, is confined to the small distance between the site of formation of this molecule in the plasma membrane and the site at which diacylglycerol interacts with protein kinase C on the cytoplasmic surface of the membrane. Prostaglandins and other metabolites of arachidonic acid which are lipid soluble but of sufficient polarity to also dissolve in water readily diffuse through membranes and aqueous regions such as the extracel-

Table 1.4 *The mobile intracellular messengers and their target proteins involved in the transfer of information contained in extracellular signals to intracellular enzymes and proteins*

Messenger	Target protein
Water-soluble diffusible messengers	
Cyclic AMP	Cyclic AMP-dependent protein kinases
	Ion channels
Cyclic GMP	Cyclic GMP-dependent protein kinases
	Ion channels
Ca^{2+}	(Ca^{2+} + calmodulin)-activated enzymes
	Ca^{2+}-activated enzymes and proteins
Inositol trisphosphate	Ca^{2+} channel in endoplasmic reticulum
Na^+, K^+, H^+, Cl^- (electrically-excitable cells)	Voltage-operated ion channels
Na^+, H^+ (non-excitable cells)	Permissive action on enzymes required for the synthesis of DNA, mRNA and protein
Fructose 2,6-bisphosphate	Allosteric sites on enzymes in pathways of intermediary metabolism
Nitric oxide (NO)	Cytoplasmic guanylate cyclase
Lipid-soluble diffusible messengers	
Diacylglycerol	(Ca^{2+} + phospholipid)-dependent protein kinases
Free fatty acids	H^+ channel in mitochondria in brown adipose tissue
Arachidonic acid metabolites	Extracellular domain of plasma-membrane receptors

lular and cytoplasmic spaces. These properties enable these molecules to move out of a cell into the extracellular medium from which they can act at receptors on the external side of the plasma membrane of the same or neighbouring cells. In addition, some arachidonic acid metabolites may interact with target enzymes within the cell and hence act as intracellular messengers. Free fatty acids have a limited role as intracellular messengers. The best example is the change in the concentration of free fatty acids which mediates the stimulation, by hormones, of mito-chondrial respiration in brown adipose tissue.

The role of metabolites in intracellular com-munication is mainly confined to the regulation of metabolic pathways. The enzymes which con-stitute a metabolic pathway can themselves be considered to be a form of intracellular com-munication. Mechanisms of metabolic regula-tion include not only those which control flux through a given pathway but also those which permit interactions between different pathways. Furthermore, the transport of metabolites and

ions from one intracellular compartment to another, for example between the cytoplasmic space and mitochondria or peroxisomes, con-veys information about the concentration of ions or metabolites in the adjacent compart-ment.

The regulation of a metabolic pathway may be exerted by the initial substrates of the path-way, by intermediate metabolites, or by products of the pathway. These regulatory metabolites may act at the active site or at an allosteric site of a regulatory enzyme. An example of this type of communication is the regulation by AMP and ATP of the pathways of glycolysis and gluconeo-genesis in the liver, and co-ordination by acetyl-CoA of the rate of gluconeogenesis with the rate of fatty-acid oxidation (Fig. 1.8).

The effect of a diffusible intracellular mess-enger on a target enzyme in the cytoplasmic space depends on both the intracellular location of the target enzyme and the concentration of the intracellular messenger at that location. There is considerable information on the chemi-

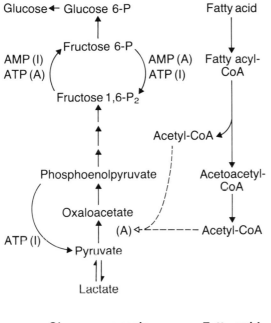

Gluconeogenesis   **Fatty-acid oxidation**

Fig. 1.8 An example of the roles of intermediary metabolites in regulation of flux through metabolic pathways and in communication between pathways. In the liver cell the rates of glycolysis and gluconeogenesis are controlled, in part, by the concentrations of ATP and AMP. ATP acts as an allosteric inhibitor (I) of the conversion of fructose 6-phosphate (fructose 6-P) to fructose 1,6-bisphosphate (fructose 1,6-P$_2$) (catalysed by phosphofructokinase) and the conversion of phosphoenolypyruvate to pyruvate (catalysed by pyruvate kinase), and as an allosteric activator (A) of the conversion of fructose 1,6-P$_2$ to fructose 6-P (catalysed by fructose 2,6-bisphosphatase). AMP acts as an allosteric activator of phosphofructokinase and an inhibitor of fructose 2,6-bisphosphatase. Acetyl-CoA co-ordinates flux through the gluconeogenic pathway with the rate of fatty-acid oxidation by acting as an allosteric activator of pyruvate carboxylase, which converts pyruvate and HCO$_3^-$ to oxaloacetate.

cal properties of diffusible molecules involved in intracellular communication and on the stereospecific binding sites for these molecules on target proteins. By contrast, relatively little information is available on the distance and direction of the flow of information within cells.

These vectorial parameters are influenced by many factors, including the overall structure of the cell, the arrangement of the various intracellular organelles, and other physical boundaries within the cytoplasmic space, the structure of the cytoskeleton and associated enzymes, and the physical properties of the chemical constituents of the cytoplasmic space. The effect of a mobile intracellular messenger on a target enzyme will also be determined by the rate of diffusion of the intracellular messenger and by the chemical half-life of this molecule.

1.9 The protein kinase network

The majority of the actions of the cyclic nucleotides, Ca^{2+}, and diacylglycerol are mediated by protein kinases. The protein kinases activated by cyclic nucleotides or Ca^{2+} are distributed at the plasma membrane and within the cytoplasmic space. Increases in cyclic nucleotides or free Ca^{2+} concentration at the plasma membrane, endoplasmic reticulum, and other intracellular sites, activate protein kinases at these sites. This may involve diffusion of the protein kinase itself as well as diffusion of the intracellular messengers within the cytoplasmic space.

A second component of the protein kinase network is linked to receptor protein–tyrosine kinases in the plasma membrane and to protein kinase C. This part of the network is independent of water-soluble diffusible intracellular messengers. The receptor protein–tyrosine kinases and protein kinase C are activated at the plasma membrane by extracellular agonists, and exert effects on target proteins located both at the plasma membrane and at intracellular sites. The transfer of many of the signals carried by the protein kinase network from the plasma membrane to sites within the cytoplasmic space probably requires other mobile protein kinases which link the plasma-membrane protein kinases to target proteins within the cell.

The transfer of information from one part of a cell to another by the network of protein kinases and by the mobile intracellular messengers is dependent on the specific conformations of the proteins, mobile intracellular messengers, and ions involved. These conformations are the basis of the mechanism by which stereospecific binding sites on intracellular enzymes and proteins recognize intracellular messengers. Changes in conformation are the basis of the process by which information is transferred from one part of a protein to another.

1.10   Communication within the nucleus

While the water- and lipid-soluble intracellular messengers, metabolites and proteins, and the protein kinase network transfer information within the cytoplasmic space and within certain organelles, different mechanisms are employed within the nucleus. These are the sequence-specific DNA-binding regulatory proteins which transfer information between genes. The sequence-specific DNA-binding receptor proteins which bind hormones and morphogens are a special class of the sequence-specific DNA-binding proteins. The sequence-specific DNA-binding receptor proteins interact specifically both with hormone or morphogen and with DNA.

Hormones which use sequence-specific DNA-binding receptor proteins include the steroid hormones, the steroid 1,25-dihydroxy cholecalciferol (the active form of vitamin D), retinol (vitamin A), and the thyroid hormones. Transfer of the information contained in these extracellular signals from the extracellular medium to the nucleus involves three main steps: movement of the hormone across the plasma membrane, movement of the hormone–receptor complex through the cytoplasmic space to the nucleus, and the binding of the hormone–receptor complex to DNA.

1.11   Newly synthesized proteins in intracellular communication

The discussion so far has focused on pathways of communication between the plasma membrane and target enzymes within the cytoplasmic space, and between hormones and specific sequences of DNA in the nucleus. The activation of certain target enzymes and the actions of hormone–receptor complexes on DNA leads to an increase in the transcription of selected genes and subsequently to increases in the rate of synthesis of a number of new proteins and enzymes. These newly synthesized proteins include enzymes and proteins located in the cytoplasmic space as well as a variety of enzymes which catalyse the synthesis of RNA, DNA, and proteins.

The proteins synthesized in response to an extracellular signal are an important component of the overall pathway by which an initial extracellular signal is translated to the final cellular response (Fig. 1.9). The specific response is determined by the nature, concentration, and final intracellular location of the proteins synthesized.

In some cell types, a given extracellular signal induces the synthesis of only one or a small number of proteins. Examples include the induction by hormones of the synthesis of specific regulatory enzymes in pathways of intermediary metabolism in liver and adipose cells, induction of the synthesis of polypeptide hormones in endocrine cells, and induction of the synthesis of a digestive enzyme (e.g. α-amylase) in exocrine cells. For responses which involve the stimulation of cell growth, the number of newly-synthesized proteins is much greater. An increase in the rate of synthesis of a large number of proteins occurs during the S phase of the cell cycle in which the synthesis of DNA is stimulated. An example of changes in the concen-

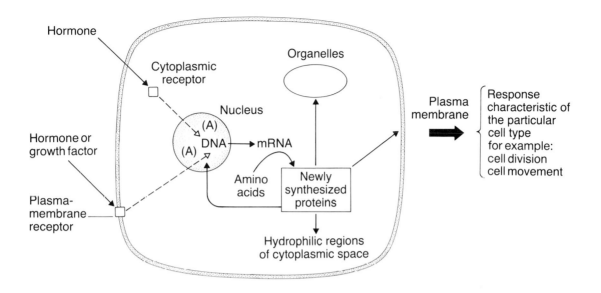

Fig. 1.9 Many extracellular signals induce the synthesis of new enzymes and other proteins. Information carried by these proteins is defined by both the catalytic activities and functions of the enzymes and proteins, and by the final location of the enzymes and proteins in hydrophilic regions of the cytoplasmic space ('soluble proteins'), organelles, and membranes.

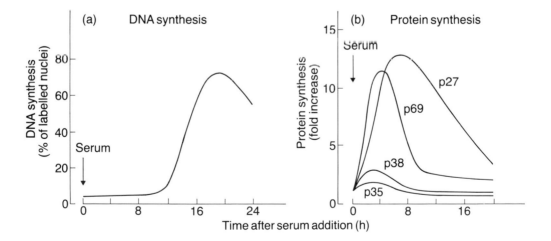

Fig. 1.10 The addition of serum to quiescent NIH-3T3 cultured fibroblasts induces (a) the synthesis of DNA and (b) the synthesis of proteins required for cell growth and division. Synthesis of the proteins was measured using cells labelled with [^{35}S]methionine and two-dimensional polyacrylamide gel electrophoresis to identify newly synthesized proteins. These have been designated proteins p27, p35, p38, and p69 according to their molecular weights. These four proteins represent a small proportion of the total number of newly synthesized proteins. From Santaren and Bravo (1986).

tration of four such proteins synthesized in cultured NIH-3T3 fibroblasts in response to serum is shown in Fig. 1.10.

In addition to the movement of proteins newly synthesized in response to the action of an extracellular signal there is a substantial flow of protein molecules from one part of a cell to another. This includes newly synthesized enzymes which move from free ribosomes in the cytoplasmic space to the correct intracellular location to replace degraded enzymes, the transport of enzymes and proteins along the nerve axoplasm, the synthesis of membrane proteins and incorporation of these proteins into the appropriate cell membrane, and the movement of proteins involved in the transport of lipids within the cell.

1.12 Amplification of the initial extracellular signal

Most of the pathways of intracellular communication amplify the initial extracellular signal. This can be pictured by considering the main steps which follow the interaction of an extracellular signal with a cell. Fig. 1.11 shows schematically the binding of a single molecule of an agonist with one molecule of a plasma-membrane receptor linked either to the generation of an intracellular messenger (Fig. 1.11(a)) or to activation of a protein–tyrosine kinase (Fig. 1.11(b)), and the binding of a hormone to a sequence-specific DNA-binding receptor protein (Fig. 1.11(c)). The binding of

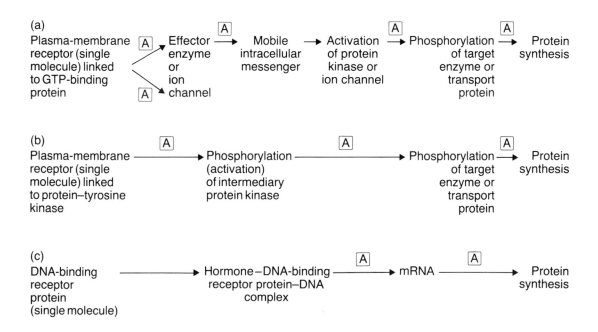

Fig. 1.11 The sites of signal amplification for the combination of an agonist with (a) a plasma-membrane receptor linked to a GTP-binding regulatory protein, (b) a plasma-membrane receptor which contains a protein–tyrosine kinase catalytic site on the cytoplasmic domain, and (c) a sequence-specific DNA-binding receptor. In each case, the interaction of one molecule of agonist with a single receptor molecule leads to the activation of many target enzymes and the synthesis of many new proteins. Steps in which the signal is amplified are indicated by 'A'.

the single molecule of agonist to the single receptor molecule leads to the activation of many molecules of target protein and the synthesis of many molecules of new protein. In the case of plasma-membrane receptors, there are several steps at which the extracellular signal is amplified (Figs 1.11(a) and (b)). The main sites of amplification in the action of the hormone–DNA-binding receptor protein complex is the synthesis of mRNA and protein (Fig. 1.11(c)).

1.13 Specificity of the pathways of intracellular communication

The number of alternative pathways available for the transfer of information within cells is small in relation to the large number of different responses which are induced by extracellular signals. For example, in many cells inositol polyphosphates, Ca^{2+}, and cyclic AMP are the major diffusible intracellular messengers employed in response to a number of extracellular signals. The small number of constituents of the pathways of intracellular communication is analogous to the small number of basic constituents involved in communication between different cells in an animal through the endocrine and nervous systems.

How does such a small number of intracellular pathways allow each of a wide variety of extracellular signals to induce specific responses? An answer to this question lies in the proposal that the elements of the pathways of intracellular communication, when combined in different ways, provide a system in which specific intracellular responses are elicited from each of a variety of extracellular signals. The main elements which are thought to provide specificity are the receptors for extracellular signals, the coupling between receptors and intracellular pathways of communication, and the interactions between these pathways. While these pathways of intracellular communication and the interaction

between them may well explain the transmission of all signals, it is likely that several intracellular messengers or processes of intracellular communication are yet to be discovered.

1.14 Summary

One view of the cells which compose a multicellular animal is that each cell functions to transfer a set of extracellular signals to induce a specific set of responses. The cell may be considered as being exposed to a milieu of extracellular signals. Pathways of intracellular communication are required to co-ordinate the basic functions of each cell and to provide links between the extracellular signals and intracellular responses.

The major forms of extracellular signals are hormones, local hormones, neurotransmitters, and metabolites. Cells receive these signals through plasma-membrane receptors, sequence-specific DNA-binding receptor proteins, and through the metabolism of certain extracellular substrates. In addition to conveying information contained in an extracellular signal from one site in a cell to another site, paths of intracellular communication also amplify the extracellular signal so that it can induce an adequate cellular response.

There have been many contributions to the discovery of pathways of intracellular communication. One of these is knowledge of the physical and chemical structure of cells. Key observations which have laid the foundation for present knowledge of the processes of intracellular communication are the discovery of cyclic AMP, elucidation of the role of Ca^{2+} in muscle contraction, the discovery of the protein kinases, and elucidation of the functions of the sequence-specific DNA-binding receptors for hormones and morphogens.

The main components of the intracellular communication systems are GTP-binding regulatory proteins at the plasma membrane, mobile intracellular messengers and metabolites, the protein kinase network, sequence-specific DNA-binding proteins, and the proteins that are synthesized in response to extracellular signals. The mobile intracellular messengers may traverse the aqueous phase of a cell, as in the case of the movement of cyclic AMP within the cytoplasmic space, or may be confined to the lipid phase, as in the case of the movement of diacylglycerol in the plasma membrane. There are two major components of the protein kinase network. One is the protein kinases which are activated by mobile intracellular messengers, the other is composed of the receptor protein–tyrosine kinases in the plasma membrane and protein kinase C. The protein–tyrosine kinases and protein kinase C are activated at the plasma membrane and may exert effects on intracellular target proteins through other protein kinases in the cytoplasmic space.

One of the unresolved problems in intracellular communication is how such an apparently small number of pathways conveys information from a large variety of extracellular signals to give specific intracellular responses. This is probably achieved through interactions between the different types of pathways of intracellular communication.

References

Banting, F. G. and Best, C. H. (1922). Internal secretion of pancreas. *J. Lab. Clin. Med.*, **7**, 251–66.

Cheung, W. Y. (1970). Cyclic 3′,5′-nucleotide phosphodiesterase. Demonstration of an activator. *Biochem. Biophys. Res. Commun.*, **38**, 533–8.

De Lorenzo, R. J. (1976). Calcium-dependent phosphorylation of specific synaptosomal fraction proteins: possible role of phosphoproteins in mediating neurotransmitter release. *Biochem. Biophys. Res. Commun.*, **71**, 590–7.

De Robertis, E. D. P. and De Robertis, E. M. F. (1987). *Cell and molecular biology* (8th edn). Lea and Febiger, Philadelphia.

Ebashi, S. and Kodama, A. (1965). A new protein factor promoting aggregation of tropomyosin. *J. Biochem.*, **58**, 107–8.

Eckhart, W., Hutchinson, M. A., and Hunter, T. (1979). An activity phosphorylating tyrosine in polyoma T antigen immunoprecipitates. *Cell*, **18**, 925–33.

Heilbrunn, L. V. (1940). The action of calcium on muscle protoplasm. *Physiol. Zool.*, **13**, 88–94.

Heilbrunn, L. V. and Wiercinski, F. J. (1947). The action of various cations on muscle protoplasm. *J. Cell. Comp. Physiol.*, **29**, 15–32.

Hokin, M. R. and Hokin, L. E. (1953). Enzyme secretion and the incorporation of ^{32}P into phospholipids of pancreas slices. *J. Biol. Chem.*, **203**, 967–77.

Inoue, M., Kishimoto, A., Takai, Y., and Nishizuka, Y. (1977). Studies on a cyclic nucleotide-independent protein kinase and its proenzyme in mammalian tissues. *J. Biol. Chem.*, **252**, 7610–16.

Jöbsis, F. F. and O'Connor, M. J. (1966). Calcium release and reabsorption in the sartorius muscle of the toad. *Biochem. Biophys. Res. Commun.*, **25**, 246–52.

Michell, R. H. (1975). Inositol phospholipids and cell surface receptor function. *Biochim. Biophys. Acta*, **415**, 81–147.

Notides, A. and Gorski, J. (1966). Estrogen-induced synthesis of a specific uterine protein. *Proc. Natl Acad. Sci. USA*, **56**, 230–5.

Old, L. J. (1987). Tumour necrosis factor: polypeptide mediator network. *Nature*, **326**, 330–1.

Payvar, F., Wrange, O., Carlstedt-Duke, J., Okret, S., Gustafsson, J., and Yamamoto, K. R. (1981). Purified glucocorticoid receptors bind selectively *in vitro* to a cloned DNA fragment whose transcription is regulated by glucocorticoids *in vivo*. *Proc. Natl Acad. Sci. USA*, **78**, 6628–32.

Rall, T. W., Sutherland, E. W., and Berthet, J. (1957). The relationship of epinephrine and glucagon to liver phosphorylase. IV. Effect of epinephrine and glucagon on the reactivation of phosphorylase in liver homogenates. *J. Biol. Chem.*, **224**, 463–75.

Rasmussen, H., Kojima, I., Kojima, K., Zawalich, W., and Apfeldorf, W. (1984). Calcium as intracellular messenger: sensitivity modulation, C-kinase pathway, and sustained cellular response. *Adv.*

Cyclic Nucleotide Protein Phosphorylation Res., **18**, 159–93.

Ridgway, E. B. and Ashley, C. C. (1967). Calcium transients in skeletal muscle fibres. *Biochem. Biophys. Res. Commun.*, **29**, 229–34.

Rodbell, M., Birnbaumer, L., Pohl, S. L., and Krans, H. M. J. (1971). The glucagon-sensitive adenyl cyclase system in plasma membranes of rat liver. V. An obligatory role for guanyl nucleotides in glucagon action. *J. Biol. Chem.*, **246**, 1877–82.

Santaren, J. F. and Bravo, R. (1986). A basic cytoplasmic protein (p27) induced by serum in growth-arrested 3T3 cells but constitutively expressed in primary fibroblasts. *EMBO J.*, **5**, 877–82.

Streb, H., Irvine, R. F., Berridge, M. J., and Schulz, I. (1983). Release of Ca^{2+} from a non-mitochondrial intracellular store in pancreatic acinar cells by inositol-1,4,5-trisphosphate. *Nature*, **306**, 67–9.

Talwar, G. P., Segal, S. J., Evans, A., and Davidson, O. W. (1964). The binding of estradiol in the uterus: a mechanism for derepression of RNA synthesis. *Proc. Natl Acad. Sci. USA*, **52**, 1059–66.

Thompson, E. B., Tomkins, G. M., and Curran, J. F. (1966). Induction of tyrosine α-ketoglutarate transaminase by steroid hormones in a newly established tissue culture cell line. *Proc. Natl Acad. Sci. USA*, **56**, 296–03.

Tipton, S. R. and Nixon, W. L. (1946). The effect of thiouracil on the succinoxidase and cytochrome oxidase of rat liver. *Endocrinology*, **39**, 300–6.

Toft, D. and Gorski, J. (1966). A receptor molecule for estrogens: isolation from the rat uterus and preliminary characterization. *Proc. Natl Acad. Sci. USA*, **55**, 1574–81.

Ullrich, A., Coussens, L., Hayflick, J. S., Dull, T. J., Gray, A., Tam, A. W., *et al.* (1984). Human epidermal growth factor receptor cDNA sequence and aberrant expression of the amplified gene in A431 epidermoid carcinoma cells. *Nature*, **309**, 418–25.

Walsh, D. A., Perkins, J. P., and Krebs, E. G. (1968). An adenosine 3',5'-monophosphate-dependent protein kinase from rabbit skeletal muscle. *J. Biol. Chem.*, **243**, 3763–5.

Further reading

Alberts, B., Bray, D., Lewis, J., Raff, M., Roberts, K., and Watson, J. D. (1989). *Molecular biology of the cell*, 2nd edn. Garland Publishing Inc., New York.

Dawkins, R. (1989). *The selfish gene*. Oxford University Press.

Morgan, N. G. (1989). *Cell signalling*. Open University Press, Milton Keynes.

Sporn, M. B. and Roberts, A. B. (1988). Peptide growth factors are multifunctional. *Nature*, **332**, 217–19.

Molecular biology of signal transduction (1988). *Cold Spring Harbor Symp. Quant. Biol.* **LIII**, 1–1031, The Cold Spring Laboratory, Cold Spring Harbor, New York, USA.

2 *Role of cell structure in intracellular communication*

2.1 Significance of cell structure in intracellular communication

A complete understanding of the pathways of intracellular communication requires knowledge of cell structure. A large number of processes take place in the cytoplasmic space and in other intracellular spaces. Each of these processes is defined by both the chemical reactions involved and the structures which influence the movement of the chemical intermediates. The structures of the cell play a major part in co-ordinating and directing the chemical reactions that take place within the cell. The role of intracellular compartmentation in this co-ordination is reasonably well understood. Less is known about the role of the microstructures within the cytoplasmic space. Nevertheless, it is believed that the microstructure plays an important part in the co-ordination of metabolic reactions, in the formation of pathways of intracellular communication, and in co-ordination between these pathways.

Some of the questions which might be asked concerning the relationship between cell structure and the pathways of intracellular communication are illustrated by consideration of an example, the stimulation by acetylcholine of the secretion of α-amylase in the pancreatic acinar cell. In this cell, the receptor for acetylcholine is located on the basal membrane whereas α-amylase is secreted at the apical surface. An electron micrograph of pancreatic acinar cells is shown in Fig. 2.1 and a schematic diagram of the lines of communication between the basal and apical surfaces in this cell is shown in Fig. 2.2.

The combination of acetylcholine with its receptor leads to increases in the concentration of free Ca^{2+} in the cytoplasmic space and in the concentration of diacylglycerol in that region of the plasma membrane which surrounds the acetylcholine receptor. The changes in these intracellular messengers activate (Ca^{2+} + calmodulin)-dependent protein kinase and protein kinase C, respectively. The phosphorylation of proteins by these protein kinases permits the movement of secretory granules to the apical membrane and the subsequent exocytosis of the vesicle contents.

In searching for a complete description of this system, the following questions can be asked. Does Ca^{2+} diffuse uniformly through the cytoplasmic space, and at what speed does it move? Is the increase in diacylglycerol concentration confined to that region of the plasma membrane in the vicinity of the acetylcholine receptor? How does protein kinase C, which is initially activated at the basal membrane, induce the movement of secretory granules at the apical membrane which is a distance of about 10 μm from the basal membrane? Does (Ca^{2+} + calmodulin)-dependent protein kinase move through the cytoplasmic space? What confines the secretory granules to the region of the cytoplasmic space near the apical membrane? These are just a few of the questions that might be asked in relation to the structural and spatial aspects of signals transmitted by acetylcholine to intracellular sites

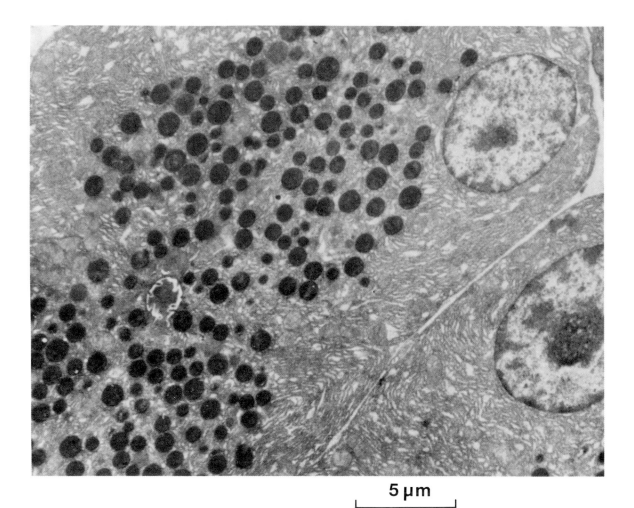

5 μm

Fig. 2.1 An electron micrograph of a region of a pancreatic acinus showing sections of the basal and apical surfaces of one pancreatic acinar cell (centre). The lumen of the pancreatic duct (centre left) and two neighbouring acinar cells (upper left and lower right-hand sides) are also shown. From Leeson and Leeson (1970). A schematic drawing of the central acinar cell is shown in Fig. 2.2.

in the pancreatic acinar cell.

In this chapter an attempt will be made to provide a framework in which the questions just posed can be answered, to create a picture of the structure of the cytoplasmic space which can serve as a context in which individual pathways of intracellular communication discussed in subsequent chapters can be viewed, to describe how information is transferred between the nucleus and the cytoplasmic space, and how structural information within a cell is specified by the

movement of proteins and organelles. The discussion in the first part of the chapter will focus on the role of intracellular structure in directing the flow of information within a cell.

2.2   Structure of the cytoplasmic space

2.2.1   *Membranes which define the cytoplasmic space*

About half the volume of a typical animal cell is occupied by organelles. The major organelles

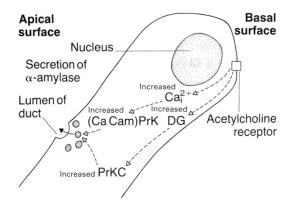

Fig. 2.2 The pathways of communication in the pancreatic acinar cell which allow the combination of acetylcholine with receptors on the basal surface of the cell to induce the release of α-amylase from secretory granules which fuse with the apical surface. The transmission of information from the basal surface to the apical surface of the cell is achieved by changes in intracellular free Ca^{2+} concentration ($[Ca^{2+}]_i$) and diacylglycerol (DG) and through the actions of (Ca^{2+} + calmodulin)-dependent protein kinase ((CaCam)PrK) and protein kinase C (PrKC). The outline of the cell was drawn from that shown in the electron micrograph of Fig. 2.1.

are the endoplasmic reticulum, Golgi apparatus, mitochondria, lysosomes, endosomes, and peroxisomes (Fig. 2.3). There are also present within the cell a number of small vesicles which transfer proteins and lipids between organelles and between the endoplasmic reticulum and the plasma membrane. The functions of these are described in Section 2.6. Each organelle and the nucleus provide a specific environment which is separate from that of the cytoplasmic space. For example, the generation of ATP in mitochondria, the degradation of proteins in lysosomes, and the storage of DNA and synthesis of RNA in the nucleus take place in specific environments which differ from that of the cytoplasmic space.

The endoplasmic reticulum is composed of one continuous membrane which constitutes about half the total area of membranes present in the cell. This membrane system ramifies through most of the cytoplasmic space. An indi-

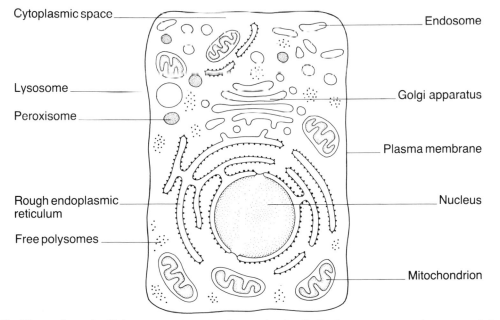

Fig. 2.3 The major subcellular compartments of an animal cell. Each compartment is separated from the rest of the cell by a selectively permeable membrane. The space enclosed by the endoplasmic reticulum, Golgi apparatus, and lysosomes is topologically the same as the extracellular space. The cytoplasmic space is defined as that part of the cell which is bounded by the plasma membrane and intracellular membranes.

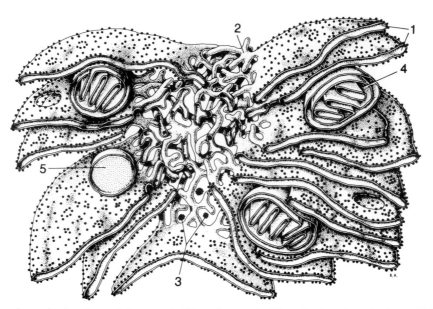

Fig. 2.4 A schematic drawing of the rough (1) and smooth (2) endoplasmic reticulum of the hepatocyte showing the ramification of this membrane system throughout the cytoplasmic space. Other structures shown are glycogen granules (3), mitochondria (4), and a lysosome (5). From Krstic (1979).

cation of the extent of this network is shown by the representation of the endoplasmic reticulum in the liver cell in Fig. 2.4. The space enclosed by the endoplasmic reticulum, as well as that enclosed by the Golgi apparatus, lysosomes, and the transport vesicles which move between these organelles and between the Golgi apparatus and the plasma membrane, is topologically the same as the extracellular space.

The cytoplasmic space is defined as the space bounded by the plasma membrane, the nuclear membrane, and the membranes of intracellular organelles. Much of the cytoplasmic space is occupied by proteins. The physical environment of water, metabolites, and ions within the cytoplasmic space differs substantially from the environment of these molecules in dilute aqueous solution. Pathways of intracellular communication involve the transfer of information from the plasma membrane to enzymes and other proteins within the cytoplasmic space, or the transfer of information from this space across the barrier of a membrane to enzymes

and other proteins within an organelle.

Five main components of the cytoplasmic space of an animal cell can be identified. These are the cytoplasmic surfaces of the plasma membrane and organelle membranes, the cytoskeleton, the microtrabecular lattice, the enzymes and other proteins which are associated with these structures, and the space between the intracellular structures and proteins.

2.2.2 *The cytoskeleton*

The cytoskeleton determines the external shape of the cell and the spatial distribution of intracellular organelles, and is responsible for movement of the external boundaries of the cell and for movement of its intracellular structures. The cytoskeleton also provides sites of attachment for a number of proteins in the plasma membrane. The main elements of the cytoskeleton are the microtubules, the intermediate filaments, and the actin filaments, which are also called the microfilaments.

The microtubules, intermediate filaments, and

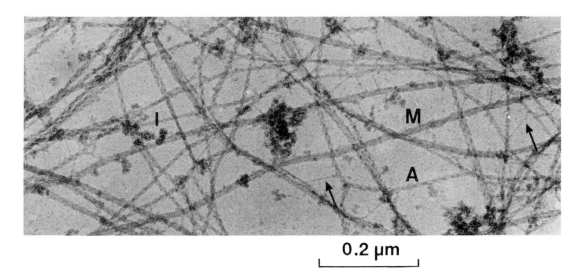

Fig. 2.5 An electron micrograph of a section of the periphery of a cultured BSC-1 cell extracted with Triton X-100, showing microtubules (M), intermediate filaments (I), and actin filaments (A). The arrows show another type of filament which connects intermediate filaments and actin microfilaments. From Schliwa (1986).

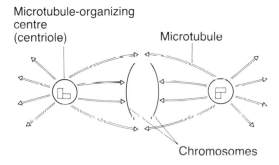

Fig. 2.6 During metaphase, microtubules are responsible for the movement of the chromosomes towards the centrioles (microtubule-organizing centres). The arrowheads represent the growing ends of microtubules.

actin filaments form an interconnected network within the cytoplasmic space. The nature of this network at the periphery of a cultured cell, revealed after extraction of the cellular membranes by the detergent Triton X-100, is shown in Fig. 2.5. The structure of the cytoskeletal network and the relative contribution to this network by each of the three main types of filament varies from one part of the cytoplasmic

space to another. The picture of the cytoskeletal network created by the electron micrograph shown in Fig. 2.5 does not reflect the dynamic nature of this network—the cytoskeleton undergoes rapid changes as a result of degradation and re-formation of the elements of which it is composed. These changes can occur within a time-scale of milliseconds.

The thickest elements which compose the cytoskeleton are the microtubules. These are hollow cylinders with an external diameter of 25 nm and an internal diameter of 15 nm. The microtubule cylinders are composed of the protein tubulin. This protein is a dimer consisting of one α and one β subunit. During mitosis, microtubules constitute the mitotic spindle (Fig. 2.6). At interphase they are observed as strands which radiate outwards from locations within the vicinity of the nucleus (Fig. 2.7).

The main functions of microtubules are to contribute to the maintenance of an asymmetric cell shape and to permit intra- and extracellular movement. The microtubules are responsible for the vectorial movement of organelles and ves-

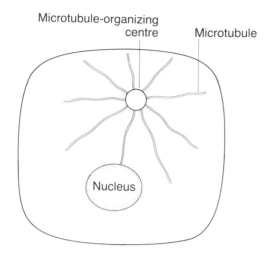

Fig. 2.7 In cells in interphase, microtubules radiate outwards from a microtubule-organizing centre towards the plasma membrane.

icles, and for the movement of chromosomes during mitosis. In cells at interphase, microtubules are attached to the endoplasmic reticulum and Golgi apparatus, and determine the spatial location of these organelles within the cytoplasmic space.

A group of proteins called the microtubule-associated proteins (MAP) bind to microtubules. While the physical and chemical properties of many of these proteins have been characterized, their biological functions are less clear. This group of proteins includes those designated MAP1, MAP2, MAP3, MAP4, and a number of other MAP proteins, the proteins dynein and kinesin, and proteins designated *tau*, STOPs and chartins. Dynein and kinesin are responsible for the movement of organelles and proteins that are attached to microtubules (Section 2.6.8).

Microtubules are constantly being degraded and re-formed. Growth is initiated at a nucleation site called a microtubule-organizing centre. One type of organizing centre is the centriole. The amount and direction of microtubule growth depends on the rate of polymerization of tubulin and the degree to which the microtu-

bule interacts with other components of the cytoskeleton.

The major role of the intermediate filaments is to contribute to the maintenance of overall cell structure. There are at least five classes of intermediate filaments. These are distinguished on the basis of the cell type in which they are present and the subunits of which the filaments are composed. The known classes of intermediate filaments are vimentin, which is present in cells of mesenchymal origin; desmin, which is present in myogenic cells; filaments composed of glial fibrillar acidic protein which are present in astroglial cells; neurofilaments, which are composed of neurofilament triplet protein; and cytokeratins which are found in differentiated epithelial cells.

In contrast to the microtubules and microfilaments, the intermediate filaments are not involved in intracellular or extracellular movement. Intermediate filaments have a diameter of 10 nm and extend from the nucleus to the plasma membrane (Fig. 2.8). Each filament is attached to the nuclear lamina from which it passes through a nuclear pore to the cytoplasmic space. At the periphery of the cell each filament is

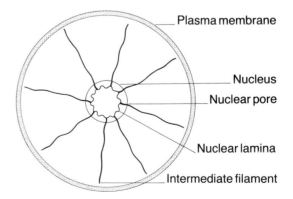

Fig. 2.8 Intermediate filaments link the nuclear lamina to the plasma membrane. These filaments, which are attached to the nuclear lamina, pass through pores in the nuclear envelope, traverse the cytoplasmic space, and are attached to the plasma membrane at the periphery of the cell.

attached to the membrane skeleton. Intermediate filaments are also associated with desmosomes.

In comparison with microtubules, intermediate filaments are relatively insoluble. Agonists that stimulate cell proliferation, for example bombesin, or the combination of platelet-derived growth factor and insulin in the case of fibroblasts, induce the phosphorylation of the components of intermediate filaments. This results in transient dissociation of the intermediate filaments into subunits which are then packed into non-filamentous spheroidal structures during mitosis. These processes may be part of a possible function of intermediate filaments in regulating the dissociation and reassembly of the nuclear lamina during mitosis.

The thinnest filaments of the cytoskeleton are the actin filaments. These have a diameter of about 7 nm. Actin filaments are chiefly located at the periphery of the cell. They are observed as parallel bundles of filaments, as stress fibres, and as annular rings (Fig. 2.9). The actin filaments provide mechanical support for cell extensions and for other cellular structures. The actin filaments are the contractile systems of non-muscle cells and are responsible for the locomotion of these cells.

Actin is the most abundant protein in cells. In each cell type actin constitutes 5–10 per cent of the total cellular protein. A large number of proteins interact with actin filaments. These proteins can be divided into three major categories: proteins which affect the rate of actin polymerization, proteins which form cross-links between actin filaments, and proteins which bind to the ends of actin filaments. Different arrangements of actin filaments allow forces to be generated linearly or in a complex three-dimensional pattern.

Actin filaments are composed of actin monomers arranged in a helix in which different surfaces of the actin monomer are exposed at

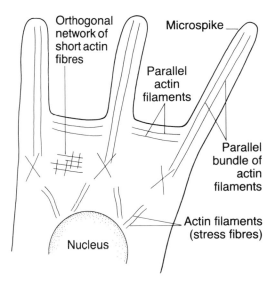

Fig. 2.9 The different arrangements of actin filaments present in a cell that is growing and moving in tissue culture. Parallel bundles of actin filaments contain α-actinin and actin-binding proteins. Stress fibres contain myosin, α-actinin, tropomyosin, and actin-binding proteins.

each end. This means that an actin filament is a polarized structure. The two ends are designated the plus end and the minus end. During growth, for example the formation of microspikes, actin filaments grow from the plus end.

The network of actin filaments is responsible for the gel-like nature of the cytoplasmic space at the periphery of a cell. This gel matrix, which is sometimes called the cortical zone, excludes organelles from the periphery of the cell but allows the diffusion of smaller particles and solutes to the plasma membrane.

It is the actin filaments that are primarily responsible for connections between the rest of the cytoskeleton and the plasma membrane. The nature of these connections has been investigated extensively in the red blood cell, because the structure of this relatively simple cell has been more amenable to analysis. In erythrocytes, actin filaments are linked to each other at the plasma membrane by the protein spectrin. This, in turn, is linked to transmembrane proteins by several other proteins, including ankyrin and a protein designated band 4.1 (Fig. 2.10). In platelets the link between the cytoskeleton and the plasma membrane involves actin, a protein called actin-binding protein, and various glycoproteins which span the plasma membrane. The main functions of the links between the cytoskeleton and the plasma membrane are the provision of a structural foundation for the plasma membrane which determines the shape of this membrane, control of the distribution of integral and peripheral plasma-membrane proteins, including receptors, and communication between the extracellular matrix and the cytoskeleton, as described in Section 2.3.

2.2.3 *The microtrabecular lattice*

Within the space between the intracellular membranes and filaments of the cytoskeleton there is probably a further fine network of filaments called the microtrabecular lattice. This lattice is shown schematically in Fig. 2.11. The microtrabecular lattice was first described by K. R. Porter and his colleagues (Wolosewick and Porter 1979) who used high-voltage electron microscopy in order to examine fine details of cell structure. Although there is a body of evidence which supports the existence of the microtrabecular lattice, there are some workers who believe that observation of the lattice is an experimental artefact.

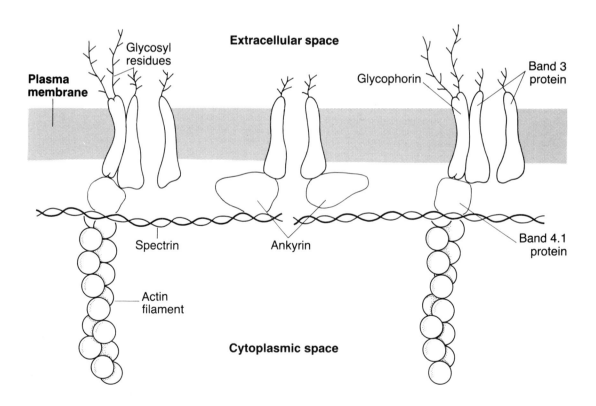

Fig. 2.10 A schematic representation of the way in which the cytoskeleton is linked to the plasma membrane of the red blood cell. Actin filaments are probably linked to a protein called band 3 and to glycophorin a, which are both integral membrane proteins, by spectrin, a protein designated band 4.1, and ankyrin. Spectrin forms a protein network on the cytoplasmic side of the membrane. From Carraway and Carraway (1989).

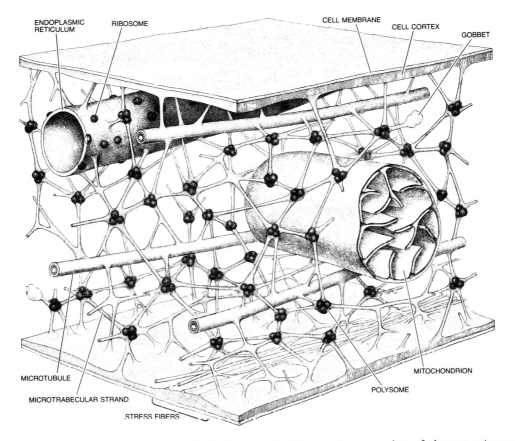

Fig. 2.11 A model of the microtrabecular lattice compiled from a large number of electron micrographs. The lattice is thought to be composed of thin strands of protein which form links between intracellular membranes, organelles, and components of the cytoskeleton. The existence of the microtrabecular lattice has not yet been established unequivocally. From Porter and Tucker (1981).

Porter (1986) and Clegg (1984) have speculated that most hydrophilic enzymes and proteins (defined experimentally as 'soluble' proteins) located within the cytoplasmic space are associated, in an ordered manner, with the microtrabecular lattice and the cytoskeleton (Fig. 2.12). This implies that the physical environment of enzymes and other proteins in the cytoplasmic space is quite different from the environment provided by a dilute aqueous solution.

Electron spin resonance spectroscopy has been used to show that the microviscosity of water in the cytoplasmic space is about five times

that of pure water. Clegg has suggested that between 4 and 40 per cent of all the water in the cytoplasmic space is bound to proteins. This is sometimes called 'bound' cell water. The idea of bound water is shown schematically in Fig. 2.12. Water which is bound in this way probably has physical properties that differ from those of the rest of the water in the cytoplasmic space. However, even this water, which is sometimes called 'bulk' cell water, probably has properties that differ from those of pure water. For example, the water molecules may form relatively stable clusters comparable in size to macromolecules and may pack together to form an in-

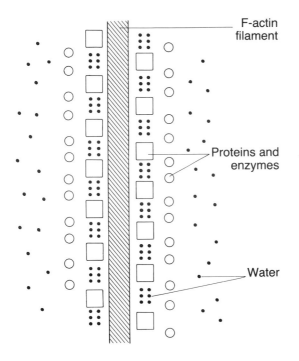

F-actin
filament

Proteins and
enzymes

Water

Fig. 2.12 A diagram of the proposals of K. R. Porter, J. Clegg, and others, which predict an ordered arrangement of protein and water molecules around strands of the microtrabecular lattice, such as an F-actin filament. A variety of different enzymes and other proteins are thought to be bound to each microtrabecular filament. Some of these proteins (represented as squares) are bound more tightly than others (represented as circles). A large proportion of the water molecules (indicated by the dots) in this microregion of the cytoplasmic space may be bound to the microtrabecular filaments, proteins and metabolites.

tegrated network of water molecules in the cytoplasmic space.

2.3 Transmission of information through changes in intracellular structure

The normal growth of a number of types of animal cell requires adherence of the cells to an extracellular matrix. This interaction between cells and extracellular matrix is required for the maintenance of tissue structure, for cell movement during morphogenesis, and for cell migration. The interaction is also important in pathological states, such as the healing of wounds and the metastasic process. The major components of the extracellular matrix are glycoproteins, proteoglycans, glycosaminoglycans, and collagen. The glycoproteins include fibronectin, laminin, elastin, and entacin. The proteins which constitute the extracellular matrix are secreted by adjacent cells, chiefly fibroblasts.

Cells attach to the extracellular matrix at sites called adhesions. The adhesive force at these sites is generated by the interaction between proteins in the plasma membrane of the cell and proteins in the extracellular matrix. The main group of plasma-membrane proteins involved in this interaction are called the integrins. Some adhesive force is also supplied by other plasma-membrane proteins, including the proteoglycan syndecan. Each integrin protein spans the plasma membrane (Fig. 2.13). The extracellular domain of the integrin molecule acts as a receptor for one or more proteins of the extracellular matrix while the cytoplasmic domain interacts with the cytoskeleton. The cytoplasmic domain is probably linked to actin filaments of the cytoskeleton through the proteins vinculin and talin.

There are a number of different integrins present in animal cells, including integrins which are receptors for fibronectin, vitronectin, laminin, and certain glycoprotein complexes. Some integrin receptors are specific for one extracellular matrix protein, for example the fibronectin and vitronectin integrin receptors, while others bind many different extracellular matrix proteins. The fibronectin integrin receptor present in avian cells was the first integrin protein to be discovered (Neff *et al.* 1982; Greve and Gottlieb 1982). Each integrin receptor is probably a heterodimer composed of one α and one β subunit. Each α and β polypeptide chain possesses a transmembrane domain, a short carboxy-terminal cytoplasmic domain and a large amino-terminal extracellular domain (Fig. 2.13). The different integrin receptors are formed by differ-

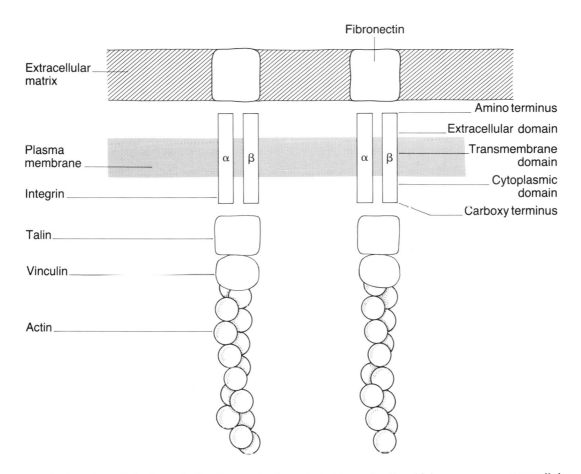

Fig. 2.13 Proteins of the integrin family couple the cytoskeleton of cells which grow on an extracellular matrix to proteins such as fibronectin present in the extracellular matrix. Integrins, which are composed of an α and a β subunit, act as receptors or sites of attachment for fibronectin and other proteins in the extracellular matrix. The link between integrin and actin is probably provided by the proteins vinculin and talin. The binding of fibronectin to integrin may induce conformational changes in the integrins, talin, vinculin, and the cytoskeleton. These may transmit information about the nature of the extracellular matrix to intracellular locations.

ent combinations of one β subunit, of which there are three known forms, and one α subunit, of which there are a large number of known forms.

Many integrin receptors recognize a specific tripeptide motif, called the RGD (arg, gly, asp) motif, which is present in extracellular-matrix proteins such as fibronectin. More than one type of integrin receptor may be present on the surface of a given cell. For example, fibroblasts possess receptors for fibronectin, laminin, and

vitronectin. The presence of different combinations of integrin receptors may be responsible for the different adhesive properties exhibited by different cell types.

There are a number of observations which indicate that information can be transferred from the extracellular matrix to intracellular sites. Firstly, the shape of cells is influenced by components of the extracellular matrix. For example, fibronectin promotes cell spreading while laminin promotes cell attachment.

Secondly, the shape adopted by a given cell may depend on whether the cell is exposed to the extracellular matrix at one surface only, or is completely surrounded by the matrix. Thirdly, in many cells, growth factors will only induce an increase in the rate of cell growth if the target cell is anchored to a solid support. Finally, some experiments indicate that the nature of the extracellular matrix and the shape of a cell both contribute to the determination of the state of differentiation of that cell.

The mechanisms by which the presence of a protein, such as fibronectin, in the extracellular matrix induces a change in intracellular function are not yet understood. The extracellular matrix protein probably induces a conformational change in the integrin receptor which, in turn, is relayed to the proteins of the cytoskeleton.

In addition to signals which carry information from the extracellular matrix to enzymes which determine the shape of the cytoskeleton and to other intracellular enzymes, there are many responses to agonists, such as those linked to the generation of an intracellular messenger or to the activation of a protein–tyrosine kinase, which involve a change in the structure of the cytoskeleton. One example is the action of an agonist on a secretory cell to cause the movement and exocytosis of secretory granules. Another example is the action of f–met–leu–phe, platelet-activating factor, leukotriene B_4, or a number of other agonists on neutrophils. Each of these agonists increases neutrophil motility by inducing actin polymerization and by increasing the amount of actin associated with the cytoskeleton. A different type of example is the observation that the ability of an extracellular signal to induce a cellular response depends on the integrity of intracellular structures. For example, the disruption of actin filaments in Swiss 3T3 mouse fibroblasts by dihydrocytochalasin inhibits the stimulation, by serum, of DNA synthesis and cell growth.

A further example of a signal which leads to alterations in the behaviour of the cytoskeleton is the phosphorylation of integrin proteins. In avian cells infected by the Rous sarcoma virus, which contains the *src* oncogene encoding a protein–tyrosine kinase, the fibronectin integrin receptor is phosphorylated on a tyrosine residue. The phosphorylated integrin shows a decreased ability to bind talin and fibronectin. These changes probably underlie alterations in adhesive properties and morphology of the transformed cells.

2.4   Movement of mobile intracellular messengers and protein kinases

The structure of the cytoplasmic space and the presence of intracellular membranes which define the subcellular compartments play an important role in directing the flow of information from extracellular signals to intracellular sites. Although the relationship between cell structure and intracellular signalling is not yet fully understood it is important to try to understand how intracellular structures might channel signals in a given direction, and how these structures may constrain the movement of the mobile components of the intracellular signalling systems.

A number of experiments indicate that the movement of ions, metabolites, and proteins through the aqueous phase of the cytoplasmic space is considerably restricted compared with the movement of these molecules in pure water. The types of constraint that limit the movement of metabolites may well impede free movement of mobile intracellular messengers and protein kinases, although there have been few direct experimental measurements of the rates of movement of these molecules in the cytoplasmic space. It is useful to consider the constraints on the movement of metabolites as an indication of the type of constraint which may apply to the movement of intracellular messengers.

An experimental demonstration of constraints imposed on the movement of metabolites is provided by experiments conducted by Clegg (1984) with cultured L cells. These cells normally metabolize glucose to CO_2 through the glycolytic pathway and citric acid cycle. The formation of $[^{14}C]CO_2$ from $[^{14}C]$glucose as a function of time is shown in Fig. 2.14 (untreated cells). When the plasma membrane of L cells is made permeable to small molecules (but not to proteins) by treatment with dextran sulphate, the permeabilized L cells still metabolize glucose to CO_2 at a substantial rate comparable to that of untreated cells (Fig. 2.14). Clegg has argued that if the environment of the cytoplasmic space were a completely aqueous one, there should be little metabolism of glucose by permeabilized cells because cofactors such as ATP and NAD would have been completely lost from the cell by diffusion. Clegg suggests that the results of the experiment shown in Fig. 2.14 indicate that there are substantial constraints on the movement of metabolites such as ATP and NAD in the cytoplasmic space.

Evidence from a variety of experimental approaches suggests that, for a number of metabolic pathways, the component enzymes are arranged in a complex. Srere (1976) and Masters and his colleagues (Clarke and Masters 1974) and many others have speculated that the enzymes of a given metabolic complex are arranged sequentially so that metabolites which are intermediates in the pathway remain associated with the enzyme complex and cannot escape into the bulk of the cytoplasmic space. Examples of these putative complexes include enzymes involved in the synthesis of DNA, RNA, amino acids, proteins, glycogen, fatty acids, purines, pyrimidines, and steroids, and enzymes which comprise the glycolytic pathway, β-oxidation pathway for fatty acids, citric acid cycle, urea cycle, and electron transport pathway. One of the consequences of the existence of these enzyme complexes may be the channelling of the metabolites of a given metabolic pathway through specific microregions of the cell.

It is not yet known whether the mobile intracellular messengers are confined to specific regions of the cytoplasmic space in the manner speculated for metabolites. Evidence that mobile intracellular messengers and protein kinases can move relatively freely through the cytoplasmic space comes from experiments in which these agents have been introduced into the cytoplasmic space by microinjection or through permeabilized plasma membranes. When introduced in this manner, the intracellular messengers or protein kinases induce predicted physiological responses in the cells. Indeed, on the basis of measured rates of diffusion of small molecules in water it can be calculated that if the cytoplasmic space were a completely

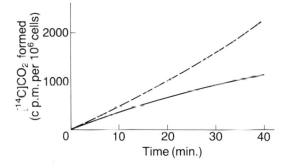

Fig. 2.14   An experiment which shows that in L cells in which the plasma membrane has been rendered permeable to metabolites but not to proteins (full curve), $[^{14}C\text{-}U]$glucose is metabolized to $[^{14}C]CO_2$ at a rate which is more than 50 per cent of the rate of glucose metabolism in untreated cells (broken curve). Both permeabilized and untreated cells were incubated in the absence of added cofactors. Glucose is metabolized to CO_2 through the glycolytic pathway and the citric acid cycle. The failure of permabilization to completely inhibit the metabolism of $[^{14}C\text{-}U]$glucose has been interpreted by Clegg as an indication that metabolites such as ATP and NAD are constrained to a location within the vicinity of the pathways that metabolize these compounds. From Mansell and Clegg (1983).

aqueous environment, the time taken for a molecule like cyclic AMP to move from the plasma membrane to the centre of a cell would be very short, about 100 ms.

The environment of the cytoplasmic space is not, however, equivalent to that of pure water. Therefore the rates of movement of mobile intracellular messengers and protein kinases in the cytoplasmic space are likely to be considerably slower than the rates of movement of these molecules in dilute aqueous solution. With the exception of Ca^{2+}, it has not been possible to measure the rates of movement of intracellular messengers and protein kinases through the cytoplasmic space. Experiments conducted with the axoplasm of the giant nerve of the squid have shown that the rate of diffusion of Ca^{2+} through the cytoplasmic space is about two orders of magnitude lower than the rate of diffusion

of Ca^{2+} in dilute aqueous solution. It is therefore probable that cells do not behave as aqueous bags that contain mobile messengers and protein kinases in dilute solution.

2.5 Transfer of information across the nuclear membrane

During interphase the contents of the nucleus and the reactions involved in the synthesis of DNA and RNA within the nucleus are shielded from the cytoplasmic space by the nuclear envelope. The main flow of information from the nucleus to the cytoplasmic space is in the form of RNA–protein complexes and ribosomes. The RNA present in RNA–protein complexes includes RNA which encodes proteins synthesized on ribosomes in the cytoplasmic space. Histones, DNA polymerases and RNA polymer-

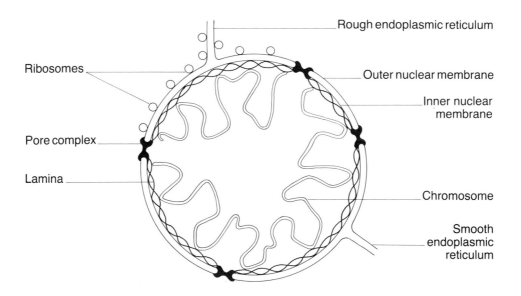

Fig. 2.15 The nuclear envelope is composed of an outer and an inner membrane and the nuclear lamina. The outer nuclear membrane is continuous with the membrane of the smooth and rough endoplasmic reticulum and possesses many of the properties of this membrane system, including the ability to bind ribosomes. The nuclear lamina is composed of proteins called lamins. These form filaments which line the nucleoplasmic surface of the inner nuclear membrane. The nuclear lamina provides an anchorage for chromosomes during interphase. The nuclear membrane is spanned by a large number of pores through which nuclear proteins, RNA–protein complexes, and ribosomes move by processes of active transport. At the interface between the inner and outer nuclear membranes and the pore complex the two membranes are joined.

ases, enzymes involved in the processing of RNA, sequence-specific DNA-binding proteins, DNA-binding receptor proteins for hormones and morphogens, and various protein–serine or protein–tyrosine kinases constitute the flow of information which moves from the cytoplasmic space to the nucleus.

The cytoplasmic side of the nuclear envelope consists of a double membrane while the inside of the envelope is composed of the nuclear lamina (Fig. 2.15). The two components of the double membrane are called the inner and outer membranes. At a number of locations, the outer membrane is continuous with the endoplasmic reticulum (Fig. 2.15). The nuclear lamina is a site of attachment of chromosomes. The lamina is a protein network composed of a class of intermediate filaments termed lamins. Several types of lamins exist. Those present in a particular nucleus depend, in part, on the animal from which the lamins are derived.

The movement of molecules across the nuclear envelope occurs through pores. These are water-filled cylindrical channels with an effective diameter of about 9 nm and a length of about 15 nm. There are probably between 3000 and 4000 pores in the nuclear envelope of an animal cell.

Each nuclear pore is created by a complex of glycoproteins. When examined by electron microscopy, the pore is seen as a hole into which eight 'spokes' face. Each spoke is probably composed of one or more polypeptide chains. At the boundary between the pore complex and the nuclear envelope, the inner and outer components of the nuclear membrane are joined (Fig. 2.15). The glycoprotein complex which constitutes a pore is very large with a total molecular mass of about $25–100 \times 10^3$ kDa. In electron micrographs of the nuclear membrane a granule is often observed in the centre of the pore. The granule may be a ribosome in transit or part of the pore complex.

The pore complex seems to act as a molecular sieve which readily allows the passive movement of molecules with molecular weights less than about 20 kDa. Metabolites, ions, and protein and RNA species with a low molecular weight probably move through nuclear pores by passive diffusion. However, proteins and RNA–protein complexes with molecular weights greater than about 20 kDa move by the process of active transport.

Nuclear proteins, which generally have molecular weights greater than 20 kDa, are directed to the nucleus by a signal sequence. The nature of this signal sequence is described in the next section. The steps in the process by which proteins are transported into the nucleus are not yet fully understood. The signal sequence probably binds to a receptor protein which is part of the nuclear-pore complex. This may lead to a conformational change in the proteins which compose the nuclear pore, an opening or gating of the channel, and movement of the protein through the pore. By this mechanism, proteins with diameters very much greater than 9 nm, the diameter of the nuclear pore, can enter the nucleus. In contrast to other newly synthesized proteins which cross membranes such as those of the mitochondria and endoplasmic reticulum to reach their final destination (described in the next section), nuclear proteins remain folded during their movement through nuclear pores. Nuclear proteins move across the nuclear membrane only in one direction: from the cytoplasmic space to the nucleus.

RNA is transported from the nucleus to the cytoplasmic space as an RNA–protein complex. These complexes, as well as ribosomes, which have a diameter of about 15 nm, probably move through the nuclear pores by a gating mechanism similar to that used for the inward flow of nuclear proteins. The movement of RNA–protein complexes and ribosomes from the nucleus to the cytoplasmic space is unidirectional.

2.6   Transmission of information which defines cell structure

2.6.1   *Signal sequences and the direction of newly synthesized proteins to specific cellular locations*

Information on cell structure is conveyed by the movement of newly synthesized proteins to their final destinations and by the movement of vesicles and organelles within the cytoplasmic space. Most proteins synthesized in animal cells are finally located in regions of the cell far removed from the ribosomes on which the proteins are synthesized. These proteins may be destined to move to an intracellular location, such as the cytoplasmic space, an intracellular membrane or the lumen of the mitochondria or peroxisomes, or to move to the extracellular space or to an intracellular space which is topologically equivalent to the extracellular space, such as the lumen of the endoplasmic reticulum, the Golgi cisternae, or lysosomes.

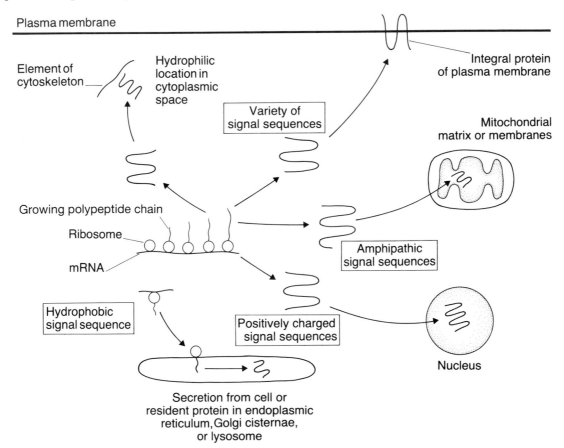

Fig. 2.16 Newly synthesized proteins are directed to their final intracellular locations by signal sequences. These are one or more distinctive sequences of amino-acid residues which are often removed once the protein has reached its final destination. Distinctive signal sequences direct proteins to the nucleus, the mitochondrial matrix, the mitochondrial membranes, the plasma membrane, hydrophilic locations in the cytoplasmic space, and the lumen of the endoplasmic reticulum. Some proteins directed to the lumen of the endoplasmic reticulum are formed into transport vesicles which mediate ultimate secretion of the proteins from the cell, while others reside in the endoplasmic reticulum or move to the Golgi apparatus or lysosomes.

Specific signal mechanisms have evolved to specify the final intracellular location of proteins (Fig. 2.16). With the possible exception of proteins located in hydrophilic regions of the cytoplasmic space (defined experimentally as 'soluble' proteins), those proteins destined for location at specific intracellular sites or for secretion from the cell contain one or more sequences of amino acids, called signal sequences, which direct the protein to its final destination. These signal sequences are sometimes called topogenic sequences. Some signal sequences are removed when the protein reaches its final destination.

The signal sequences seem to define a gross physical property, such as an amphipathic domain in the case of proteins destined for the mitochondria, a positively charged domain in the case of proteins directed to the nucleus or an hydrophobic domain in the case of secreted proteins. The interaction of one of these proteins with the target membrane appears to depend on the overall colligative property of the signal sequence rather than on the specific sequence of amino-acid residues which compose the signal sequence.

2.6.2 *Mechanisms which direct newly synthesized proteins to their intracellular locations*

Newly synthesized proteins destined for intracellular locations are synthesized on polysomes (free ribosomes) located in the cytoplasmic space. These newly synthesized proteins may be ultimately located in hydrophilic regions of the cytoplasmic space, in intracellular membranes such as those of the mitochondria and peroxisomes (but not the endoplasmic reticulum), in the plasma membrane, and in intermembrane spaces such as the mitochondrial matrix, nucleus, and the lumen of peroxisomes. While some plasma membrane proteins are synthesized on free ribosomes, many are synthesized on ribosomes attached to the endoplasmic reticulum

(Section 2.6.3).

Proteins destined for location in hydrophilic regions of the cytoplasmic space, for example the enzymes lactate dehydrogenase and hexokinase, probably contain some form of signal sequence that defines their final destination. However, little is known about the nature of these putative signal sequences. Once synthesized, the proteins undergo rapid folding to a stable form in which hydrophobic segments are buried. In this protected form the proteins then move to their final destination.

Proteins destined for location as integral proteins in the plasma membrane, the mitochondrial membranes, and for location in the mitochondrial matrix are partially folded during their synthesis on polysomes in order to protect their hydrophobic regions. Each partially folded protein probably combines with another protein called a chaperone protein and is guided to its destination by the signal sequence (Fig. 2.17). At the target membrane the newly synthesized protein binds to a receptor, is unfolded, and is translocated through the membrane in a process which derives energy from the hydrolysis of ATP. The signal sequence may be removed by the action of a peptidase called a leader peptidase.

Chaperone molecules probably stabilize newly synthesized proteins in a partially folded state. During and after its synthesis, a polypeptide chain begins to fold. In folding, the protein moves through a series of conformational states from one of highest free energy and maximum flexibility to one of lowest free energy and minimum flexibility. A relatively open and more flexible form of the protein is required for translocation through a membrane. The binding of a chaperone molecule to a newly synthesized protein probably maintains the protein in a more flexible conformation. One group of proteins which are candidates for chaperone molecules are the heat-shock or stress proteins. These have molecular weights of 25, 70, and 90 kDa. One

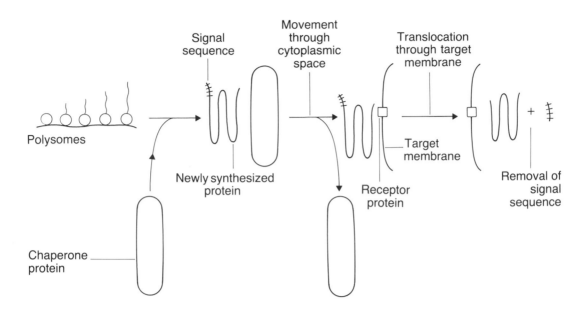

Fig. 2.17 Proteins destined for location in the nucleus, mitochondrial matrix, mitochondrial membranes, or plasma membranes are synthesized on free polysomes. Each protein is directed to its final location by a signal sequence within the newly synthesized polypeptide chain. The newly synthesized protein probably combines with another protein, called a chaperone protein, which stabilizes the conformation of the newly synthesized protein in a more flexible and less tightly folded state. The signal sequence is recognized by a receptor protein on the appropriate target membrane. Binding of the signal sequence to the receptor protein is accompanied by dissociation of the chaperone protein and initiation of translocation of the newly synthesized protein through the target membrane.

of these proteins, hsp90, binds to the steroid-hormone receptor in the cytoplasmic space (described in more detail in Chapter 10). Heat-shock proteins were first identified in cells by their presence at increased concentrations after an increase in temperature from 37 °C to 43 °C.

The acylation and farnesylation of some membrane-bound proteins probably plays a role in targeting these proteins to the cytoplasmic face of the plasma membrane. The farnesyl moiety is a 15-carbon molecule which contains three isoprene units. Farnesyl pyrophosphate is an intermediate in the pathway for the synthesis of squalene and cholesterol from mevalonate.

Acylation or farnesylation is essential for the plasma membrane location of the *src* protein–tyrosine kinase and the low molecular weight GTP-binding proteins encoded by the *ras* genes. The properties of the several members of the

ras protein family are described in Chapter 3. The mature *src* protein contains one myristyl group attached to the amino-terminal glycine. All mature *ras* proteins contain one farnesyl group attached to cys 186 and may also contain one palmitoyl group attached to cys 181. The mature H-*ras* protein contains an additional palmitoyl group attached to cys 184. The farnesyl and palmitoyl groups are attached in two post-translational steps (Fig. 2.18). Attachment of the farnesyl group is associated with removal of the last three amino acids ala–ala–X (X can be one of a number of amino acids) from the cys–ala–ala–X motif at the carboxy terminus. This reaction is catalysed by a carboxypeptidase and is succeeded by carboxymethylation of the α-carbon atom of cys 186.

The acyl and farnesyl groups on the *src* and *ras* proteins probably strengthen the hydropho-

Extracellular space

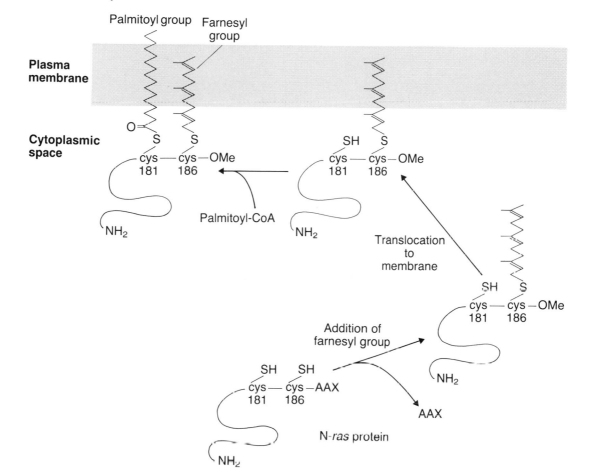

Fig. 2.18 The presence of a farnesyl group on cys 186 and a palmitoyl group on cys 181 of the N-*ras* protein probably plays a role in targeting this protein to the plasma membrane and in attaching the protein to the membrane. The farnesyl and palmitoyl groups are added in two steps. Addition of the farnesyl group is associated with proteolytic cleavage of a cys–ala–ala–X motif (X is any amino acid) at the carboxy terminus to yield the tripeptide ala–ala–X (AAX) and with carboxymethylation of the α-carboxyl group of cys 186.

bic interaction of these proteins with the plasma membrane. Oncogenic forms of the *src* and *ras* proteins which can transform established cultured cell lines are also acylated and farnesylated. If the structure of the protein is altered by site-directed mutagenesis so that the protein cannot be acylated, the resulting altered forms of the oncogenic proteins cannot transform cells.

The complete role of the acyl groups that are linked to proteins attached to the plasma mem-

brane is not yet fully understood. For example, it is not yet clear why the acyl group attached to any given protein is of a specific type and fatty-acid chain length. Moreover, there are also a number of other cellular proteins that are acylated but are not located at the plasma membrane. This suggests that acyl groups may serve functions other than directing and attaching proteins to the plasma membrane.

Signal sequences which designate the location

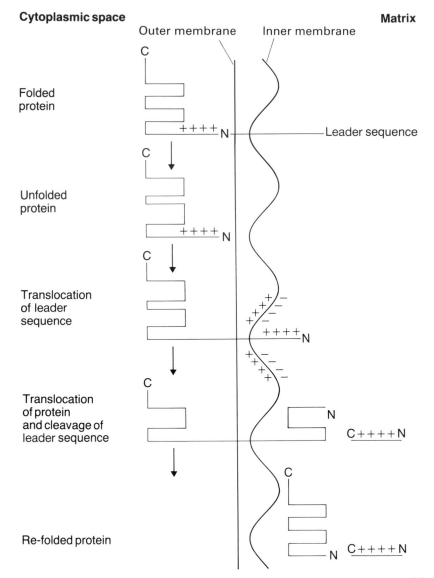

Fig. 2.19 A positively charged signal sequence (the leader sequence) at the amino terminus (N) directs proteins synthesized on free polysomes in the cytoplasmic space to the mitochondrial matrix. The leader sequence interacts with a site on the outer mitochondrial membrane. After the protein unfolds the force exerted on the positively charged leader sequence by the electrochemical gradient across the inner membrane translocates the protein into the matrix. Translocation takes place at a site where the inner and outer mitochondrial membranes are closely associated. Within the matrix the leader sequence is cleaved and the protein re-folds.

of a protein in the mitochondrial matrix are called transit or leader peptides. Leader sequences are highly basic (positively charged) and amphipathic, and are of a variable length and sequence. The leader sequence is attached to the amino terminus of the protein. The movement of a protein, synthesized on a polysome, from the cytoplasmic space adjacent to the mitochondrial outer membrane, to the mitochondrial matrix, first involves unfolding of the protein

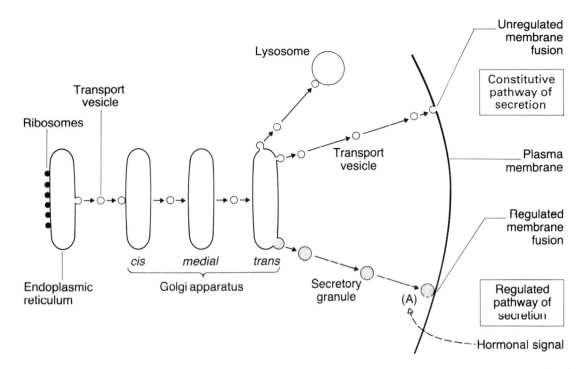

Fig. 2.20 Proteins destined for secretion are synthesized on ribosomes attached to the rough endoplasmic reticulum and are translocated to the lumen of the endoplasmic reticulum during synthesis. After transfer to the *cis, medial,* and *trans* Golgi cisternae, the proteins are then transferred to the plasma membrane by one of two pathways. The constitutive secretory pathway employs transport vesicles and is present in all cells. Cells such as pancreatic acinar cells, which have a specific secretory function, possess a second secretory pathway called the regulated secretory pathway. In this pathway proteins which are to be transferred from the *trans* Golgi cisternae to the plasma membrane are concentrated in secretory granules. The movement and exocytosis of secretory granules is dependent on activation (A) by an extracellular signal such as a hormone. Some proteins synthesized on the rough endoplasmic reticulum are not excreted but are retained in the endoplasmic reticulum or Golgi cisternae, or are transferred to lysosomes where they form the protein components of these vesicles.

(Fig. 2.19). The positively charged leader sequence then moves into the mitochondrial matrix across both the outer and inner membranes at a point where these membranes are in contact. The energy for translocation of the leader sequence is derived from the electrochemical gradient across the inner mitochondrial membrane. After cleavage of the leader sequence and translocation of the protein across the membrane, the protein re-folds in the mitochondrial matrix, combines with a chaperone protein and moves to its destination.

Some mitochondrial proteins encoded by

nuclear genes are located in the inner or outer mitochondrial membrane, or in the intermembrane space. Proteins destined for location in the intermembrane space contain two leader sequences. These proteins are first translocated to the mitochondrial matrix by a mechanism similar to that shown in Fig. 2.19 then move outwards through the inner membrane to the intermembrane space. Proteins destined for location in the inner membrane probably follow a similar pathway but are retained in the membrane.

As described earlier, proteins destined for

location in the nucleus (presumably all nuclear proteins) are directed to nuclear pores by signal sequences. The amino acids which constitute the signal sequence may be located at the amino terminus, carboxy terminus, or interior of the polypeptide chain. Unlike most other signal sequences, nuclear protein signal sequences are not cleaved after the protein has moved across the nuclear membrane. This may allow the protein to be relocated in the nucleus again after a round of cell division in which the nuclear membrane has been broken down and reformed.

2.6.3 *Mechanisms which direct newly synthesized proteins to extracellular spaces and the plasma membrane*

Proteins destined for secretion to the extracellular space or for location in spaces topologically identical to the extracellular space, and some proteins destined for location in the plasma membrane are synthesized on ribosomes attached to the rough endoplasmic reticulum. Proteins located in spaces topologically similar to the extracellular space include those which reside in the endoplasmic reticulum or Golgi system, lysosomal hydrolases and other proteins which reside in the lysosomes, and proteins contained in any vesicles which can be formed from, or fused with, the endoplasmic reticulum or Golgi system. All these proteins, together with proteins destined for secretion, are translocated to the lumen of the rough endoplasmic reticulum during their synthesis.

For each of these proteins, synthesis of the polypeptide chain occurs while the ribosome is attached to the endoplasmic reticulum. During synthesis, the polypeptide chain enters the lumen of this organelle. If the protein is destined for secretion from the cell or for location in the Golgi cisternae or lysosomes it is then transferred from the lumen of the endoplasmic reticulum to the Golgi system. Proteins destined for secretion move to the plasma membrane while those destined for lysosomes move to these organelles. Proteins which are components of the endoplasmic reticulum are retained in this organelle.

Some integral membrane proteins are also delivered to the plasma membrane through the secretory pathway as components of transport vesicles which fuse with the plasma membrane. These proteins possess signal sequences which direct them to the plasma membrane and help to determine the correct orientation of the protein in this membrane. Proteins which span the membrane once with the carboxy terminus facing the cytoplasmic space have a cleavable signal sequence while proteins which span the membrane more than once have multiple signal sequences. Proteins which span the membrane once with the amino terminus facing the cytoplasmic space have no identifiable signal sequence although they may possess other properties which direct them to the plasma membrane.

There are two pathways for the secretion of proteins, called the regulated and constitutive pathways (Fig. 2.20). In each of these pathways, proteins to be secreted are transferred in transport vesicles from the lumen of the endoplasmic reticulum to the *trans* Golgi cisternae. In the regulated pathway, proteins, metabolites, such as neurotransmitters, and ions which are to be secreted are packaged into vesicles called secretory granules in the *trans* Golgi cisternae. The secretory granules are then delivered to the plasma membrane and the contents released by exocytosis. In the regulated secretory pathway, secretion only occurs in response to an extracellular signal such as a hormone. This pathway of secretion is present only in specialized secretory cells, for example, pancreatic acinar cells which secrete amylase, platelets which secrete a variety of proteins and metabolites, and nerve cells which secrete neurotransmitters.

The constitutive pathway of secretion is not regulated by extracellular signals and is present in all cells. Thus, specialized secretory cells possess both the regulated and constitutive pathways while other cells possess only the constitutive secretory pathway. In the constitutive pathway, proteins are packaged into vesicles, called transport vesicles, in the *trans* Golgi cisternae. The constitutive pathway is responsible for a continuous traffic of transport vesicles from the *trans* Golgi region to the plasma membrane.

The constitutive secretory pathway is also called the bulk-flow pathway or default pathway of secretion. The latter term refers to the hypothesis that recognition processes positively select proteins which originate in the lumen of the endoplasmic reticulum for translocation to all other cellular destinations but allows all non-selected proteins to be secreted.

The movement of proteins synthesized on the rough endoplasmic reticulum to their appropriate final destination depends as much on the

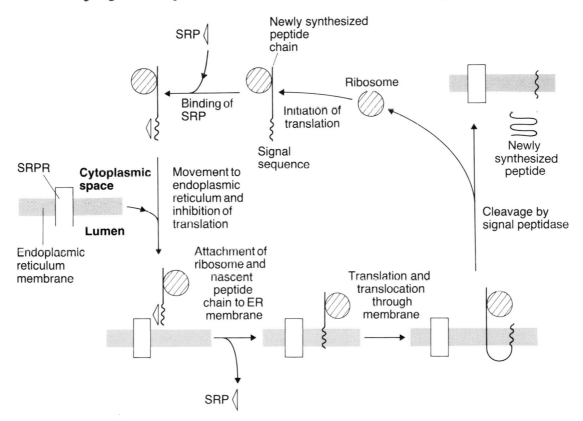

Fig. 2.21 Proteins synthesized on the rough endoplasmic reticulum possess a hydrophobic signal sequence which is present on the nascent polypeptide chain initially synthesized on a free ribosome. The signal sequence has a high affinity for a protein called a signal recognition protein (SRP) to which it binds. The formation of this complex results in an inhibition of mRNA translation. The ribosome–mRNA–nascent polypeptide chain–SRP complex then binds to the membrane of the rough endoplasmic reticulum (ER) as a result of interaction between the SRP and a SRP receptor protein (SRPR) present in the endoplasmic reticulum membrane. This allows attachment of the nascent polypeptide chain to the endoplasmic reticulum membrane, probably at a site separate from the SRPR, continuation of mRNA translation, and translocation of the newly synthesized polypeptide chain through the membrane of the endoplasmic reticulum. After completion of translocation, the ribosome dissociates and the signal sequence is cleaved by a signal peptidase.

sorting of the proteins in the endoplasmic reticulum and Golgi system as on the mechanisms by which the proteins are moved from the lumen of the endoplasmic reticulum through the cell. These sorting processes determine which proteins remain in the endoplasmic reticulum and Golgi system, and which proteins are transferred to lysosomes, transport vesicles of the constitutive secretory pathway or to secretory granules of the regulated secretory pathway.

The process of sorting probably depends on the three-dimensional structure and certain amino acid sequences on the protein to be sorted. It is likely that these properties allow the protein to be recognized by a receptor protein in the membrane of the vesicle in which the newly synthesized protein is to reside or to which the newly synthesized protein is to be transferred. In the case of integral plasma membrane proteins, multiple sorting signals, including covalently-bound glycosyl-phosphatidylinositol, direct these proteins to the plasma membrane. In polarized cells that possess both apical and basal membranes, the glycosyl-phosphatidylinositol moiety may be responsible for directing a given protein to the apical membrane. The translocation of newly synthesized proteins from the ribosome in the cytoplasmic space to the lumen of the endoplasmic reticulum, and the transfer of proteins from the lumen of the endoplasmic reticulum to the extracellular medium by the constitutive and regulatory pathways of secretion, will now be considered in more detail.

2.6.4 *Transfer of newly synthesized proteins to the lumen of the endoplasmic reticulum*

The signal sequence of proteins destined for the lumen of the endoplasmic reticulum consists of a hydrophobic chain of about 20 amino-acid residues attached to the amino terminus of the protein. The central region of this sequence, called the H-region, consists of 8–18 consecutive uncharged amino-acid residues. The presence of this signal sequence on a nascent polypeptide chain is recognized by a protein called the signal recognition protein (SRP). The SRP, which is an oligomer composed of six polypeptide chains and one molecule of RNA, can be considered as a dissociable subunit of the ribosome. The signal sequence of the nascent peptide binds to the SRP to form a complex which consists of the ribosome, nascent peptide, SRP, mRNA, and tRNA (Fig. 2.21).

The signal sequence binds to a 54 kDa subunit of the SRP. Interaction of the signal sequence with the 54 kDa SRP subunit probably occurs in the carboxyl half of the subunit in a region called the M domain which is enriched in methionine residues. The predicted tertiary structure of the 54 kDa SRP subunit contains four amphipathic helices. One face of each helix is hydrophobic and is composed of methionine residues while the other face contains patches of polar residues. A hydrophobic region of the signal sequence probably binds to the hydrophobic methionine region of the M domain of the 54 kDa SRP subunit.

Interaction of the nascent polypeptide chain with the SRP inhibits further mRNA translation and allows the ribosome to bind to a receptor, called the signal recognition protein receptor (SRPR), on the membrane of the endoplasmic reticulum. Another name for the receptor protein is the docking protein. The SRPR, which is a heterodimer composed of an α and a β subunit, is found only on the endoplasmic reticulum membrane.

After combination of the ribosome–SRP complex with the SRPR, the SRP is released and the ribosome is probably transferred to another site on the endoplasmic reticulum membrane. This enables the hydrophobic peptide signal sequence to enter the membrane. Location of the ribosome complex at this second site may involve another protein which destabilizes the phospholipid bilayer and allows insertion of the

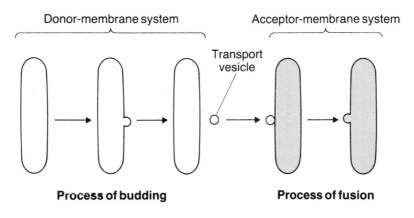

Fig. 2.22 The transfer of proteins from one membrane system (the donor) to a second membrane system (the acceptor), for example, the membrane systems described in Fig. 2.20, is achieved by entrapment of the protein inside a transport vesicle. These vesicles are formed by budding from the donor membrane. They transfer their contents to the acceptor-membrane system by fusion. The composition and concentration of the contents of the transport vesicle reflect those of the lumen of the donor-membrane system.

polypeptide chain through the phospholipid bilayer or through a pore.

The 54 kDa subunit of the SRP and the SRPR both contain binding sites for GTP. The GTP-binding site in the 54 kDa SRP subunit is located in the amino-terminal half of the molecule called the G domain. GTP may be required for the binding of the SRP to the SRPR and for interaction of the nascent polypeptide chain with the endoplasmic reticulum membrane. After binding of the ribosome–SRP complex to the SRPR, hydrolysis of GTP may lead to conformational changes in the SRP and the SRPR which result in the firm attachment of the ribosome to the endoplasmic reticulum.

Once docked at the correct site, translation of the mRNA and synthesis of the polypeptide chain continues. At the same time, the polypeptide is translocated through the membrane and the signal peptide cleaved by a peptidase (Fig. 2.21).

2.6.5 *Formation and fusion of transport vesicles in the constitutive secretory pathway*
In the constitutive pathway of secretion, newly synthesized protein destined for secretion from the cell is transferred from the lumen of the endoplasmic reticulum in turn to the *cis* Golgi compartment, then to the *medial* Golgi compartment, the *trans* Golgi compartment, and finally to the plasma membrane (Fig. 2.20). The transfer from one membrane system to another is achieved by transport vesicles. These are formed by membrane budding and fusion (Fig. 2.22). In these processes, protein is transferred from one membrane compartment to another without passing across a membrane. The contents entrapped in the transport vesicle reflect the contents of the lumen of the organelle from which the vesicle is formed.

Transport vesicles move along microtubules between the endoplasmic reticulum, Golgi compartments, and plasma membrane in a process which requires ATP. The fusion of a transport vesicle with an acceptor membrane requires the presence of a low molecular weight GTP-binding protein. The nature and properties of the low molecular weight GTP-binding proteins are described in more detail in Chapter 3. The fusion process is inhibited by GTPγS, an analogue of GTP.

The low molecular weight GTP-binding protein is probably required to direct the transport vesicle to a recognition protein (docking protein) which identifies the correct acceptor membrane for that particular transport vesicle (Fig. 2.23). The hydrolysis of GTP may act as a switch to ensure that the transport vesicle binds tightly to the correct acceptor membrane. The role of the low molecular weight GTP-binding proteins in the process by which a transport vesicle identifies the correct acceptor membrane is not completely understood. However, this process of recognition is of sufficient importance to warrant a description of how the low molecular weight GTP-binding protein is thought to act.

The GTP switch probably acts in the following way. Both correct (cognate) and incorrect (non-cognate) transport vesicles bind rapidly to the recognition protein in a given acceptor membrane. The rate of dissociation of the correct transport vesicle from the recognition protein is slow compared with the rate of dissociation of the incorrect vesicle. For the correct vesicle, the additional time spent bound to the recognition protein in the membrane allows GTP to be hydrolysed, conformational changes to occur in the GTP-binding protein and in the recognition protein, and the vesicle to be locked to the membrane. A critical factor in this recognition process is the relationship between the rate of GTP hydrolysis and the time the transport vesicle spends attached to the membrane before the hydrolysis of GTP.

The fusion of transport vesicles with the *cis* and *medial* Golgi membranes requires a protein called N-ethylmaleimide-sensitive fusion protein (NSF). This protein was discovered through its sensitivity to inhibition by N-ethylmaleimide. The NSF is a tetramer composed of subunits with a molecular weight of 76 kDa. The NSF is probably a component of a protein complex that is assembled and disassembled in a cyclic fashion in order to ensure the efficient fusion between the transport vesicle and its target membrane.

The transfer of proteins from the lumen of the endoplasmic reticulum to the plasma membrane through the constitutive secretory pathway requires Ca^{2+}. This may be required for the movement of transport vesicles along microtubules and for the fusion of vesicles to acceptor membranes.

2.6.6   *Formation and fusion of secretory granules*

The formation of secretory granules at the *trans* Golgi compartment in the pathway of regulated secretion involves aggregation and concentration of the proteins that are to be included in the secretory granule and addition of the non-protein components of the granule, such as neurotransmitters. In contrast to transport vesicles formed in the constitutive secretory pathway, the concentration of a given protein in secretory granules is very much greater than the concentration of the same protein in the lumen of the Golgi compartment. The newly formed secretory granule is covered by a coat which is composed of the protein clathrin. The secretory granules move to the plasma membrane along microtubules.

The interaction of secretory granules with the plasma membrane and release of the granule contents to the extracellular space require a change in the structure of the cytoskeleton adjacent to the plasma membrane. The secretory granules are initially held away from the membrane by the cortical mesh of actin filaments (Fig. 2.24). This mesh is composed of F-actin which is cross-linked and stabilized by spectrin and α-actinin. The primary intracellular signal for the change in cytoskeletal structure appears to be an increase in the concentration of free Ca^{2+} in the vicinity of the granule. Ca^{2+} probably exerts its effects by binding to the Ca^{2+}-binding proteins chromobindin, calpactin, and synexin. This causes the dissociation of actin from spec-

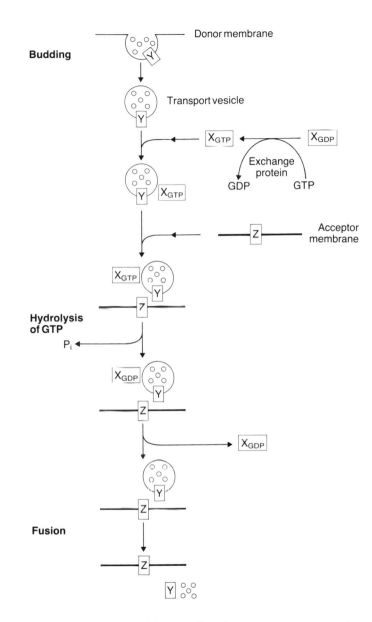

Fig. 2.23 The process by which a transport vesicle recognizes the correct acceptor membrane probably involves a low molecular weight GTP-binding protein, designated here as protein X, and specific proteins, designated here as Y and Z, in the membrane of the vesicle and in the acceptor membrane, respectively. The sequence of events which is thought to occur is as follows. GTP binds to the guanine nucleotide binding site of protein X and a molecule of X-GTP binds to protein Y on the surface of the transport vesicle. Although the vesicle–Y–X-GTP complex has a relatively low affinity for protein Z, a complex between the vesicle–X-GTP and protein Z is formed. The subsequent hydrolysis of GTP is thought to induce conformational changes in proteins X and Y which increases the affinity of protein Y for protein Z, and hence results in a much tighter association between the vesicle and the acceptor membrane. This allows dissociation of X-GDP from the membrane and fusion of the transport vesicle with the membrane. X-GTP is regenerated by the action of a GTP exchange protein.

trin, activation of the enzyme gelsolin, and the capping and shortening of actin filaments. These changes are accompanied by the phosphorylation of myosin light chains. The result is a decrease in viscosity of the actin-filament network which allows the secretory granules to move to the plasma membrane (Fig. 2.24). The granules then fuse with the membrane and release their contents by exocytosis.

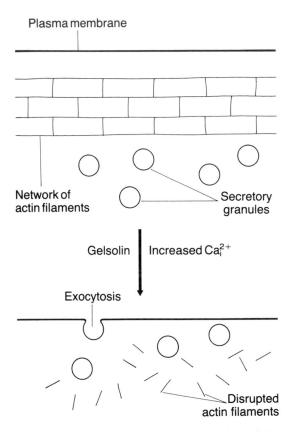

Fig. 2.24 An increase in the concentration of free Ca^{2+} in the cytoplasmic space adjacent to the plasma membrane is probably the main signal which initiates the movement of secretory granules to the plasma membrane and the subsequent exocytosis of the granules. At resting intracellular free Ca^{2+} concentrations, secretory granules are held away from the plasma membrane by the network of actin filaments. In conjunction with gelsolin, an increased concentration of free Ca^{2+} induces solubilization of the actin network which, in turn, allows the granules to interact with the plasma membrane.

2.6.7 *Endocytosis*

The outward movement of secretory granules and transport vesicles from the perinuclear space to the plasma membrane, which was described earlier, is part of a two-way traffic between these two intracellular locations (Fig. 2.25). The other component of this two-way traffic is the inward movement of endocytotic vesicles. The process of endocytosis is most clearly described for the transport of receptors from the plasma membrane to lysosomes or the Golgi apparatus (Chapter 3). In addition to its role in regulating the concentration of plasma-membrane receptors, endocytosis probably also serves other functions. These include the return of membrane material from the plasma membrane to the Golgi apparatus. This balances the movement of membrane material to the plasma membrane in the process of secretion.

The process of endocytosis is complex and not yet completely understood. Endosomes are formed at the plasma membrane by the inward budding of this membrane (Fig. 2.25). The formation of an endocytotic vesicle involves the attachment of clathrin protein to the cytoplasmic face of the membrane. Together with proteins called adaptins, clathrin concentrates receptor proteins in coated pits, which are the precursors of endosomes. The proteins and lipids present in peripheral endosomes are passed either to perinuclear endosomes, which may interact with the *trans* Golgi system to deliver proteins for recycling to the plasma membrane in transport vesicles, or to endolysosomes, the precursors of lysosomes. The fusion of endosomes with each other or with acceptor membranes, such as the Golgi system or an endolysosome, requires an N-ethylmaleimide-sensitive protein. This may be identical to the NSF protein required for the fusion of transport vesicles to the *medial* and *trans* Golgi membranes.

As described earlier, newly synthesized lyso-

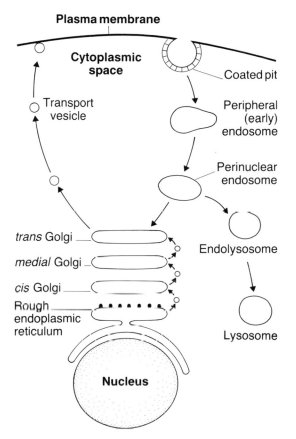

Fig. 2.25 In most animal cells there is a continuous traffic of vesicles in both directions between the plasma membrane and the perinuclear space. Outward traffic consists chiefly of transport vesicles formed at the *trans* Golgi cisternae. Inward movement chiefly consists of endosomes formed at the plasma membrane by the process of endocytosis. Some endosomes fuse with the *trans* Golgi network while the contents of others are transferred to lysosomes.

somal hydrolases are transported from the *trans* Golgi cisternae to endolysosomes by transport vesicles. The signal which directs these enzymes to the endolysosome is probably a mannose-6-phosphate moiety which recognizes mannose-6-phosphate receptors in the membrane of endolysosomes.

In cell-free experimental systems, the fusion of endocytotic vesicles with acceptor membranes is inhibited by the p34[cdc2] protein kinase which

plays a central role in the control of the cell cycle (Chapter 10). This inhibition may be a reflection of a mechanism which operates during mitosis to allow the division of single intracellular organelles, such as the endoplasmic reticulum and Golgi apparatus, into two, during cell division. During mitosis these organelles are disassembled into small vesicles preceding the equal proportioning of the membrane material from each organelle between daughter cells and the re-assembly of the organelle in each daughter cell.

2.6.8   *Movement of organelles between the nucleus and the plasma membrane*

The traffic of vesicles and organelles between the perinuclear space and the plasma membrane is most clearly apparent between the cell body and the synaptic terminus in nerve cells. In the nerve cell, ribosomes are located only in the cell body, so that proteins destined for location or secretion at the synaptic terminus must be carried over a long distance. The movement of organelles and vesicles in nerve cells is called axonal transport. This type of transport has been studied extensively using video-enhanced contrast microscopy.

The component of axonal transport which is outward from the cell body is called anterograde movement. This is composed of the relatively slow movement of microtubules, neurofilaments, actin filaments, other cytoskeletal proteins and enzymes, and the relatively fast movement of transport vesicles, secretory granules, and mitochondria. Proteins and enzymes move at a rate of about 1–5 nm per day whilst the membrane-bounded vesicles move at a rate of about 400 nm per day. The anterograde movement of a protein, transport vesicle, or organelle takes place along a microtubule to which the protein, vesicle, or organelle is attached. The microtubule network provides a highway for the movement of these particles. The movement is catalysed by the enzyme kinesin which utilizes energy released by the hydrolysis of ATP to move particles along the microtubule.

The inward component of axonal transport, called retrograde transport, is composed chiefly of endocytotic vesicles and ageing mitochondria. These move along microtubules at a rate of about 200–300 nm/day. A single microtubule can facilitate the movement of vesicles or organelles in both the retrograde and anterograde directions. Movement in the retrograde direction is catalysed by the protein dynein. Samples of the extracellular fluid are incorporated into endocytotic vesicles and are transported to the cell body. The formation of endocytotic vesicles and their retrograde movement may allow the cell body to gain information about the chemical environment of the extracellular space.

2.7 Summary

The nature of a given signal transmitted within an animal cell is determined by the chemical composition of the signalling molecules and the physical structure of the pathway along which the signalling molecules pass. Animal cells are subdivided into a number of membrane-bound compartments. These include the nucleus, mitochondria, and peroxisomes, and the endoplasmic reticulum, Golgi system, and lysosomes which are topologically similar to the extracellular space. Most of the pathways of intracellular communication pass through the cytoplasmic space while some pass into the nucleus and intracellular organelles.

The cytoplasmic space is highly structured. The basic framework is provided by the cytoskeleton which consists of microtubules, intermediate filaments, and actin filaments. Within this network is the microtrabecular lattice. The components of the cytoskeleton probably bind proteins, enzymes, and water in an ordered manner.

Some information is conveyed across the plasma membrane and within cells by changes in the shape of the cytoskeleton. The cytoskeleton is linked to proteins in the extracellular matrix by membrane-spanning proteins called integrins which span the plasma membrane. Proteins in the extracellular matrix, such as fibrinogen, probably influence the behaviour of cells by changing the conformations of integrins and the cytoskeleton. Many extracellular signals which lead to the generation of an intracellular messenger or the activation of a protein kinase induce changes in the structure of the cytoskeleton.

Subcellular structures may help to channel signals through pathways of intracellular communication in the same way that multienzyme complexes probably direct the flow of metabolites along metabolic pathways. Intracellular messengers, protein kinases, and sequence-specific DNA-binding proteins appear to be able to diffuse freely through most of the cytoplasmic space, although it is unlikely that the rate at which they move is the same as that in a pure aqueous environment.

Many signals in the form of proteins and RNA cross the nuclear envelope which lies between the cytoplasmic space and the nucleus. These molecules pass through nuclear-pore complexes which act as molecular sieves. Nuclear proteins are targeted to the nucleus by signal sequences which probably recognize receptors on the pore complex. Combination of the signal sequence with the pore complex opens the pore and allows the protein to move into the nucleus. RNA, in the form of RNA–protein complexes, and ribosomes move out of the nucleus through pores by a process of active transport. The movement of each type of macromolecule through nuclear pores is unidirectional.

The movement of newly synthesized proteins to their final destination in the cell and the movement of organelles and membrane-bound vesicles between specific intracellular locations conveys information about cell structure from one part of the cell to another. Hydrophilic proteins which are destined for location in the cytoplasmic space, and proteins destined for location in the nucleus, mitochondrial matrix, mitochondrial membranes, and plasma membrane are synthesized on free ribosomes. These proteins are directed to membranes or membrane-bound spaces by signal sequences. These sequences of amino-acid residues bind to receptor proteins on target membranes. The newly synthesized protein is then unfolded, translocated through the membrane and, in most cases, the signal sequence is removed by a specific peptidase.

Proteins that are secreted from the cell, together with those that reside in the endoplasmic reticulum and Golgi apparatus, and lysosomal hydrolases, are synthesized on ribosomes attached to the rough endoplasmic reticulum. The nascent polypeptide chain is directed to the endoplasmic reticulum by a signal sequence, a signal recognition protein, and a receptor for the signal recognition protein. The nascent peptide chain is then translocated to the lumen of the endoplasmic reticulum.

Proteins destined for secretion are transferred sequentially from the endoplasmic reticulum to the *cis*, *medial*, and *trans* Golgi cisternae then to the plasma membrane. The transfer of protein from one membrane system to another involves budding of the donor membrane, the formation of a small membrane-bound vesicle called the transport vesicle which contains the newly synthesized protein, and fusion of the vesicle with the acceptor membrane. Recognition by the vesicle of the correct acceptor membrane involves a low molecular weight GTP-binding protein. This pathway, which is present in all cells, is called the constitutive secretory pathway. Some cells possess an additional pathway of protein secretion called the regulated secretory pathway.

The latter pathway involves the formation of secretory granules which only fuse with the plasma membrane in response to an extracellular signal.

Within the cytoplasmic space there is a constant traffic of transport vesicles, mitochondria, and proteins from the Golgi system to the plasma membrane. A traffic of endosomes formed by endocytosis of the plasma membrane moves in the opposite direction. All these vesicles, organelles, and proteins move along microtubules. In nerve cells, in which the distances along these pathways is large, the movement of membrane vesicles, organelles, and proteins is called 'axonal transport'.

References

Carraway, K. L. and Carraway, C. A. C. (1989). Membrane–cytoskeleton interactions in animal cells. *Biochim. Biophys. Acta*, **988**, 147–71.

Clarke, F. M. and Masters, C. J. (1974). On the association of glycolytic components in skeletal muscle extracts. *Biochim. Biophys. Acta*, **358**, 193 207.

Clegg, J. S. (1984). Properties and metabolism of the aqueous cytoplasm and its boundaries. *Am. J. Physiol.*, **246**, R133–51.

Greve, J. M. and Gottlieb, D. I. (1982). Monoclonal antibodies which alter the morphology of cultured chick myogenic cells. *J. Cell. Biochem.*, **18**, 221–9.

Krstíc, R. V. (1979). *Ultrastructure of the mammalian cell: an atlas*, pp. 98–9. Springer, Berlin.

Leeson, T. S. and Leeson, C. R. (1970). *Histology* (2nd edn), p. 316. W. B. Saunders, Philadelphia.

Mansell, J. L. and Clegg, J. S. (1983). Cellular and molecular consequences of reduced cell water content. *Cryobiology*, **20**, 591–612.

Neff, N. T., Lowrey, C., Decker, C., Tovar, A., Damsky, C., Buck, C., and Horwitz, A. F. (1982). A monoclonal antibody detaches embryonic skeletal muscle from extracellular matrices. *J. Cell Biol.*, **95**, 654–66.

Porter, K. R. (1986). Structural organization of the cytomatrix. In *The organization of cell metabolism* (ed. G. R. Welch and J. S. Clegg), pp. 9–26. Plenum,

New York.

Porter, K. R. and Tucker, J. B. (1981). The ground substance of the living cell. *Sci. Am.*, **244**, 40–51.

Schliwa, M. (1986). The cytoskeleton: an introductory survey. In *Cell biology monographs* (ed. M. Alfert, W. Beermann, L. Goldstein, and K. R. Porter), Vol. 13. Springer, Vienna.

Srere, P. A. (1976). Apparent K_ms and apparent concentrations: an apparent conundrum. In *Gluconeogenesis, its regulation in mammalian species* (ed. R. W. Hanson, and M. A. Mehlman), pp. 153–61. Wiley, New York.

Wolosewick, J. J. and Porter, K. R. (1979). Microtrabecular lattice of the cytoplasmic ground substance: artifact or reality. *J. Cell Biol.*, **82**, 114–39.

Further reading

Alberts, B., Bray, D., Lewis, J., Raff, M., Roberts, K., and Watson, J. D. (1989). *Molecular biology of the cell* (2nd edn), Ch. 8. Garland, New York.

Balch, W. E. (1989). Biochemistry of interorganelle transport: a new frontier in enzymology emerges from versatile *in vitro* model systems. *J. Biol. Chem.*, **264**, 16965–8.

Bershadsky, A. D. and Vasiliev, J. M. (1988). *Cytoskeleton*. Plenum, New York.

Burridge, K., Fath, K., Kelly, T., Nuckolls, G. and Turner, C. (1988). Focal adhesions: transmembrane junctions between the extracellular matrix and the cytoskeleton. *Ann. Rev. Cell Biol.*, **4**, 487–525.

Carraway, K. L. and Carraway, C. A. C. (1989). Membrane–cytoskeleton interactions in animal cells. *Biochim. Biophys. Acta*, **988**, 147–71.

Clegg, J. S. (1984). Properties and metabolism of the aqueous cytoplasm and its boundaries. *Am. J. Physiol.*, **246**, R133–51.

Gerace, L. and Burke, B. (1988). Functional organization of the nuclear envelope. *Ann. Rev. Cell Biol.*, **4**, 335–74.

Grand, R. J. A. (1989). Acylation of viral and eukaryotic proteins. *Biochem. J.*, **258**, 625–38.

Kellermayer, M. and Hazlewood, C. F. (1986). Restricted motion of cellular K^+ in permeabilized cells. In *The organization of cell metabolism* (ed. G. R. Welch and J. S. Clegg), pp. 75–8. Plenum, New York.

Kelly, R. B. (1990). Microtubules, membrane traffic, and cell organization. *Cell*, **61**, 5–7.

Mastro, A. M. and Hurley, D. J. (1986). Diffusion of a small molecule in the aqueous compartment of mammalian cells. In *The organization of cell metabolism* (ed. G. R. Welch and J. S. Clegg), pp. 57–74. Plenum, New York.

Negendank, W. and Edelmann, L. (1988). *The state of water in the cell*. Scanning Microscopy International, AMF O'Hare (Chicago), Illinois.

Pelham, H. R. B. (1989). Control of protein exit from the endoplasmic reticulum. *Ann. Rev. Cell Biol.*, **5**, 1–23.

Porter, K. R. (1984). The cytomatrix: a short history of its study. *J. Cell Biol.*, **99**, 3S–12S.

Springer, T. A. (1990). The sensation and regulation of interactions with the extracellular environment: the cell biology of lymphocyte adhesion receptors. *Ann. Rev. Cell Biol.*, **6**, 359–402.

Srere, P. A. (1987). Complexes of sequential metabolic enzymes. *Ann. Rev. Biochem.*, **56**, 89–124.

Srivastava, D. K. and Bernhard, S. A. (1987). Biophysical chemistry of metabolic reaction sequences in concentrated enzyme solution and in the cell. *Ann. Rev. Biophys. Biophys. Chem.*, **16**, 175–204.

Watterson, J. G. (1987). A role for water in cell structure. *Biochem. J.*, **248**, 615–17.

3 The plasma-membrane receptors and GTP-binding proteins

3.1 Plasma-membrane receptors involved in intracellular communication

Receptors involved in the transmission of signals across the plasma membrane belong to one of a number of plasma-membrane receptor subgroups. Other types of receptor include those for antigens and those required for the uptake of metals and metabolic substrates such as the iron–transferrin complex and low-density lipoproteins (LDL). All known plasma-membrane receptors for extracellular signals are proteins.

Each receptor protein consists of several regions called domains, and each domain is often encoded by a discrete exon. Each receptor may be considered a patchwork of domains that are related in structure to domains present in other receptors and in other proteins. For example, certain domains in the LDL receptor are related in sequence to domains of enzyme components of the blood-clotting system, the complement system, and the precursor of epidermal growth factor (EGF). The full significance of this remarkable observation is not yet understood but it probably reflects the fact that in the evolution of proteins it has been easier to duplicate and modify existing genes than to develop entirely new ones.

The idea that external signals such as hormones, local hormones, and neurotransmitters, which alter the activity of target cells, bind to specific receptors on the cell surface, was first proposed by Langley at the beginning of this century (Langley 1906). Similar ideas were proposed by Ehrlich at about the same time to explain the action of drugs (Ehrlich 1913). Lang-

Table 3.1 *Classification of plasma membrane receptors on the basis of stereospecific structure of agonists and antagonists*

Broad class of agonist	Specific agonists for which there are distinct receptors
Acetylcholine	Acetylcholine (muscarinic, nicotinic)
Catecholamines	Adrenalin, noradrenalin (α_1, α_2; β_1, β_2) Dopamine (D_1, D_2)
Low-molecular-weight peptides	Vasopressin (V_1, V_2) Bombesin Angiotensin II Atrial natriuretic peptide Substance P f–met–leu–phe
Polypeptides and proteins	Glucagon Insulin, insulin-like growth factors Epidermal and platelet-derived growth factors Nerve growth factor Thrombin Colony-stimulating factor Calcitonin Thyroid-stimulating hormone Thyrotropin-releasing hormone (thioliberin) Gonadotropin-releasing hormone
Prostanoids	Prostaglandin E_2 Thromboxane A_2 Prostacyclin Leukotrienes

Table 3.2 *Classification of plasma-membrane receptors on the basis of the mechanism by which receptors are coupled to effector enzymes or ion channels*

Receptor subgroup	Examples of agonists
Receptor protein is an ion channel (agonist-gated channel)	Acetylcholine (nicotinic, Na^+) Glycine (Cl^-) γ-Aminobutyric acid (A) (Cl^-)
Cytoplasmic domain of receptor protein has protein–tyrosine kinase activity	Epidermal growth factor, platelet-derived growth factor, insulin
Cytoplasmic domain of receptor couples with a protein–tyrosine kinase which has no extracellular or membrane-spanning domains	Antigens (CD4 and CD8 receptors on T cells)
Cytoplasmic domain of receptor protein has phosphoprotein–tyrosine phosphatase activity	CD45 (leukocyte cell-surface protein) LAR (leukocyte common-antigen related protein)
Cytoplasmic domain of receptor has guanylate cyclase activity	Atrial natriuretic peptide
Receptor protein couples with enzyme or ion channel through GTP-binding protein	α-Adrenergic agonists Vasopressin (V_1 and V_2) Glucagon
Receptor protein couples with an integral membrane protein	Interleukin-6

ley's initial deduction was strengthened by evidence from a number of other experiments for stereospecificity in the interaction between extracellular agonists and components of the cell surface.

Observations on the stereospecificity of the interaction of agonists with cells led to the development of a system for distinguishing between different receptors. This system takes into account the stereospecificity of the binding site on a given receptor for a range of both agonists and antagonists (Ehrenpreis *et al.* 1969; Patil and La Pidus 1972). Receptors were first classified into subgroups on this basis. Examples of some families of receptors presently defined in this way are listed in Table 3.1.

Another way of classifying receptors utilizes knowledge of the mechanism by which the agonist–receptor complex transmits information to alter the function of intracellular proteins. On this basis plasma-membrane receptors can be divided into at least seven families (Table 3.2).

These are

1. Agonist-gated ion channels.
2. Receptors which possess protein–tyrosine kinase activity in the cytoplasmic domain.
3. Receptors which couple with a protein–tyrosine kinase which has no extracellular or membrane-spanning domains.
4. Receptors with a phosphoprotein–tyrosine phosphatase catalytic site on the cytoplasmic domain.
5. The receptor for atrial natriuretic peptide which possesses a guanylate cyclase catalytic site on the cytoplasmic domain.
6. Receptors linked to an effector enzyme or ion channel through an oligomeric GTP-binding regulatory protein (G protein).
7. Receptors which couple with an integral membrane protein.

The general structures of members of each of these families of receptors are shown in Fig. 3.1 and examples of receptors in each group are

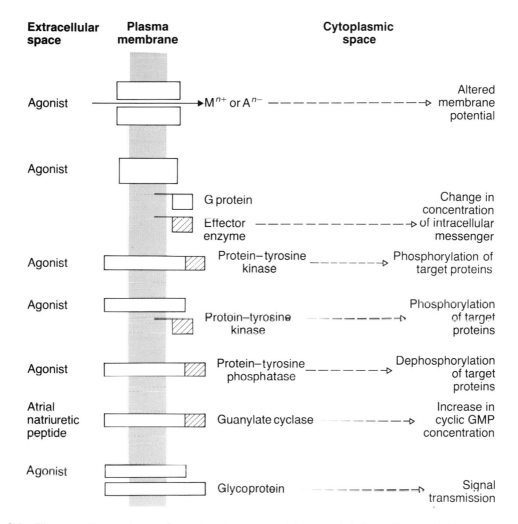

Fig. 3.1   The seven known types of receptor structure which transmit information carried by agonists across the plasma membrane.

listed in Table 3.2. Only a few phosphoprotein–tyrosine phosphatase receptors have so far been described. The properties of these enzymes are described in more detail in Chapter 4 in the section on phosphoprotein–tyrosine phosphatases.

The ion channel of the agonist-gated ion channel receptor is an integral part of the receptor protein (Fig. 3.1). The response elicited by the agonist is mediated by a change in the intracellular concentrations of Na^+ or Cl^-. The protein–

tyrosine kinase catalytic site is part of the protein–tyrosine kinase receptor polypeptide chain and is located on the cytoplasmic face of the plasma membrane (Fig. 3.1). Likewise, the guanylate cyclase catalytic site is part of the cytoplasmic domain of the atrial natriuretic peptide receptor (Fig. 3.1). Three separate proteins constitute each receptor system which is coupled to an effector protein through a G protein (Fig. 3.1). These are the receptor protein, the G protein, and the effector enzyme or ion channel.

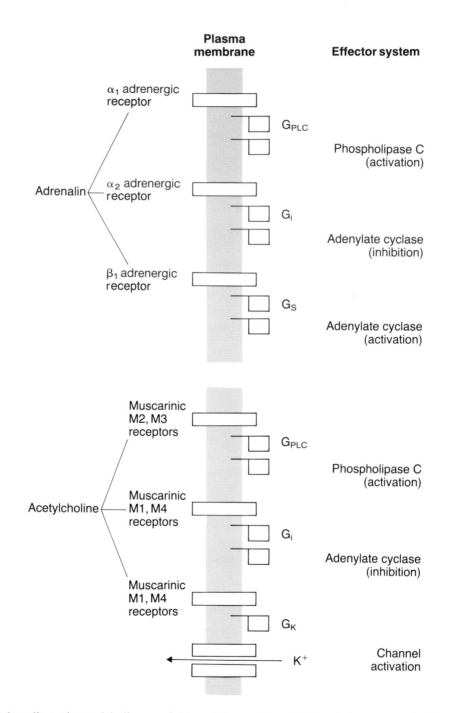

Fig. 3.2 Adrenalin and acetylcholine can initiate different lines of intracellular communication by binding to different receptor sub-types which are coupled through different G proteins to different effector proteins. In addition to the interaction of acetylcholine with muscarinic acetylcholine receptors shown here, this agonist also binds to nicotinic acetylcholine receptors. The muscarinic receptor sub-types which couple with specific effector proteins have not been completely defined.

The G protein and the effector protein are located on the cytoplasmic face of the plasma membrane (Fig. 3.1).

The most clearly defined examples of receptors which couple to a protein–tyrosine kinase that has no extracellular or membrane-spanning domains are the antigen receptors CD4 and CD8 on T-lymphocytes. These receptor proteins interact with the p56 *Lck* protein–tyrosine kinase.

Relatively little is known about the mechanism of action of the last-mentioned family of receptors, those in which the receptor protein couples to an integral membrane protein. Members of the cytokine family of agonists, which includes the interleukins and prolactin, probably belong to this receptor family. In the case of interleukin-6 the integral membrane protein is a 130 kDa glycoprotein, gp130. The signal transmitted as a result of interaction between the interleukin-6 receptor and gp130 may involve the phosphorylation of target proteins on tyrosine residues.

An examination of Table 3.1 shows that a given agonist can bind to more than one type of receptor. As a result, the same agonist can activate different membrane-transduction systems and hence different pathways of intracellular communication. For example, adrenalin binds to at least three receptor sub-types (Fig. 3.2) and acetylcholine can probably bind to several types of nicotinic acetylcholine receptor and to at least five types of muscarinic acetylcholine receptor. Three of the different muscarinic-coupling systems are shown in Fig. 3.2. The response of a given cell to adrenalin or acetylcholine depends, in part, on the number of each receptor sub-type present in that cell. The picture which is emerging, although not yet complete, is one in which there are a large number of receptor sub-types, each coupled to a specific intracellular pathway, available for the actions of a given agonist.

In the first half of this chapter, the structures of the major families of plasma-membrane receptors will be described together with the less well-understood processes which control the number of receptors of a given type accessible to an agonist on the plasma membrane of a cell. The second half of the chapter will describe the structures of the G proteins and the ideas about how these G proteins interact with receptors and effector proteins. Since another group of monomeric GTP-binding regulatory proteins has a number of properties in common with the oligomeric G proteins, their structures and properties will also be considered here even though they probably do not have the same biological functions as the oligomeric G proteins.

3.2   Structure of the plasma-membrane receptors

3.2.1   *Isolation of receptors*

For more than 50 years after the development of the concept of the receptor by Langley, the term 'receptor' remained an operational definition because techniques needed to study the structure of receptors were not available. Evidence for the presence in the plasma membrane of specific molecules with receptor function was obtained when receptor proteins were first extracted from membranes. Initially, extraction was achieved using organic solvents (De Robertis *et al.* 1967). However, organic solvents frequently denature proteins and ligand-binding activity was often destroyed. The use of organic solvents has been superseded by detergents (Changeux *et al.* 1970). Detergents solubilize receptors by selectively replacing planar sheets of membrane lipid with small curved detergent micelles, the exteriors of which are hydrophilic. This often allows the retention of ligand binding by the solubilized receptor. The receptors for acetylcholine (nicotinic) and insulin were among the first to be purified.

Rapid advances in the elucidation of the structures of plasma-membrane receptors and the proteins and enzymes with which they interact have been largely due to improved understanding of solubilization, the application of affinity chromatography and other new techniques for the purification of proteins, new techniques for the determination of amino-acid sequences of small amounts of polypeptides, and techniques for the isolation of the genes which encode receptor proteins. The structures of many agonist-gated ion channel receptors, receptors coupled to G proteins, receptors which possess tyrosine kinase activity, and the guanylate cyclase atrial natriuretic peptide receptor have been determined.

3.2.2 *General features of receptor structure*

The extracellular domains of most receptor proteins are hydrophilic, are glycosylated, and contain the binding site for the agonist. The transmembrane domain is composed of one or more short strands of polypeptide chain and has a pronounced hydrophobic character. Each of these membrane-spanning sequences consists of about 20 predominantly non-polar and uncharged amino-acid residues arranged in an α-helical configuration (Fig. 3.3). The transmembrane domains of the protein–tyrosine kinase receptors and receptors linked to G proteins generally lack charged residues. However, the transmembrane domains of agonist-gated receptors do possess charged residues. These are thought to face away from the lipid and towards a pore or channel and probably play a crucial role in regulating the passage of ions.

The cytoplasmic domain of receptor proteins is hydrophilic and contains the site which interacts with a G protein or the protein–tyrosine kinase or guanylate cyclase active site. The cytoplasmic domain of most receptors also contains a number of serine or threonine residues which can be phosphorylated by protein kinases

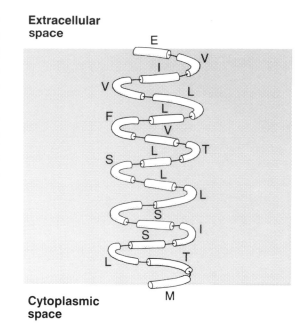

Fig. 3.3 The structure of one hydrophobic membrane-spanning sequence of a receptor protein. The amino-acid residues which span the membrane are arranged in an α-helical configuration and are indicated using the one-letter code: E, glu; V, val; I, ile; L, leu; F, phe; T, thr; S, ser; and M, met. From Stevens (1985).

(Section 3.6 of this chapter). A number of receptor polypeptide chains contain covalently bound fatty-acid moieties, chiefly myristic and palmitic acids. These may be involved in the interaction of the receptor protein with the membrane.

The molecular weights and subunit structures of representatives of each of the main families of plasma-membrane receptors are shown in Table 3.3. As mentioned earlier, plasma-membrane receptors are assembled from combinations of the transcription products of a number of exonic regions of DNA which are often related in sequence to domains of other proteins. The structures of three of the major families of receptor will now be considered in more detail. The structure of the atrial natriuretic peptide receptor which possesses guanylate

Table 3.3 *Molecular weights and subunit structures of some plasma-membrane receptors*

Receptor subgroup	Receptor	Molecular weight (kDa)	Number of polypeptide chains
Agonist-gated ion channel	Acetylcholine (nicotinic)	275	Five
	γ-Aminobutyric acid (A)	220	Two
Coupled to enzyme or ion channel by G protein	Acetylcholine (muscarinic)	70	One
	β_1-Adrenergic	64	One
	α_1-Adrenergic	80	One
	α_2-Adrenergic	60	One
	Glucagon	120	Two
	Vasopressin (V_1)	76	Two
Protein–tyrosine kinase activity on cytoplasmic domain	Epidermal growth factor	170	One
	Insulin	320	Four
	Platelet-derived growth factor	180	One
Guanylate cyclase activity on cytoplasmic domain	Atrial natriuretic peptide	120–180	One

cyclase activity is described in Chapter 5 in relation to the formation of cyclic GMP, and the structures of receptors with phosphoprotein–tyrosine phosphatase activity in Chapter 4.

3.2.3 *Agonist-gated ion channels*

The agonist-gated ion channels are the largest receptor molecules. The agonist is usually a small molecule such as acetylcholine or glycine. The nicotinic acetylcholine receptor has been investigated most extensively. In response to the binding of acetylcholine, this receptor admits a pulse of Na^+ to the cytoplasmic space (Fig. 3.4). The overall shape of the nicotinic acetylcholine receptor, as revealed by electron image analysis, is shown in Fig. 3.5. The molecular structure of this receptor was first elucidated by Numa, Heinemann, Changeux, and their colleagues (Noda *et al.* 1983; Claudio *et al.* 1983; Devillers-Thiery *et al.* 1983). The protein is an oligomer composed of four different subunits combined in the ratio α_2:β:γ:Δ. Each subunit has a molecular weight of about 55 kDa and is encoded by a separate gene. However, there is considerable homology between the amino-acid sequences of the different subunits.

Each of the subunits of the nicotinic acetylcholine receptor oligomer spans the membrane four times (Fig. 3.6). The subunits are arranged, in turn, to form a water-filled pore or channel through which Na^+ ions move, following the binding of acetylcholine to the extracellular domain of the α subunit. The plan view of the quaternary structure of the receptor–channel complex is shown in Fig. 3.7. Each M2 strand has a number of charged amino-acid side chains.

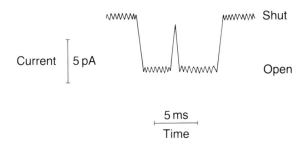

Fig. 3.4 A transient increase in Na^+ movement (downward deflection) through the Na^+ channel of the nicotinic acetylcholine receptor is induced by the binding of acetylcholine. Current through the membrane (carried by Na^+) has been measured by the patch-clamp technique. Two transient increases in current, separated by a very brief interval, are shown. From Colquhoun and Sakmann (1985).

The inside of the pore formed by the oligomeric protein is probably composed of the M2 strand from each of the subunits so that the five M2 strands line the pore with charged residues facing the interior of the pore (Finer-Moore and Stroud 1984). The structures of the γ-aminobutyric acid (A)-gated Cl⁻ channel and the glycine-gated Cl⁻ channel are similar to that of the nicotinic acetylcholine receptor, although each of the three receptors has a different number of subunits.

3.2.4 Receptors which interact with G proteins

The primary structures of only a few of the plasma-membrane receptors which couple with effector enzymes or ion channels are known in detail, although the number of different receptors in this group is large (Table 3.4). The amino-acid sequences of the muscarinic acetylcholine receptor (Kubo et al. 1986), the β-adrenergic receptor (Dixon et al. 1986; Yarden et al. 1986) and the photoreceptor rhodopsin (Ovchinnikov 1982) were among the first to be elucidated. These molecules are each composed of a single polypeptide chain which spans the membrane seven times (Fig. 3.8).

The stereospecific binding site for the agonist is a sequence, or group of sequences, of amino acids in the extracellular domain of a G protein-coupled receptor. One approach which has been employed to give a more precise location of the catecholamine binding site on the β-adrenergic receptor is the use of a radioactively labelled agonist which can be covalently attached to the receptor. This approach has shown that the catecholamine binding site is formed by the juxtaposition of membrane-spanning sequences 3, 4, 5, and 7.

Site-directed mutagenesis has been used to search for regions of the cytoplasmic amino-acid sequences of the β_2-adrenergic receptor which interact with the α subunit of G proteins. The results of these experiments suggest that the amino-terminal segment of the cytoplasmic tail

Table 3.4 *Enzymes and ion channels which are coupled to receptors through G proteins*

Enzyme or ion channel	Receptor
Adenylate cyclase	β-Adrenergic agonist
	Glucagon
	Vasopressin (V_2)
	Prostaglandin E_2
Cyclic GMP phosphodiesterase	Rhodopsin
Phosphatidylinositol 4,5-bisphosphate-specific phospholipase C	Acetylcholine (muscarinic)
	Vasopressin (V_1)
	α_1-Adrenergic agonist
	Thrombin
Phospholipase A_2	α_1-Adrenergic agonist
NADPH oxidase	f–met–leu–phe
K⁺ channels	Acetylcholine (muscarinic)
Voltage-operated Ca^{2+} channels	α_2-Adrenergic agonist

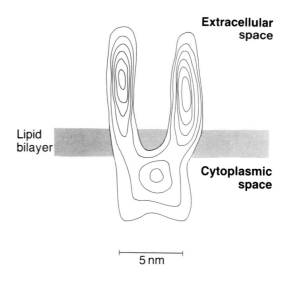

Fig. 3.5 Cross-section of the nicotinic acetylcholine receptor in a plane perpendicular to the plane of the plasma membrane, as revealed by electron imaging. From Brisson and Unwin (1985).

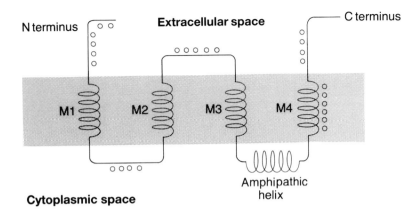

Fig. 3.6 The arrangement of the polypeptide chain of one subunit of the nicotinic acetylcholine receptor in the phospholipid bilayer. The four membrane-spanning sequences are designated M1 to M4. The loops on both the extracellular and cytoplasmic domains contain amino-acid residues which are charged (indicated by OOO). Transmembrane strand M2 may form the boundary to the water-filled channel through which Na^+ ions move. Each of the four different types of subunit ($\alpha,\beta,\gamma,\Delta$) which constitute the oligomeric receptor has a structure similar to the one shown. Adapted from Stevens (1985).

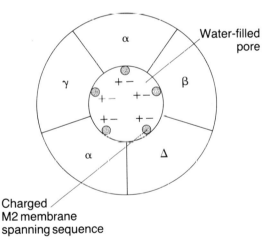

Fig. 3.7 The quaternary structure of the nicotinic acetylcholine receptor as viewed from above the plane of the membrane. Each of the five subunits ($\alpha,\alpha,\beta,\gamma,\Delta$) is arranged around a central water-filled channel. The tertiary structure of each individual subunit is shown in Fig. 3.6. Strand M2, which contains charged amino-acid residues, lines the pore. Adapted from Stevens (1985).

and the carboxy-terminal segment of cytoplasmic loop 3 of the β_2-adrenergic receptor contribute to the binding site which interacts with G_s. Amino-acid residues in cytoplasmic loop 2 and

cys 341, which is near the carboxy terminus, may also participate in the formation of this binding site.

3.2.5 *Receptors which contain a protein–tyrosine kinase domain*

Receptors which possess a protein–tyrosine kinase catalytic site on the cytoplasmic domain (protein–tyrosine kinase receptors) have only one membrane-spanning sequence per subunit, and most have only one subunit (Table 3.3). Agonists which interact with these receptors are usually polypeptide hormones or growth factors (e.g. insulin or epidermal growth factor (EGF)). The primary structures of the receptors for insulin, EGF, and platelet-derived growth factor (PDGF) are shown in Fig. 3.9. The amino-acid sequences of the receptors for insulin and EGF were determined by Ullrich and his colleagues (Ullrich *et al.* 1984, 1985). There is considerable homology between the amino-acid sequences of each of the protein–tyrosine kinase receptors. The extracellular domain of these receptors contains covalently bound carbohydrate moieties and a number of cysteine residues which are

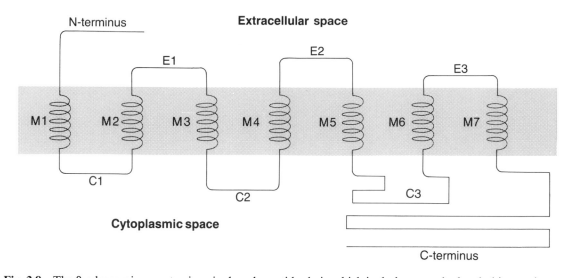

Fig. 3.8 The β-adrenergic receptor is a single polypeptide chain which includes seven hydrophobic membrane-spanning sequences. Each membrane-spanning sequence consists of about 20 amino-acid residues arranged in an α-helical configuration, as shown in Fig. 3.3. The extracellular domain of the receptor contains the binding site for catecholamines and is comprised of the amino terminus and three hydrophilic loops (E1, E2, and E3). The intracellular domain, which includes the site which interacts with the G protein, is comprised of the carboxy terminus and three hydrophilic loops (C1, C2, and C3).

characteristic of this type of receptor. There is probably considerable β-pleated sheet structure in the extracellular domain. Some of the sub-structures of the extracellular domain may be designed to protect the extracellular components of the receptor from hydrolysis by extracellular enzymes.

The membrane-spanning sequence of protein–tyrosine kinase receptors is usually flanked by one or more basic amino acids which probably interact with the charged head groups of the membrane phospholipid. A proline residue is frequently present close to the membrane on the extracellular side. These proline sequences may serve to break the α-helical structure of the membrane-spanning sequence and to anchor the receptor in the membrane.

The extracellular and intracellular domains of the EGF receptor are composed of 621 and 542 amino acids, respectively. The residues involved in the binding of ATP in the protein–tyrosine kinase domain are lysine 721 and a nearby

sequence gly–X–gly–X–phe–gly–X–val. A group of tyrosine residues, which can be phosphorylated by the EGF receptor protein–tyrosine kinase, and threonine 654, which is phosphorylated by protein–serine kinases, are situated in the cytoplasmic domain of the EGF receptor.

The mechanism by which information is transmitted from the stereospecific binding site for a growth factor or hormone on the extracellular domain of the receptor to activate the protein–tyrosine kinase in the cytoplasmic domain is of considerable interest. It is puzzling how the signal can be transmitted through the single membrane-spanning sequence. This may be achieved by a conformational change within the membrane-spanning sequence of the receptor molecule. The results of some experiments conducted with the EGF receptor suggest that transmission of the conformational change across the membrane requires the association of receptors (Fig. 3.10).

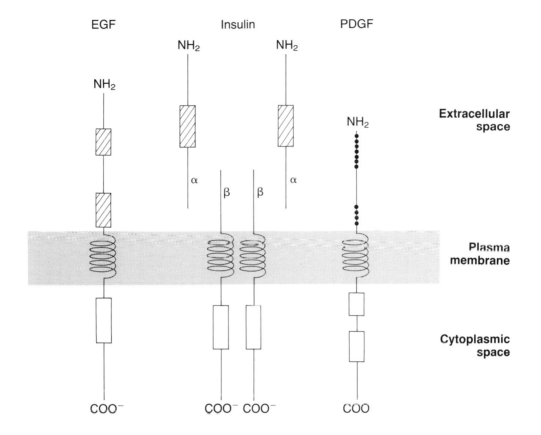

Fig. 3.9 The primary structures of the receptors for EGF, insulin, and PDGF, each of which possesses a cytoplasmic protein–tyrosine kinase domain. For each of these receptors, the amino terminus is outside the cell and the carboxy terminus is in the cytoplasmic space. Each polypeptide chain has only one membrane-spanning sequence. The insulin receptor is a tetramer composed of two different polypeptide chains (α and β) joined by disulphide bridges. The EGF and PDGF receptors are single polypeptide chains. The extracellular domain of each receptor includes the binding site for the agonist and a number of regions rich in cysteine. These are shown as solid circles or hatched rectangles. The catalytic site of the protein–tyrosine kinase enzyme in the cytoplasmic domain is shown as an open rectangle. From Yarden *et al.* (1986).

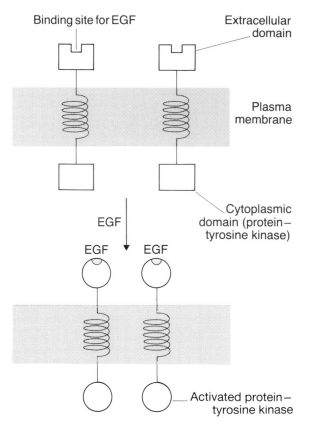

Binding site for EGF

Extracellular domain

Plasma membrane

Cytoplasmic domain (protein–tyrosine kinase)

EGF

EGF   EGF

Activated protein–tyrosine kinase

Fig. 3.10 The binding of EGF to its receptors causes association of the receptor–EGF complexes. This may be a step in the mechanism by which the binding of EGF to the external domain activates the protein–tyrosine kinase in the cytoplasmic domain. The affinity for EGF of the oligomeric receptors is greater than that of the monomeric receptors.

3.3 Regulation of the concentration of plasma-membrane receptors and termination of the signal

3.3.1 *Experimental observation of changes in the numbers of plasma-membrane receptors*

Changes in the concentration of plasma-membrane receptors and in the ability of these receptors to couple with intracellular effector systems constitute an important mechanism by which the actions of agonists on target cells are regulated and by which the signal carried by an

agonist is switched off. The mechanisms which control the number of receptors on the plasma membrane are complex and are presently only partly understood.

At the time when knowledge of receptor structure began to rapidly expand it was observed that for some receptors, like the insulin receptor, the number of receptors available to the agonist changes under different physiological conditions. For many agonists, the maintenance of an increased concentration of the agonist in the extracellular medium for periods longer than several minutes causes a desensitization of the target cell to the action of that agonist. In some cases this also desensitizes the cell to the actions of other agonists. The terms 'homologous' and 'heterologous' have been used by some investigators to describe desensitization by a given agonist which affects the actions of that agonist alone (homologous) or the actions of other agonists (heterologous).

The observed decrease in the number of receptors accessible to agonist is often described rather loosely as the 'down regulation' of receptors. There are also many examples in which the maintenance of a decreased concentration of an agonist in the extracellular fluid leads to an increase in the number of receptors available to bind the agonist. This is termed the 'up regulation' of receptors.

3.3.2 *Mechanisms which control receptor concentration*

The concentration of plasma-membrane receptors that are accessible to an agonist at any given time is determined by the relative rates of a number of intracellular processes (Fig. 3.11). These include the endocytosis of receptors, the return of endocytosed receptors to the plasma membrane, the transfer of receptors to lysosomes, the degradation of receptors, and the synthesis of new receptors. Another process which is thought to occur in some cells in response

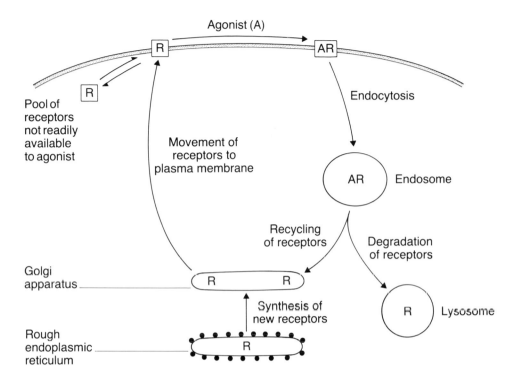

Fig. 3.11 The concentration of plasma-membrane receptors available for interaction with an agonist depends on the relative rates of several intracellular processes. These are endocytosis of the agonist–receptor complex, recycling of receptors from endosomes to the plasma membrane, degradation of the receptors in lysosomes, and the synthesis of new receptors. In some cells receptors for some agonists may also be converted from a form available to the agonist to a form which is located near the plasma membrane but which is unavailable to the agonist.

to certain agonists is the conversion of receptors at the plasma membrane from a form readily available to the agonist to a form located near the plasma membrane but less readily available or unavailable to the agonist. However, this mechanism is not yet understood.

Desensitization is often associated with a decrease in the number of receptors accessible to the agonist on the plasma membrane. The effect of agonist concentration on the number of available receptors is due principally to changes in either the rate of endocytosis of the receptor–agonist complex or the rate at which endocytosed receptors are recycled back to the plasma membrane. Uncoupling of the receptor

from the effector system can also lead to desensitization. As described later (Section 3.6), phosphorylation of either the receptor or, for G protein-coupled receptors, the G protein with which it interacts can cause this uncoupling.

Most or all intracellular responses induced by agonists which bind to plasma-membrane receptors are conveyed to intracellular enzymes or proteins during the period in which the agonist is bound to its receptor on the plasma membrane. While it has been suggested that certain intracellular responses induced by insulin may be conveyed after the hormone–receptor complex has entered the cytoplasmic space, there is no firm evidence to support this suggestion.

3.3.3 *Endocytosis of agonist–receptor complexes and degradation of receptors*

The processes involved in the endocytosis of agonist–receptor complexes have been studied using radioactively labelled agonists and the techniques of autoradiography and electron microscopy. These experiments have shown, for example, that significant quantities of ^{121}I are accumulated intracellularly following the addition of [^{121}I] insulin to lymphocytes. Most of this radioactivity is detected in the lysosomes (Fig. 3.12).

Many plasma-membrane receptors are endocytosed after combination with an agonist, and subsequently the agonist and a proportion of the receptors are degraded. Receptors for which this has been most clearly demonstrated include those for insulin, EGF, platelet-derived growth factor (PDGF), and nerve growth factor (NGF). Although the full physiological implications are not yet understood it is believed that the endocytosis of receptors is involved in switching off the signal conveyed by the agonist and in regulating the response of the target cell to the agonist through the number of available receptors.

Rates of internalization of agonist–receptor complexes vary markedly for different receptors. For example, 50 per cent of insulin receptors are internalized within 30 min. of the addition of the hormone to hepatocytes. On the other hand, for the interaction of EGF with fibroblasts, 90 per cent of the EGF receptors are internalized within about 2 min.

A large number of steps are involved in the uptake of agonist–receptor complexes. These are summarized in Fig. 3.13. In the absence of an agonist, receptors are distributed reasonably evenly on the surface of the cell. Combination of the agonist with receptors induces aggregation of the receptors which, in turn, move into structures called coated pits. Coated pits are 50–150 nm in diameter. The shape and size of each coated pit is determined by an hexagonal protein lattice which forms on the cytoplasmic side of the plasma membrane. The lattice network is composed of polymers of two different protein complexes, assembly factor and clathrin. Assembly factor consists of heavy (100–115 kDa) and light (50 kDa) chains. Clathrin is composed of heavy chains (180 kDa) and at least

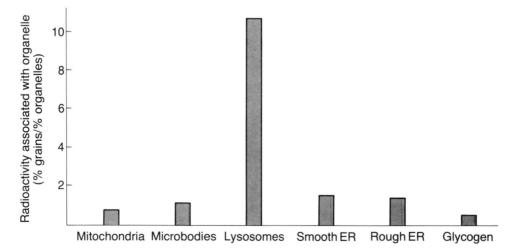

Fig. 3.12 The distribution of radioactivity between intracellular organelles in hepatocytes incubated with [^{121}I]insulin for 30 min. The majority of radioactivity is associated with the lysosomes. ER represents the endoplasmic reticulum. From Carpentier *et al.* (1979).

three types of light chain (33–36 kDa). These form structures which are pentagonal and hexagonal in shape.

Coated pits that contain receptors form endocytotic vesicles which subsequently fuse with endosomes (Fig. 3.13). These are polymorphic organelles with an internal pH of about 5. The low pH of the endosome often causes dissociation of the agonist–receptor complex. Agonist molecules within the endosome are transferred to lysosomes while the receptors are either transferred to lysosomes or are recycled to the plasma membrane via the Golgi apparatus (Fig. 3.13). Transfer to the lysosomes involves the formation of a multi-vesicular body. Degradation of receptor and agonist occurs in the lysosomes.

The proportion of endocytosed receptors which are degraded varies with the type of receptor and physiological state of the target cells. For the insulin receptor, it has been estimated that each receptor is recycled to the plasma membrane about 200 times before it is degraded.

3.4 The GTP-binding regulatory proteins

3.4.1 *Discovery of the oligomeric G proteins*
The role of oligomeric GTP-binding regulatory proteins (G proteins) in coupling between receptors and effector enzymes or ion channels was briefly discussed at the beginning of this chapter. The requirement for GTP in the actions of hormones and other agonists on the plasma membrane was first demonstrated by Rodbell and his colleagues. They found that the activation of adenylate cyclase by adrenalin in adipocyte membranes is stimulated by GTP (Rodbell *et al.* 1971). Subsequently, Cassel and Selinger (1976) observed that catecholamines stimulate the hydrolysis of GTP in turkey erythrocyte membranes. These and other experiments suggested that the activation of adenylate cyclase by agonist–receptor complexes requires the interaction of GTP with a neighbouring protein

located in the plasma membrane. This protein was later called a GTP-binding regulatory protein.

Direct evidence for a role for a G protein in the activation of adenylate cyclase was obtained when Ross and Gilman (1977) reconstituted the receptor–adenylate cyclase system in a synthetic phospholipid membrane using partially purified preparations of the β-adrenergic receptor, a G protein, and adenylate cyclase. The subsequent development of methods for the purification of G proteins (Schleifer *et al.* 1980) allowed investigation of their molecular mechanism of action.

3.4.2 *The oligomeric G proteins*
Animal cells contain a number of different G proteins. Each type of G protein links a given type of receptor to a given effector enzyme or ion channel. This coupling occurs on the cytoplasmic face of the plasma membrane and is often represented by a scheme like that shown in Fig. 3.14. This scheme represents a static picture of the relationship between the receptor, G protein, and effector protein. The real picture more likely involves movement of all three proteins in the plane of the membrane and collisions between components of the system, as described later (Section 3.4.4).

G proteins can be divided into three groups on the basis of knowledge of their structure and function. The first group consists of three members, the structure and function of which have both been well characterized. These are G_s (stimulatory) and G_i (inhibitory), which couple receptors to adenylate cyclase, and G_t (transducin), which couples rhodopsin to cyclic GMP phosphodiesterase (Table 3.5). There is one G protein, G_o, in the second group. Knowledge of the structure of this protein is reasonably complete whereas the cellular function has not been defined. For G proteins in the third group there is considerable information on the function but little knowledge of structure. G proteins

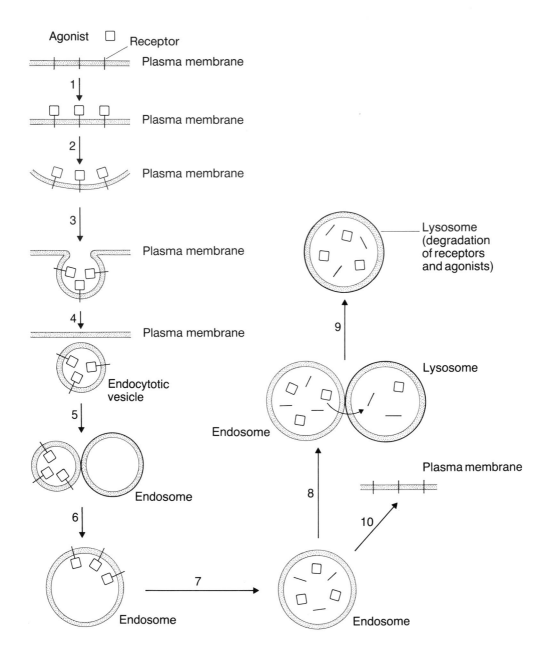

Fig. 3.13 Pathways for the endocytosis, degradation and, intracellular translocation of agonist–receptor complexes. The steps shown are 1: combination of the agonist with a receptor; 2: movement of the agonist–receptor complexes to a coated pit; 3: endocytosis of the coated pit; 4: formation of an endocytotic vesicle near the plasma membrane; 5: fusion of the endocytotic vesicle with an endosome; 6: mixing of the contents of the endocytotic vesicle and those of the endosome; 7: dissociation of the agonist–receptor complex; 8: transfer of agonist and some receptors to lysosomes; 9: degradation of receptors and agonists; 10: recycling of some receptors to the plasma membrane.

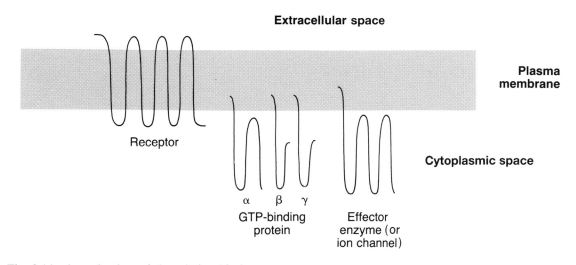

Fig. 3.14 A static view of the relationship between a receptor, a G protein, and an effector enzyme at the cytoplasmic face of the plasma membrane. Coupling between the receptor, G protein, and effector protein requires a collision between the receptor and the G protein and a collision between the α subunit of the G protein and the effector protein.

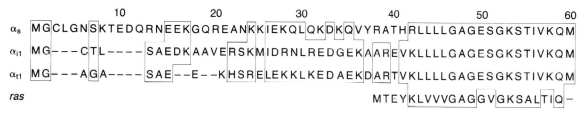

Fig. 3.15 Amino-acid sequences at the amino terminus of the α subunits of three oligomeric G proteins, α_s, α_{i1}, and α_{t1} and at the amino terminus of the protein encoded by the cHa *ras* gene. The region shown is part of the GTP-binding site. Homologous residues are enclosed in boxes. In the first 60 residues of α_s there are two short inserted sequences (3–5 and 9–12) which are absent from the other α subunit polypeptide chains.

Table 3.5   *The well characterized oligomeric G proteins of the plasma membrane, and examples of their receptors and effector enzymes*

G Protein	Examples of receptor	Effector protein
G_s	Adrenergic agonists (β) Glucagon Vasopressin (V_2) Olfactory	Adenylate cyclase (activated)
G_i	Adrenergic agonists (α_2) Acetylcholine (M) Somatostatin	Adenylate cyclase (inhibited)
Transducin$_1$ (G_{t1})	Rhodopsin	Cyclic GMP phosphodiesterase (activated)
Transducin$_2$ (G_{t2})	Cone opsins	Cyclic GMP phosphodiesterase (activated)

in this group include those which couple receptors to phosphatidylinositol 4, 5-bisphosphate (PtdIns 4, 5 P_2)-specific phospholipase C, phospholipase A_2, K^+ channels, or Ca^{2+} channels.

3.4.3 Structures of the oligomeric G proteins

The G proteins are isolated as heterotrimers which consist of the subunits α, β, and γ. The molecular weights of the heterotrimers are about 90 kDa. The α, β, and γ subunits have molecular weights of 39–45, 35–37 and 8 kDa, respectively. The α subunit contains the binding site for GTP and the catalytic activity responsible for the hydrolysis of this nucleotide. This subunit also contains sites which interact with the βγ complex, with the receptor, and with the effector enzyme or ion channel.

A number of experiments indicate that each subunit (α, β, or γ) of a G protein is attached to the cytoplasmic side of the plasma membrane as shown in schematic form in Fig. 3.14. None of the subunits contains a membrane-spanning sequence. The α subunit is attached to the membrane through an acylated cysteine residue near the carboxy terminus of the polypeptide chain. One of the functions of the β and γ subunits, which have both hydrophilic and hydrophobic sequences, may be to assist in anchoring the α subunits to the plasma membrane.

The α subunits of each of the different G proteins have slightly different molecular weights and different amino-acid sequences. It is these differences in the structure of the α subunits which appear to be chiefly responsible for the different properties of the individual oligomeric G proteins. A further level of structural complexity is indicated by the detection of two different α subunits in preparations of G_s and three in preparations of G_i. Notwithstanding these differences, there is considerable homology between the amino-acid sequences of all the α subunits. Fig. 3.15 shows a comparison of the sequences for a short section of the amino terminus mini of the α_s, α_i and α_t polypeptide chains. Regions of the α subunits are also homologous with the *ras* proteins, as described in Section 3.5.2.

The region of the α subunit which is thought to interact with the polypeptide chain of the receptor is an amphipathic α-helix located at the carboxy terminus of the α subunit. A long sequence of amino-acid residues between residues 60 and 208 may interact with the effector enzyme. The amino-acid sequences of these two regions of the α subunit are found to be highly conserved between α subunits from different G proteins and between α subunits of the same G protein from different species of animal. A possible site which is responsible for interaction of the α subunit with the βγ complex is a sequence of amino acids at the amino terminus.

In contrast to differences in the molecular weights of the different species of α subunit, the molecular weights of β_s, β_i, and β_t are similar. However, the β subunits are not all identical and at least three genes encoding a β-subunit polypeptide have been detected. A number of antibodies have been raised against selected amino-acid sequences within α- and β-subunit polypeptides. These antibodies have proved useful in identification of the type of subunit present in a given membrane.

3.4.4 Activation of the oligomeric G proteins by the agonist–receptor complex and GTP

The transfer of information across the plasma membrane from the receptor for a given agonist to a specific effector enzyme requires the movement of the receptor, G protein, and effector enzyme. This movement occurs both within the plane of the membrane and on the cytoplasmic surface of the membrane. The major interactions are between individual receptor molecules, between receptors and G proteins, between different subunits of G proteins, and between α subunits of G proteins and effector enzymes.

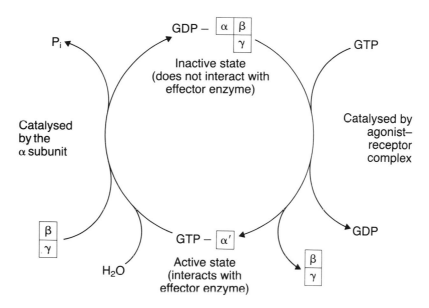

Fig. 3.16 The cycle in which the active form of the α subunit of a G protein is switched on and off. The agonist–receptor complex catalyses the activation, by GTP, of the α subunit of the oligomeric G protein. Interaction of the agonist–receptor complex with the oligomeric G protein alters the conformation of the α subunit and enhances the exchange of GTP for GDP. The short lifetime of the active form of the α subunit, α'^{GTP}, is terminated by the hydrolysis of GTP. This reaction is catalysed by the α subunit itself. During its lifetime, one molecule of α'^{GTP} probably interacts with many molecules of effector enzyme.

Whilst it has clearly been shown that receptors move in the plane of the plasma membrane, experimental observation of the interaction between components of the G proteins and effector enzymes on the cytoplasmic face of the membrane has not yet been possible.

The initial events in the activation of the G proteins are the formation of the agonist–receptor complex and the interaction of this complex with inactive α^{GDP} βγ oligomer. This leads to the exchange of GDP for GTP and dissociation of the αβγ oligomer to release α'^{GTP} and the βγ complex (Fig. 3.16). The rate-limiting step in this process is the dissociation of GDP. During this sequence of events, the α subunit undergoes a conformational change to a form (α') which interacts with the effector enzyme and induces a change in the conformation and activity of the effector enzyme.

The active conformation of the α subunit is converted to the inactive conformation by the hydrolysis of GTP. This reaction is catalysed by the α subunit itself and is accompanied by the combination of α^{GDP} with the βγ complex to re-form α^{GDP} βγ (Fig. 3.16). Each molecule of α'^{GTP} is probably in the active conformation for several seconds before the GTP is hydrolysed.

It is likely that the agonist–receptor complex acts in a catalytic manner during activation of the G proteins so that, at the molecular level, the complex of one agonist and one receptor molecule interacts with many αβγ oligomers within a period of a few seconds. In the plasma membranes of some cell types, the number of molecules of α subunit greatly exceeds the number of molecules of the βγ complex. In these systems, one βγ complex may catalyse the binding of GTP to many α subunits. Moreover, each α'^{GTP} subunit may interact with many effector enzyme molecules within its lifetime.

Some experiments indicate that α'^{GTP} subunits are released from the plasma membrane into the cytoplasmic space following the binding of an agonist with its receptor. Rodbell (1985) has speculated that in addition to the activation of effector enzymes attached to the cytoplasmic face of the plasma membrane, α'^{GTP} subunits which are released from the plasma membrane diffuse into the cytoplasmic space and interact with other effector enzymes located within this space. However, there is no strong evidence to support this idea.

Experimental evidence which indicates that G proteins do indeed interact with receptors was first obtained in studies with isolated plasma-membrane preparations. The addition of GTP or GDP was found to lower the affinity for an agonist of a receptor coupled to a G protein. On the other hand, it was observed that addition

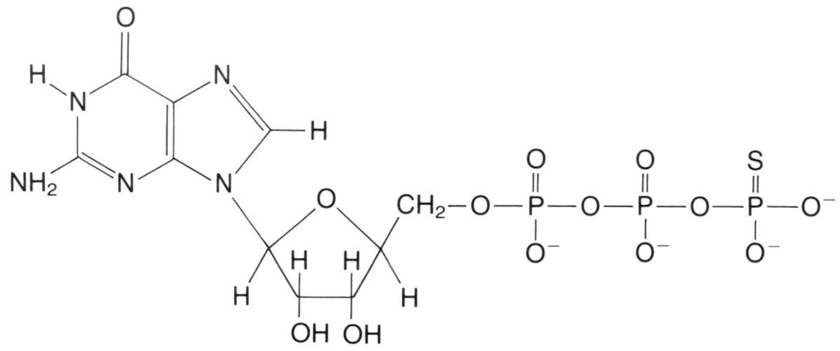

Guanosine 5'[γ-thio]trisphosphate
(guanosine 5'-(3-O-thio)triphosphate)

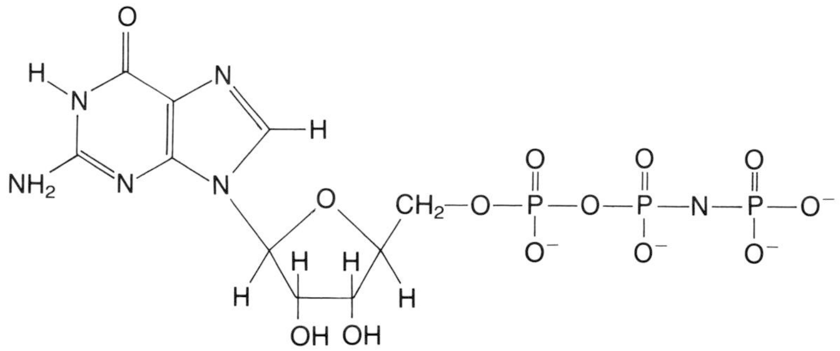

Guanyl-5'-yl βγ-8-imidodiphosphate

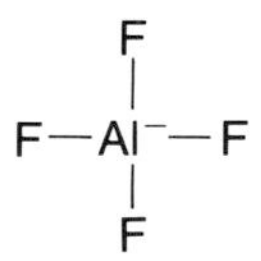

AlF_4^-

Fig. 3.17 Structures of guanosine 5'[γ-thio]trisphosphate (GTPγS) and guanyl-5'-y1βγ-8-imidodiphosphate (Gpp[NH]p), two slowly hydrolysable analogues of GTP which activate G proteins, and the structure of AlF_4^-, which also activates G proteins. Each of these compounds binds to the GDP-binding site of a G protein and converts α^{GDP} to an active form, $\alpha'^{GTP\gamma S}$, $\alpha'^{Gpp[NH]p}$ or $\alpha'^{AlF_4^-}$. The α subunit–GTP analogue complex probably remains in the active form for a substantial period of time, and can activate many effector enzymes.

of the agonist enhances the combination of GTP with $\alpha^{GDP}\beta\gamma$ and increases the rate of hydrolysis of GTP by the GTPase active site of the α subunit. The agonist increases the affinity of the GTPase for GTP without changing the maximum velocity of the reaction.

Experimental investigation of the function of G proteins has been greatly assisted by the use of non-hydrolysable analogues of GTP. The most useful of these have been guanosine 5′[γ-thio]triphosphate (GTPγS) and guanyl-5′-yl βγ-8-imido diphosphate (Gpp[NH]p) (Fig. 3.17). These molecules can replace GTP in the activation of G proteins. Moreover, they induce the formation of the active conformation of the α subunit ($\alpha'^{GTP\gamma S}$ or $\alpha'^{Gpp[NH]p}$) in the absence of an agonist. Since these analogues are not readily hydrolysed, most of the α subunits are trapped in the active conformation. This active conformation can also be achieved with AlF_4^- (Fig. 3.17) which is thought to mimic the structure of the critical terminal phosphate moiety of GTP and, like GTPγS and Gpp[NH]p, can not be hydrolysed. AlF_4^- can be formed from endogenous Al^{3+} when NaF is added to intact cells or plasma-membrane preparations.

3.4.5 Interaction of activated oligomeric G proteins with effector enzymes or ion channels

The interaction of α'^{GTP} with effector proteins has been studied most extensively in two systems—the activation of cyclic GMP phosphodiesterase by light and the regulation of the activity of adenylate cyclase by hormones and neurotransmitters.

The absorption of light alters the conformation of rhodopsin so that part of the cytoplasmic domain of this molecule interacts with transducin ($\alpha_t^{GDP}\beta_t\gamma_t$). This, in turn, catalyses activation of the α subunit of transducin as follows:

$$\alpha_t^{GDP}\beta_t\gamma_t + GTP \rightleftharpoons \alpha_t'^{GTP} + \beta_t\gamma_t.$$

Activated rhodopsin

The activated conformation of the α subunit, $\alpha_t'^{GTP}$, activates cyclic GMP phosphodiesterase.

In most cells, adenylate cyclase can couple to a group of different receptors, each of which can increase cyclic AMP formation, and also to a group of receptors each of which can inhibit the formation of the cyclic nucleotide (Fig. 3.18). This coupling is achieved through the stimulatory G protein, G_s, and the inhibitory G protein, G_i. Inhibition by a given agonist is almost always observed in the presence of a second agonist which stimulates adenylate cyclase. In most membranes, the amount of G_i greatly exceeds that of G_s.

The cycle of reactions which leads to the activation of adenylate cyclase is shown on the right-hand side of Fig. 3.19. The species which interacts with adenylate cyclase is $\alpha_s'^{GTP}$. The initial event in the mechanism by which agonists inhibit

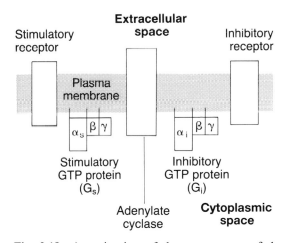

Fig. 3.18 A static view of the components of the membrane-transducing system through which agonists regulate adenylate cyclase activity in animal cells. The activation of adenylate cyclase by an appropriate agonist involves binding of the agonist to its receptor, called a stimulatory receptor, which, in turn, interacts with the G protein, G_s, which stimulates adenylate cyclase. Inhibition of the enzyme involves the binding of an appropriate agonist to its receptor, called an inhibitory receptor, which, in turn, interacts with the G protein, G_i, which inhibits adenylate cyclase.

adenylate cyclase is dissociation of the $\alpha_i^{GDP}\beta_i\gamma_i$ oligomer, shown in the left-hand side of Fig. 3.19. This releases the α subunit in its activated conformation, $\alpha_i'^{GTP}$ and the complex $\beta_i\gamma_i$. Inhibition of adenylate cyclase probably occurs by two mechanisms. The $\beta_i\gamma_i$ complexes released from $\alpha_i\beta_i\gamma_i$ may bind to $\alpha_s'^{GTP}$ and inhibit activation of the enzyme by this subunit. Adenylate cyclase may also be inhibited directly by $\alpha_i'^{GTP}$. Evidence for this last conclusion comes, in part, from studies with a mutant line (designated cyc⁻) of S49 cells. The mutant cells contain α_i, β, and γ subunits but do not contain α_s. However, adenylate cyclase is still inhibited by agonists which interact with inhibitory receptors in these mutant cells.

3.4.6 *Early ideas on the role of phospholipid methylation in the activation of adenylate cyclase*

In 1980 it was assumed that the interaction of receptors with G proteins and adenylate cyclase takes place predominantly in the hydrophobic domain of the membrane. One hypothesis which sought to explain how this interaction is facilitated following combination of an agonist with the receptor is based on the methylation of phospholipids. The idea was developed by Axelrod and his colleagues (Hirata and Axelrod 1980). These workers had observed that a number of agonists enhance the methylation by *S*-adenosylmethionine of phosphatidylethanolamine to form phosphatidylcholine. The three methylation reactions are catalysed by phospholipid methyltransferases 1 and 2 (Fig. 3.20). These enzymes are present in the plasma membrane, as well as at other intracellular locations. Some experiments indicate that phospholipid methyltransferases 1 and 2 are located at the cytoplasmic and extracellular surfaces of the plasma membrane, respectively.

Axelrod and his colleagues proposed that the combination of an agonist with its receptor activates the phospholipid methyltransferases and

increases the rate of conversion of phosphatidylethanolamine present in the inner leaflet of the bilayer to phosphatidylcholine. It was further proposed that the newly synthesized phosphatidylcholine is transferred to the outer bilayer where its presence increases the fluidity of the membrane and enhances coupling of the receptor to the G protein and adenylate cyclase. Axelrod and his colleagues also proposed that an increase in phospholipid methylation was part of the mechanism by which agonists stimulate plasma-membrane Ca^{2+} inflow and phospholipase A_2.

At the time it was proposed, the phospholipid methylation hypothesis stimulated further investigation of the factors which influence the mobility of membrane polypeptides involved in signal transduction. However, these experiments showed that it is unlikely that phospholipid methylation plays a direct role in the mechanisms by which agonist–receptor complexes activate effector enzymes. Moreover, as explained earlier, the major interactions between receptors and G proteins and between G proteins and effector enzymes have now been shown to take place in the cytoplasmic space on the inside of the plasma membrane. Furthermore, more recent experiments have shown that stimulation of the activity of phospholipid methyltransferase by agonist–receptor complexes is a consequence of the phosphorylation of these enzymes by cyclic AMP-dependent and (Ca^{2+} +calmodulin)-dependent protein kinases and by protein kinase C.

3.4.7 *Use of bacterial toxins in elucidation of the functions of oligomeric G proteins*

The activity of a number of the G proteins is altered by certain bacterial toxins. Two of the most important are the toxin from *Vibrio cholerae*, cholera toxin, and the toxin from *Bordatella pertussis*, pertussis toxin. These toxins have been useful tools in the elucidation of some of

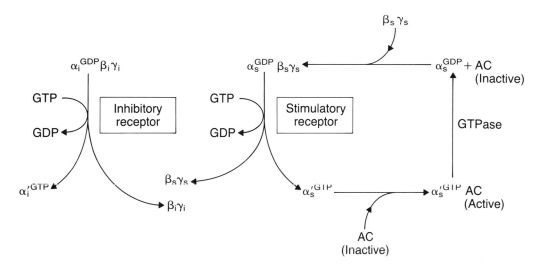

Fig. 3.19 Actions of the stimulatory and inhibitory oligomeric G proteins in the regulation of adenylate cyclase. The binding of an agonist to a stimulatory receptor leads to exchange of GTP for GDP on oligomeric $\alpha_s\beta_s\gamma_s$, dissociation of the active form of the α subunit, $\alpha_s'^{GTP}$, and interaction of $\alpha_s'^{GTP}$ with adenylate cyclase, AC. This results in the activation of adenylate cyclase. The binding of an agonist to an inhibitory receptor leads to dissociation of oligomeric $\alpha_i\beta_i\gamma_i$. This probably causes an inhibition of adenylate cyclase by two mechanisms. In the first, the $\beta_i\gamma_i$ complex released from $\alpha_i\beta_i\gamma_i$ binds to $\alpha_s'^{GTP}$ and inhibits the activation of adenylate cyclase by $\alpha_s'^{GTP}$. In the second, $\alpha_i'^{GTP}$ directly interacts with adenylate cyclase and inhibits the activity of this enzyme.

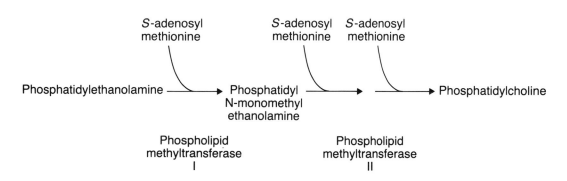

Fig. 3.20 Conversion of phosphatidylethanolamine to phosphatidylcholine by enzyme-catalysed methylation. The three methyl groups are donated by *S*-adenosyl-L-methionine. Addition of the first is catalysed by phospholipid methyltransferase I, and addition of the second and third by phospholipid methyltransferase II.

the cellular functions of G proteins. The reaction catalysed by both cholera and pertussis toxin is the ribosylation of an amino-acid residue in the α subunit (Fig. 3.21). The donor of the ribose group is NAD^+. The action of cholera toxin on G_s was discovered by Moss and Vaughan (1977). They found that the ribosylated form of G_s which results from the action of this toxin is active in the absence of agonists and GTP. Later, Katada and Ui (1982) showed that the ribosylation of G_i by pertussis toxin inhibits the action of G_i.

Cholera toxin ribosylates the α subunits of G_s and G_t on an arginine residue. Ribosylation only occurs when the α subunit is dissociated from the oligomer. The reaction requires an additional protein, ADP-ribosylation factor, which is one of the monomeric GTP-binding proteins discussed in the next section. Ribosylation by cholera toxin results in stimulation of

the ability of the α subunit to activate an effector enzyme so that activation can occur in the absence of the agonist–receptor complex. The ribosylated α subunit has a decreased affinity for the βγ complex. Cholera toxin has been used in the identification of a role for G_s in the actions of certain agonists, and as a means of bypassing receptors in the activation of adenylate cyclase.

Pertussis toxin ribosylates the α subunits of G_i, G_o, and G_t on a cysteine residue. In contrast to the action of cholera toxin, ribosylation by pertussis toxin occurs only when the α subunit is present as part of the αβγ oligomer. ADP-ribosylation factor is not required. The ribosylation of $α_i$ by pertussis toxin results in a decrease in the ability of agonists to inhibit adenylate cyclase activity. In some types of cell, pertussis toxin also ribosylates the putative G protein which is coupled to PtdIns 4, 5 P_2-specific phospholipase C. This results in an inhibition of the stimu-

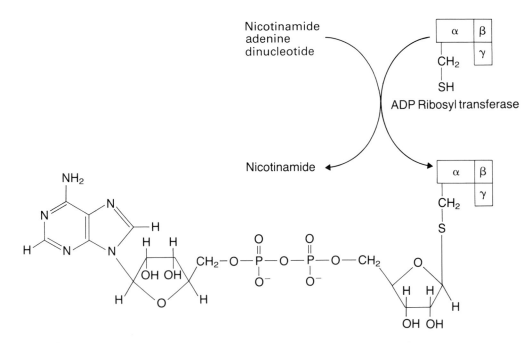

Fig. 3.21 Ribosylation of the α subunit of a G protein, catalysed by the ADP-ribosyltransferase present in pertussis toxin. The oligomeric G protein, and not the free α subunit, is the substrate for the pertussis toxin ribosyltransferase.

lation by agonists of this phospholipase. Like cholera toxin, pertussis toxin has been useful in identifying the class of G protein involved in the action of a given agonist.

3.5   The monomeric GTP-binding proteins

3.5.1   *The multiplicity of monomeric GTP-binding proteins*

Some years after the discovery of the oligomeric G proteins, a number of monomeric GTP-binding proteins were identified. The functions of many of these monomeric GTP-binding proteins have not yet been clearly defined. Some monomeric GTP-binding proteins are probably involved in the coupling of receptors to effector proteins at the cytoplasmic face of the plasma membrane, although the nature of this coupling differs from the nature of coupling mediated by the oligomeric G proteins. Many monomeric GTP-binding proteins have functions which do not involve coupling with plasma membrane receptors. However, in view of similarities between monomeric GTP-binding proteins and the α subunits of the oligomeric G proteins, the properties and possible functions of the monomeric GTP-binding proteins will be considered here.

The monomeric GTP-binding proteins are isolated from cells as single polypeptide chains with molecular weights in the range 20 to 25 kDa. As many as ten of these proteins have been detected in a single type of cell. The number of different monomeric GTP-binding proteins in a given cell may be even higher than this. The monomeric GTP-binding proteins include the protein products of the mammalian *ras, ral, rho, rap, rac,* and *rab* gene families, the yeast YP2 (YPT 1) and SEC 4 genes, and the *Drosophila* D-*ras*3 gene as well as the ADP-ribosylation factor mentioned earlier in connection with the action of pertussis toxin. One group of monomeric GTP-binding proteins, which may include

proteins encoded by some of the genes just mentioned, is involved in the movement of transport vesicles from the endoplasmic reticulum to the Golgi apparatus and plasma membrane, and in the movement of endocytotic vesicles from the plasma membrane to the Golgi apparatus (Chapter 2, Section 2.6.5). Some monomeric GTP-binding proteins are located at the plasma membrane while others are found associated with the Golgi apparatus and other intracellular structures.

The proteins encoded by the *ras* genes have received the most attention because mutated forms of these genes, the *ras* oncogenes, can transform cultured cell lines (Chapter 11). There are three closely related mammalian *ras* genes. These are the H-, K-, and N-*ras* genes which each contain four coding exons. The intervening DNA sequences are located at identical positions in each of the three genes. Alternate splicing of two forms of the fourth coding exon of the K-*ras* gene produces two different polypeptides designated K-*ras*1 and K-*ras*2. Genes with considerable homology with the mammalian H-*ras*, K-*ras*, and N-*ras* genes have been detected in other eukaryotic cells (Table 3.6). Another

Table 3.6   *Genes of the* ras *family with considerable homology with the mammalian H-, K-, and N-*ras *genes*

Gene	Organism
H-*ras*	Chicken
D*ras*1	*Drosophila melanogaster*
D*ras*2/64B	
D*ras*3	
Apl-*ras*	Snail (*Aplysia*)
Dd*ras*	Slime mould (*Dictyostelium discoideum*)
RAS1	Yeast (*Saccharomyces cerevisiae*)
RAS2	
SP RAS	Yeast (*Schizosaccharomyces pombe*)

ras-related gene, the mammalian R-*ras* gene, contains six exons.

Like the α subunits of the oligomeric G proteins, the monomeric GTP-binding proteins possess a site which binds GDP or GTP. When a molecule of GTP is bound to this site it is hydrolysed, although the rate of hydrolysis is slower than the rate of GTP hydrolysis catalysed by the α subunit of oligomeric G proteins. For a number of the monomeric GTP-binding proteins, a protein which specifically binds to the GTP-binding protein and stimulates the hydrolysis of GTP has been isolated from cell extracts. These proteins, which have been called GTPase activating proteins (GAP), probably interact with the monomeric GTP-binding proteins in intact cells although the physiological role of this interaction is not understood.

3.5.2 *Structures of the* ras *proteins*

The *ras* proteins were the first monomeric GTP-binding proteins to be discovered and their structures have been well characterized. The H-*ras*, K-*ras*1, and N-*ras* proteins are each composed of 189 amino acids while the K-*ras*2 protein is composed of 188 amino acids. Each of these *ras* proteins has a molecular weight of 21 kDa. There is a large degree of homology between the first 165 amino-acid residues at the amino terminus of the polypeptides encoded by the H-*ras*, K-*ras*1, K-*ras*2, and N-*ras* genes (Fig. 3.22). However, there are considerable differences in the amino-acid sequences at the carboxy terminus of these polypeptides.

The primary structures of the monomeric GTP-binding proteins are similar to those of ribosomal elongation factor EF-1 and ribosomal initiation factor eIF-2 from animal cells and initiation factor EF-Tu from bacterial cells. These well characterized proteins are components of multienzyme complexes which catalyse the initiation and elongation of polypeptide chains. The roles played by EF-1, eIF-2, and EF-Tu require the binding and hydrolysis of

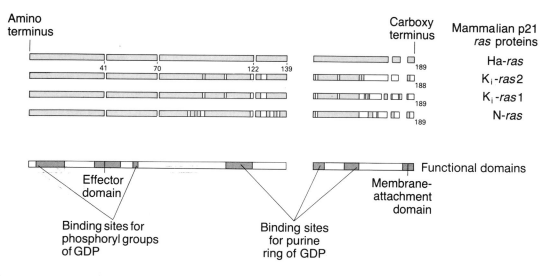

Fig. 3.22 Homologies between the amino-acid sequences of proteins encoded by the mammalian *ras* genes. The amino-acid sequence of each of the Ki-*ras*2, Ki-*ras*1, and N-*ras* proteins has been compared with that of the Ha-*ras* protein. Regions in which the amino-acid sequence of a given protein is identical to that of the Ha-*ras* protein are indicated by the shaded regions. The numbers at the carboxy terminus represent the number of amino-acid residues in each polypeptide. The functional domains of the *ras* proteins are shown at the bottom. From Hanley and Jackson (1987).

GTP. Regions of the *ras* proteins, especially those within the GTP-binding site, show considerable homology with amino-acid sequences of the ribosomal elongation and initiation factors and also with the α subunits of the oligomeric G proteins (Fig. 3.15). This homology was first observed in 1980 by Shih and his colleagues.

Within each *ras* protein, a guanine nucleotide binding domain, a domain which is the putative effector binding site, and a domain at which the protein is attached to the membrane, have been identified (Fig. 3.22). The guanine nucleotide binding domain is composed of groups of amino-acid sequences located at both the amino and carboxy terminus of the protein. Cys 186, to which a farnesyl moiety is covalently attached, cys 181 to which a palmitic acid residue may be covalently attached, and nearby amino acids at the carboxy terminus of the *ras* protein constitute the membrane attachment domain. The mechanism of attachment of the lipid moie-

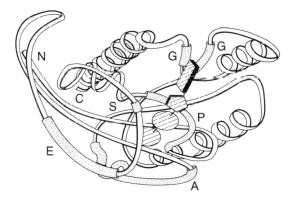

Fig. 3.23 The tertiary structure of the GDP-binding pocket of the c-H-*ras* protein determined using X-ray crystallography. The regions of the polypeptide chain which bind the guanine base, the ribose moiety, and the phosphate groups are indicated by the letters G, S, and P, respectively. The region which is thought to interact with an effector protein is indicated by the letter E. This consists of residues 32–40. The letters C and N denote the carboxy and amino termini, respectively, and the letter A designates the region which binds to the anti-*ras* protein antibody Y13-259. From de Vos *et al.* (1988).

ties to the *ras* protein and the possible functions of these groups are described in Chapter 2 in relation to the targeting of *ras* proteins to the plasma membranes (Section 2.6.2).

Elucidation of the tertiary structure of the *ras* proteins by X-ray crystallography was facilitated by knowledge of the structure of bacterial initiation factor EF-Tu. The structure of the catalytic site of the *ras* protein and its relationship to the guanine nucleotide molecule are shown in Fig. 3.23. Four key amino-acid residues in the *ras* protein are responsible for binding the guanine nucleotide. A region which interacts with other proteins, such as the *ras* GTPase activating protein, is composed of amino-acid residues 32–40 on the amino-terminal side of the nucleotide-binding site (Fig. 3.23).

3.5.3 *Cellular functions of the* ras *proteins*

All mammalian cells contain significant amounts of each of the H-, K-, and N-*ras* proteins, although the relative concentrations vary from one cell type to another. High concentrations of *ras* proteins are found both in many proliferating cells and in a number of mature differentiated cells. The latter include cells of the nervous system, pancreas, kidney, thymus, digestive tract, smooth muscle, and fibroblasts. The concentration of *ras* proteins in nerve cells is considerably higher than that in other types of cell.

Knowledge of the cellular functions of the *ras* proteins has come from experiments conducted with purified *ras* proteins and with antibodies to these proteins. Anti-*ras* antibodies were first prepared by Scholnick and his colleagues (Furth *et al.* 1982). One of the most widely used of these is the monoclonal antibody Y13-259. This antibody not only binds to each of the H-, K-, and N-*ras* proteins at the site shown in Fig. 3.23 but it also inhibits the cellular functions of these proteins. The results of the experiments conducted with pure *ras* proteins and with antibody Y13-

Table 3.7 *Intracellular pathways which require the action of a* ras *protein as revealed by the microinjection into cells of an antibody to* ras *proteins, which inhibits the function of these proteins*

Cell	Stimulus to Cell	Response
Nerve (PC12)	NGF	Cell differentiation (extension of neurites)
Oocyte	Insulin	Cell maturation
Fibroblasts (NIH-3T3)	Serum, PDGF, EGF, phorbol 12-myristate 13-acetate	Cell division
Fibroblasts (NIH-3T3)	Introduction of the *src, fes*, or *fms* oncogene	Cell transformation

259 have shown that the *ras* proteins are required in the intracellular processes by which some extracellular agonists, some intracellular stimuli, such as the actions of oncogenes which encode certain protein–tyrosine kinases, and phorbol ester activators of protein kinase C induce cell proliferation or differentiation (Table 3.7).

Attempts to delineate the cellular functions of the *ras* proteins began with the observations that the *ras* proteins are homologous to the α subunit of the oligomeric GTP-binding regulatory proteins and bind and hydrolyse GTP, albeit at a relatively slow rate. On the basis of this circumstantial evidence it was proposed that *ras* proteins link receptors to unknown effector enzymes at the cytoplasmic face of the plasma membrane in a manner similar to the oligomeric G proteins. Other circumstantial evidence which seemed to support this idea was knowledge of the function of the RAS2 gene in the yeast, *Saccharomyces cerevisiae*. In this organism the products of the RAS2 gene are required for the activation of adenylate cyclase. In mutants of *Saccharomyces cerevisiae* which lack the RAS2 gene, mammalian *ras* proteins can substitute for the RAS2 gene product in the activation of adenylate cyclase.

Early experiments conducted with lines of cultured animal cells, for example NIH-3T3 fibroblasts, transformed by a *ras* oncogene suggested that *ras* proteins might link receptors to PtdIns 4,5 P_2-specific phospholipase C or to phosphatidylcholine-specific phospholipase C. However, it was later shown that it is most unlikely that, in animal cells, *ras* proteins link receptors to adenylate cyclase, phospholipase C or, indeed, any other effector enzyme in a manner analogous to the oligomeric G proteins.

An important discovery which has helped point the way to a better understanding of the cellular functions of the *ras* proteins was the isolation, from cell extracts, of a GTPase activating protein (*ras* GAP) which interacts specifically with normal *ras* proteins and causes a stimulation of at least 100-fold in their GTPase catalytic activity (Trahey and McCormick 1987). The much lower intrinsic GTPase activity of oncogenic *ras* proteins is not stimulated by GAP. As described in Chapter 4 (Section 4.8.2) the *ras* GAP protein binds to certain protein–tyrosine kinases, such as the platelet derived growth factor (PDGF) receptor, and may be part of the signal transduction pathways initiated by activation of the protein–tyrosine kinase.

Two types of observation indicate that the binding and hydrolysis of GTP is a necessary step in the cellular function of *ras* proteins. Firstly, the introduction to cells by microinjection of anti-*ras* antibodies which inhibit the binding of guanine nucleotides to *ras* proteins inhibits the ability of *ras* oncogenes to transform cells. Secondly, mutant forms of *ras* proteins which cannot bind guanine nucleotides are unable to transform NIH-3T3 cells.

Although considerable knowledge of the *ras* proteins has accumulated during the past ten years, the cellular functions of these proteins are not yet known. A *ras* protein is required for the transmission of both extracellular and intracellular signals, such as those described in Table 3.7. Moreover, it seems clear that the action of the *ras* proteins involves the binding and hydrolysis of GTP, possibly in a reaction sequence similar to that described in the next section, and in which the *ras* GTPase activating protein participates. The transmission of intracellular signals in animal cells by *ras* proteins may involve the regulation of membrane fusion, changes in the structure of the cytoskeleton, or the coupling of plasma-membrane receptors to effector enzymes by a mechanism which differs from that of the oligomeric G proteins.

A considerable advance in knowledge of the cellular functions of the *ras* proteins has come from studies of development of the vulva in the nematode *Caenorhabditis elegans*. Genetic techniques have identified a number of genes which encode proteins necessary for the normal development of the vulva. Two of these genes, called *let* 23 and *let* 60, encode a protein–tyrosine kinase with homology to the epidermal growth factor (EGF) receptor protein–tyrosine kinase and a protein of the *ras* family (the *let* 60 *ras* protein). The *let* 23 protein–tyrosine kinase and *let* 60 *ras* GTP-binding protein are probably responsible for the transmission of an extracellular signal released from a neighbouring anchor cell which directs the vulva precursor cell to differentiate to a vulval cell. This signal is received by the *let* 23 protein–tyrosine kinase receptor in the plasma membrane of the vulval precursor cell and is transmitted to target proteins within the vulval precursor cell by the *let* 23 protein–

tyrosine kinase and the *let* 60 *ras* protein.

3.5.4   Mechanism of action of the monomeric GTP-binding proteins

The mechanisms of action of the monomeric GTP-binding proteins are probably similar to those of ribosomal elongation factor EF-1 and ribosomal initiation factor eIF-2. As described in Section 3.5.2, the structures of the monomeric GTP-binding proteins are similar to those of factors EF-1 and eIF-2. Moreover, like EF-1 and eIF-2, there are specific GTPase activating proteins which interact with the monomeric GTP-binding proteins.

Elongation factor EF-1 is required for the binding of the amino-acid–tRNA complex to the A site of the ribosome–mRNA complex in the process of protein synthesis. As shown in Fig. 3.24, EF-1^{GTP} binds to the amino-acid–tRNA complex which, in turn, binds to the A site on the ribosome–mRNA complex. (Elongation factor EF-1 itself also binds to a specific site on the ribosome.) If the amino-acid–tRNA species is the incorrect one, as specified by the mRNA, it rapidly dissociates without hydrolysis of the GTP bound to EF-1. However, if the correct amino-acid–tRNA species binds to the A site of the ribosome, its rate of dissociation is much slower so that during the time in which the amino-acid–tRNA–EF-1 complex resides on the ribosome the GTP is hydrolysed.

The hydrolysis of GTP alters the conformation of EF-1, reduces the affinity of EF-1 for the amino-acid–tRNA complex, allows EF-1^{GDP} to dissociate from the ribosome, and leaves the amino-acid–tRNA complex attached to the A site on the ribosome. The amino acid is subsequently transferred to, and elongates, the polypeptide chain on the P site of the ribosome. The exchange of GTP for GDP on EF-1^{GDP} is catalysed by an enzyme called T_s. In this system, the hydrolysis of GTP acts as a switch which ensures that only the correct amino acid is bound

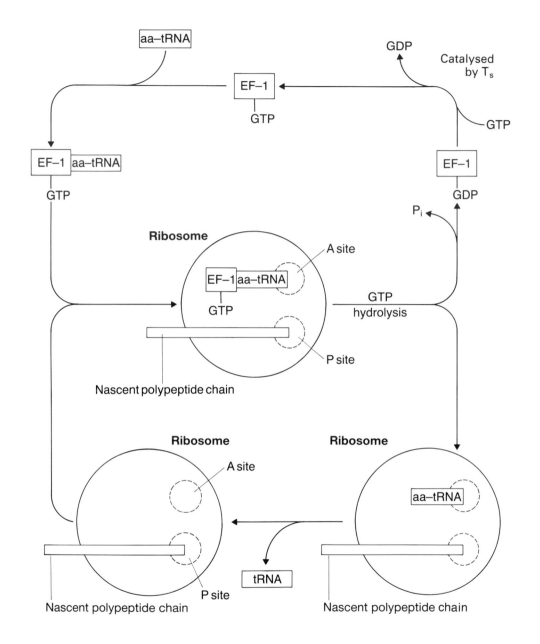

Fig. 3.24 The role of the binding and hydrolysis of GTP in the process by which mammalian elongation factor EF-1 mediates the selection and binding to the A site of the ribosome–mRNA complex of an amino-acid–tRNA species (aa–tRNA). EF-1^{GTP} binds an amino-acid–tRNA species which, in turn, binds to a ribosome so that the amino-acid–tRNA species is located at the A site on the ribosome. Hydrolysis of GTP is catalysed by EF-1. Energy released in this hydrolysis reaction induces the release of EF-1^{GDP} from the ribosome and the transfer of the aa–tRNA species from the A to the P site on the ribosome. The exchange of GDP for GTP on EF-1 is catalysed by an enzyme called T_s.

to the A site on the ribosome. A similar cycle and switch mechanism operated by the hydrolysis of GTP probably occurs in the process by which monomeric GTP-binding proteins are thought to act in the recognition, by transport vesicles, of the correct acceptor membrane (Chapter 2, Section 2.6.5).

An important difference between the mechanisms of action of the monomeric GTP-binding proteins and the mechanism of action of the oligomeric G proteins is highlighted by the action of the slowly hydrolysable analogue of GTP, GTPγS. Whereas, as described earlier, GTPγS activates the oligomeric G proteins, this same compound inhibits the function of many monomeric GTP-binding proteins. Thus many of the monomeric GTP-binding proteins are activated by the hydrolysis of GTP whereas the oligomeric

G proteins are inactivated by the hydrolysis of this nucleotide triphosphate.

3.6   Regulation of agonist action by phosphorylation of receptors and GTP-binding proteins

The actions of some agonists which bind to plasma-membrane receptors are modulated by phosphorylation of the cytoplasmic domain of their receptors, or by the phosphorylation of G proteins which can couple with these receptors. The phosphorylation of receptors is catalysed by a number of different protein kinases (Table 3.8). Receptors phosphorylated by protein kinase C and by cyclic AMP-dependent protein kinase include those for EGF, insulin, and α- and β-adrenergic agonists (Table 3.8).

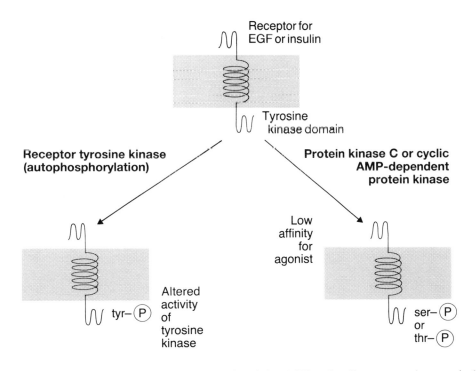

Fig. 3.25 Phosphorylation of the cytoplasmic domain of the EGF or insulin receptor by protein kinase C or by cyclic AMP-dependent protein kinase alters the affinity of the receptor for its agonist. Autophosphorylation of a tyrosine residue near the carboxy terminus is thought to be an important regulator of the activity of the protein–tyrosine kinase.

Phosphorylation of the receptors for insulin and EGF by protein kinase C converts these receptors from a form with a high affinity for the agonist to a form with a low affinity for the agonist (Fig. 3.25). Several sites on the cytoplasmic domain of the EGF receptor are phosphorylated. The phosphorylation of one of these, threonine 654, which is located 10 amino-acid residues from the membrane bilayer, is probably responsible for the change in agonist affinity. A number of experiments indicate that it is the combination of EGF with high-affinity sites on the EGF receptor which is responsible for transmission of the effects of EGF to intracellular enzymes. For example, the binding of EGF to the high-affinity receptors correlates well with

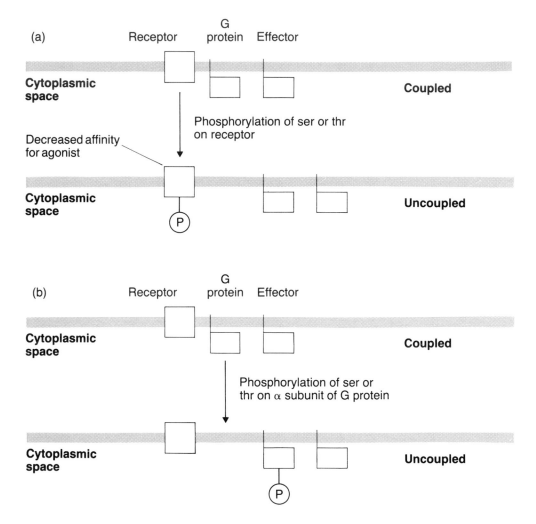

Fig. 3.26 Modulation of the action of an agonist at a receptor coupled to a G protein by phosphorylation of the receptor or G protein catalysed by protein kinase C or by cyclic AMP-dependent protein kinase. (a) Phosphorylation of the receptor often leads to a decrease in the affinity of the receptor for its agonist and to an uncoupling of the link between the receptor and G protein. (b) Phosphorylation of the α subunit of the G protein often leads to an uncoupling of the link between the G protein and the receptor and effector enzyme.

Table 3.8 *Examples of the regulation of the function of plasma-membrane receptors by phosphorylation*

Receptor	Protein kinase
β-Adrenergic	cAMP-dependent protein kinase Protein kinase C β-Adrenergic receptor kinase
α₁-Adrenergic	Protein kinase C
Rhodopsin	Rhodopsin kinase
Nicotinic acetylcholine	Protein kinase C cAMP-dependent protein kinase Protein kinase C
Insulin	Insulin receptor tyrosine kinase Protein kinase C cAMP-dependent protein kinase (or an intermediary kinase)
IGF-1	IGF-1 receptor tyrosine kinase Protein kinase C
EGF	EGF receptor tyrosine kinase Protein kinase C cAMP-dependent protein kinase
PDGF	PDGF receptor kinase

the stimulation, by the growth factor, of the initiation of DNA synthesis and mitogenesis. In the short term, the phosphorylation of the insulin or EGF receptors by protein kinase C does not change the total number of receptors available to the agonist. However, over a longer period of time phosphorylation of receptors may increase the rate of receptor endocytosis.

As shown in Table 3.8, the protein–tyrosine kinase receptors can also be phosphorylated on tyrosine residues by the receptor-protein–tyrosine kinase itself. This autophosphorylation of the EGF and insulin receptors is thought to be important in regulation of the activity of the receptor-activated protein–tyrosine kinase towards its cellular substrates (Fig. 3.25).

Phosphorylation of α₁- and β-adrenergic receptors by protein kinase C or by cyclic AMP-dependent protein kinase leads to an uncoupling of the link between the receptor and the G pro-

tein and to a decrease in the affinity of the receptor for the agonist (Fig. 3.26(a)). The link between the β-adrenergic receptor and its G protein is also uncoupled by phosphorylation of the receptor by another protein kinase, called the β-adrenergic receptor kinase, which appears to be specific for this receptor protein.

The α subunits of oligomeric G proteins are phosphorylated by protein kinase C and by some other protein kinases. This probably reduces the ability of the G protein to interact with the effector enzyme (Fig. 3.26(b)) and hence reduces the transmission of the signal, carried by an agonist, to intracellular sites.

3.7   Summary

Many extracellular signals are received by animal cells through receptor proteins located in the plasma membrane. These proteins can be classified on the basis of the stereospecificity of the receptor for agonists or on the basis of the mechanism by which the receptor transmits the signal to sites within the cell. There are at least seven families of receptors: agonist-gated ion channels; receptors which possess a protein–tyrosine kinase or phosphoprotein–tyrosine phosphatase catalytic site in the cytoplasmic domain; receptors which couple to a protein–tyrosine kinase which does not possess a membrane-spanning domain; receptors which couple to effector proteins through oligomeric GTP-binding regulatory proteins (G proteins); receptors which couple to an integral membrane glycoprotein; and the receptor for atrial natriuretic peptide, which contains a guanylate cyclase catalytic site on the cytoplasmic domain. Some agonists can bind to several different receptor proteins or to one type of receptor protein which interacts with a number of different effector systems.

The primary structures of many receptors have been determined. All receptors contain an extracellular domain, which is usually glycosylated and includes the stereospecific binding site for the agonist, a membrane-spanning domain which is composed of one or more hydrophobic α-helical sequences composed of about 20 amino acids, and a cytoplasmic domain. The agonist-gated ion channels are large molecules composed of either several subunits or of one subunit which contains repeated polypeptide motifs. Each subunit or motif contains several membrane-spanning sequences which usually possess a few charged amino acids. These charged residues surround a central pore through which ions pass in response to the binding of the agonist. Receptors which possess a protein–tyrosine kinase catalytic site on the cytoplasmic domain have only one membrane-spanning sequence per subunit and most have only one subunit. Receptors which couple to an effector protein through a G protein possess seven membrane-spanning sequences and a cytoplasmic domain which contains one or more sites which can interact with G proteins. The receptor for atrial natriuretic peptide consists of an extracellular domain, a single membrane-spanning sequence, and a cytoplasmic domain which contains the guanylate cyclase catalytic site.

There are complex, and not yet fully understood, mechanisms which regulate the number of receptors on the plasma membrane and which switch off the signal carried by the agonist. For many agonists, the continued presence of the agonist leads to desensitization of the response of the target cell to the agonist. This is due either to a decrease in the concentration of plasma-membrane receptors available to the agonist, or to an uncoupling of the receptor and effector proteins. The endocytosis of receptors and the synthesis of new receptors are the two main mechanisms by which the concentration of receptors on the plasma membrane is controlled. Endocytosed receptors are either degraded by lysosomes or are recycled to the plasma membrane. Most or all cellular responses induced by agonist–receptor complexes are initiated while the complex is stationed at the plasma membrane.

There are many different G proteins which couple different receptors to specific effector proteins such as adenylate cyclase. Considerable information has been obtained about the structure and function of G_s and G_i, the stimulatory and inhibitory proteins which couple receptors to adenylate cyclase, and about transducin, G_t, which couples rhodopsin to cyclic GMP phosphodiesterase. Each G protein is composed of three subunits, designated α, β, and γ, which are each attached to the cytoplasmic face of the plasma membrane. The α subunit binds GDP or GTP, and interacts with the receptor and effector proteins. Differences in the amino-acid sequences of the α subunit account for most of the differences between the different G proteins.

In response to interaction with the agonist–receptor complex, each G protein undergoes a cycle of activation and inactivation. This involves movement of the receptor, G protein, and effector protein in the plane of the membrane. Activation, which is catalysed by the agonist–receptor complex, involves the displacement of bound GDP by GTP and dissociation of the oligomer to yield a free α subunit and a βγ complex. The free α subunit, or possibly in a few cases, the βγ complex, interacts with the effector protein. Inactivation of the G protein involves the hydrolysis of GTP and re-association of the α and βγ subunits. Future expansion of knowledge of G proteins is likely to include elucidation of the structures of a number of newly discovered G proteins, determination of the tertiary structures of the G proteins, and elucidation of the nature of the molecular interactions which occur between G proteins, receptors, and effector proteins.

Another group of GTP-binding proteins have molecular weights in the range of 20–30 kDa and are monomeric. Their primary amino-acid sequences are similar to those of the α subunits of the oligomeric G proteins. The monomeric GTP-binding proteins include proteins encoded by the *ras* and a number of *ras*-related genes, and GTP-binding proteins involved in the fusion of transport vesicles to membranes. Each monomeric GTP-binding protein hydrolyses GTP at a slow rate but this is greatly accelerated by another protein called a GTPase activating protein. The monomeric GTP-binding proteins are probably involved in many intracellular processes including the movement of membrane vesicles within the cytoplasmic space and the fusion of vesicles to membranes. They may utilize GTP as a switch in a cycle of reactions analogous to those catalysed by initiation and elongation factors with which the monomeric GTP-binding proteins have many similarities.

The actions of agonists which bind to plasma-membrane receptors are modulated by phosphorylation of the cytoplasmic domain of the receptor or by the phosphorylation of G proteins. The cytoplasmic domain of the protein–tyrosine kinase receptors is often phosphorylated on tyrosine residues by the receptor protein–tyrosine kinase. The cytoplasmic domains of other plasma-membrane receptors are phosphorylated on serine or threonine residues by protein kinase C, cyclic AMP-dependent protein kinase, and by some other protein kinases which appear to be specific for a given receptor protein. The α subunits of G proteins can be phosphorylated by protein kinase C and some other protein kinases.

References

Brisson, A. and Unwin, P.N.T. (1985). Quaternary structure of the acetylcholine receptor. *Nature*, **315**, 474–7.

Carpentier, J-L., Gorden, P., Freychet, P., Le Cam, A., and Orci, L. (1979). Lysosomal association of internalized ^{125}I-insulin in isolated rat hepatocytes. *J. Clin. Invest.* **63**, 1249–61.

Cassel, D. and Selinger, Z. (1976). Catecholamine-stimulated GTPase activity in turkey erythrocyte membranes. *Biochim. Biophys. Acta*, **452**, 538–51.

Changeux, J.-P., Kasai, M., Huchet, M., and Meunier, J. C. (1970). Extraction à partir du tissu électrique de gymnote d'une protéine présentant plusieurs propriétés caractéristiques du récepteur physiologique de l'acetyl choline. *Crit. Rev. Acad. Sci. (Paris)*, **270**, 2864–7.

Claudio, T., Ballivet, M., Patrick, J., and Heinemann, S. (1983). Nucleotide and deduced amino acid sequences of *Torpedo californica* acetylcholine receptor γ subunit. *Proc. Natl Acad. Sci. USA*, **80**, 1111–15.

Colquhoun, D. and Sakmann, B. (1985). Fast events in single-channel currents activated by acetylcholine and its analogues at the frog muscle end-plate. *J. Physiol. (London)*, **369**, 501–57.

De Robertis, E., Fiszer, S., and Soto, E. F. (1967). Cholinergic binding capacity of proteolipids from isolated nerve-ending membranes. *Science*, **158**, 928–9.

Devillers-Thiery, A., Giraudat, J., Bentaboulet, M., and Changeux, J.-P. (1983). Complete mRNA coding sequence of the acetylcholine binding α-subunit of *Torpedo marmorata* acetylcholine receptor. A model for the transmembrane organisation of the polypeptide chain. *Proc. Natl Acad. Sci. USA*, **80**, 2067–71.

Dixon, R. A. F., Kobilka, B. K., Strader, D. J., Benovic, J. L., Dohlman, H. G., Frielle, T. *et al.* (1986). Cloning of the gene and cDNA for mammalian β-adrenergic receptor and homology with rhodopsin. *Nature*, **321**, 75–9.

Ehrenpreis, S., Fleisch, J. H., and Mittag, T. W. (1969). Approaches to the molecular nature of pharmacological receptors. *Pharmacol. Rev.*, **21**, 131–81.

Ehrlich, P. (1913). Chemotherapeutics: scientific principles, methods and results. *Lancet*, **ii**, 445–51.

Finer-Moore, J. and Stroud, R. M. (1984). Amphipathic analysis and possible formation of the ion channel in an acetylcholine receptor. *Proc. Natl Acad. Sci. USA*, **81**, 155–9.

Furth, M. E., Davis, L. J., Fleurdelys, B., and Scolnick, E. M. (1982). Monoclonal antibodies to the p21 products of the transforming gene of Harvey murine sarcoma virus and of the cellular *ras* gene family. *J. Virol.*, **43**, 294–304.

Hanley, M. R. and Jackson, T. (1987). The *ras* gene: transformer and transducer. *Nature*, **328**, 668–9.

Hirata, F. and Axelrod, J. (1980). Phospholipid methylation and biological signal transmission. *Science*, **209**, 1082–90.

Katada, T. and Ui, M. (1982). ADP ribosylation of the specific membrane protein of C6 cells by islet-activating protein associated with modification of adenylate cyclase activity. *J. Biol. Chem.*, **257**, 7210–16.

Kubo, T., Kazuhiko, F., Mikami, A., Maeda, A., Takahashi, H., Mishina, M., *et al.* (1986). Cloning, sequencing and expression of complementary DNA encoding the muscarinic acetylcholine receptor. *Nature*, **323**, 411.

Langley, J. N. (1906). On nerve endings and on special excitable substances in cells. *Proc. Roy. Soc.*, **B78**, 170–94.

Moss, J. and Vaughan, M. (1977). Mechanism of action of choleragen. Evidence for ADP-ribosyltransferase activity with arginine as an acceptor. *J. Biol. Chem.*, **252**, 2455–7.

Noda, M., Takahashi, H., Tanabe, T., Toyosato, M., Kikyotani, S., Furutani, Y., *et al.* (1983). Structural homology of *Torpedo californica* acetylcholine receptor subunits. *Nature*, **302**, 528–32.

Ovchinnikov, Y. A. (1982). Rhodopsin and bacteriorhodopsin: structure–function relationships. *FEBS Lett.*, **148**, 179–91.

Patil, P. N. and LaPidus, J. B. (1972). Stereoisomerism in adrenergic drugs. *Ergebn. Physiol.*, **66**, 213–60.

Rodbell, M., Birnbaumer, L., Pohl, S. L., and Krans, H. M. J. (1971). The glucagon-sensitive adenyl cyclase system in plasma membranes of rat liver. V. An obligatory role of guanyl nucleotides in glucagon action. *J. Biol. Chem.*, **246**, 1877–82.

Rodbell, M. (1985). Programmable messengers: a new theory of hormone action. *Trends Biochem. Sci.*, **10**, 461–4.

Ross, E. M. and Gilman, A. G. (1977). Reconstitution of catecholamine-sensitive adenylate cyclase activity: interaction of solubilized components with receptor-replete membranes. *Proc. Natl Acad. Sci. USA*, **74**, 3715–19.

Schleifer, L. S., Garrison, J. C., Sternweis, P. C., Northup, J. K., and Gilmand, A. G. (1980). The regulatory components of adenylate cyclase from uncoupled S49 lymphoma cells differs in charge from the wild-type protein. *J. Biol. Chem.*, **255**, 2641–4.

Shih, T. Y., Papageorge, A. G., Stokes, P. E., Weeks, M. O., and Scolnick, E. M. (1980). Guanine nucleotide binding and autophosphorylating activities associated with the p21^{src} protein of Harvey murine sarcoma virus. *Nature*, **287**, 686–91.

Stevens, C. F. (1985). AChR structure: a new twist in the story. *Trends Neurosci.*, **8**, 1–2.

Trahey, M. and McCormick, F. (1987). A cytoplasmic protein stimulates normal N-*ras* p21 GTPase, but does not affect oncogenic mutants. *Science*, **238**, 542–5.

Ullrich, A., Coussens, L., Hayflick, J. S., Dull, T. J., Gray, G., Tam, A. W., *et al.* (1984). Human epidermal growth factor receptor cDNA sequence and aberrant expression of the amplified gene in A431 epidermoid carcinoma cells. *Nature*, **309**, 418–25.

Ullrich, A., Bell, J. R., Chen, E. Y., Herrera, R., Petruzzelli, L. M., Dull, T. J. *et al.* (1985). Human insulin receptor and its relationship to the tyrosine kinase family of oncogenes. *Nature*, **313**, 756–61.

de Vos, A. M., Tong, L., Milburn, M. V., Matias, P. M., Jancarik, J., Noguchi, S., *et al.*, (1988). Three-dimensional structure of an oncogene protein: catalytic domain of human c-H-*ras* p21. *Science*, **239**, 888–93.

Yarden, Y., Rodriguez, H., Wong, S. K-F., Brandt, D. R., May, D. C., Burnier, J. *et al.* (1986). The avian beta-adrenergic receptor: primary structure and membrane topology. *Proc. Natl Acad. Sci. USA*, **83**, 6795–9.

Further reading

Bourne, H. R., Sanders, D. A., and McCormick, F. (1991). The GTPase superfamily: conserved structure and molecular mechanism. *Nature*, **349**, 117–27.

Bretscher, M. S. (1985). The molecules of the cell membrane. *Sci. Am.*, **253**, 86–90.

De Robertis, E. (1975). Synaptic receptor proteins. Isolation and reconstitution in artificial membranes. *Rev. Physiol. Biochem. Pharmacol.*, **73**, 9–38.

Dohlman, H. G., Caron, M. G., and Lefkowitz, R. J. (1987). A family of receptors coupled to guanine nucleotide regulatory proteins. *Biochemistry*, **26**, 2657–64.

Gilman, A. G. (1987). G. proteins: transducers of receptor-generated signals. *Ann. Rev. Biochem.*, **56**, 615–49.

Goldstein, J. L., Brown, M. S., Anderson, R. G. W., Russell, D. W., and Schneider, W. J. (1985). Receptor-mediated endocytosis: concepts emerging from the LDL receptor system. *Ann. Rev. Cell. Biol.*, **1**, 1–39.

Greenwald, I. and Broach, J. R. (1990). Cell fates in *C. elegans*: In medias *ras*. *Cell*, **63**, 1113–16.

Houslay, M. D. and Milligan, G. (1990). *G-proteins as mediators of cellular signalling processes*. Wiley, Chichester.

Staros, J. V., Cohen, S., and Russo, M. W. (1985). Epidermal growth factor receptor: characterization of its protein kinase activity. In *Molecular mechanisms of transmembrane signalling* (ed. P. Cohen and M. D. Housley), pp. 253–77. Elsevier, Amsterdam.

Wileman, T., Harding, C., and Stahl, P. (1985). Receptor-mediated endocytosis. *Biochem, J.*, **232**, 1–14.

Yarden, Y., Escobedo, J. A., Kuang, W-J., Yang-Feng, T. L., Daniel, T. O., Tremble, P. M. *et al.* (1986). Structure of the receptor for platelet-derived growth factor helps define a family of closely related growth factor receptors. *Nature*, **323**, 226–32.

4 *The protein kinases and phosphatases*

4.1 Regulation of cell function by protein phosphorylation

The network of protein kinases and phosphoprotein phosphatases is a comprehensive set of pathways by which information is transferred between intracellular sites in animal cells. The existence of protein kinases with a regulatory function was first indicated by the observations of Fischer and Krebs (1955) and Rall *et al.* (1957) of the presence in animal cells of both an active phosphorylated and an inactive dephosphorylated form of the enzyme glycogen phosphorylase. The first protein kinase enzyme to be discovered, cyclic AMP-dependent protein kinase, was isolated about ten years later (Huijing and Larner 1966; Walsh *et al.* 1968). Subsequently the large number of other protein kinases and the phosphoprotein phosphatases were discovered.

Protein kinases catalyse the transfer of a phosphate moiety from $MgATP^{2-}$ to a serine, threonine, or tyrosine residue in the polypeptide chain of a target protein, the substrate (Fig. 4.1). This results in the formation of a covalent bond in

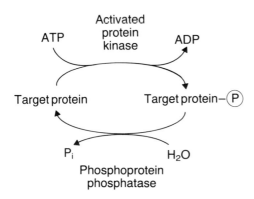

Fig. 4.1 The reversible phosphorylation of a target protein catalysed by a protein kinase and phosphoprotein phosphatase. The phosphorylated target protein may have higher or lower activity than the non-phosphorylated enzyme.

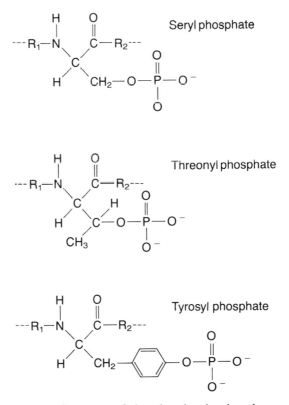

Fig. 4.2 Structures of phosphorylated serine, threonine, and tyrosine residues in the polypeptide chains of target proteins which have been phosphorylated by a protein kinase.

which the phosphate group is esterified to the hydroxyl side chain of the acceptor amino-acid residue (Fig. 4.2). Phosphorylation of this amino-acid residue alters the conformation of the target protein and causes either an activation or an inhibition of the function of the target protein.

An example of enzyme inhibition induced by phosphorylation is the phosphorylation of acetyl-CoA carboxylase by AMP-activated protein kinase. This decreases by about 80 per cent the maximum velocity of the reaction at saturating concentrations of the allosteric activator citrate and increases by five-fold the apparent dissociation constant for citrate (Fig. 4.3).

The co-ordinate control of glycogenolysis in the liver by glucagon, which increases the intracellular cyclic AMP concentration, provides an example in which both activation and inhibition of enzyme activity are induced by the same protein kinase. The phosphorylation of glycogen phosphorylase kinase by cyclic AMP-dependent protein kinase results in an activation of this enzyme which, in turn, phosphorylates and activates glycogen phosphorylase. This leads to an increase in glycogenolysis. The phosphorylation of glycogen synthetase by cyclic AMP-dependent protein kinase leads to an inhibition of

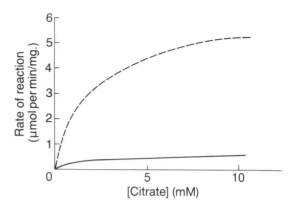

Fig. 4.3 The phosphorylation of acetyl-CoA carboxylase by AMP-activated protein kinase causes a decrease of about 80 per cent in the maximum velocity and a five-fold increase in the apparent dissociation constant for the activator, citrate. Phosphorylated enzyme: full line; non-phosphorylated enzyme: broken line. From Davies *et al.* (1990).

activity of glycogen synthetase and hence to inhibition of glycogen synthesis. Thus the net effect of the action of glucagon is to stimulate glycogen breakdown. Generally, enzymes involved in catabolic (degradative) processes are activated by phosphorylation whereas those involved in anabolic (biosynthetic) processes are inhibited by phosphorylation.

The phosphate moiety covalently bound to phosphorylated target proteins is removed by

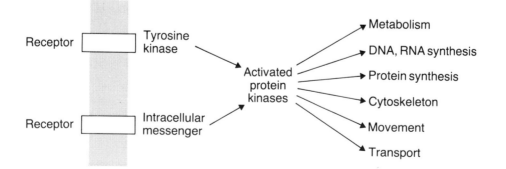

Fig. 4.4 A network of protein kinase enzymes transfers information between mobile intracellular messengers or plasma-membrane receptors and intracellular target proteins. Protein kinases in the cytoplasmic space are activated allosterically by either a mobile intracellular messenger or by phosphorylation catalysed by a plasma-membrane protein–tyrosine kinase.

hydrolysis with water in a reaction catalysed by a phosphoprotein phosphatase (Fig. 4.1). Each cell possesses many different protein kinases and phosphoprotein phosphatases which act on a large number of different target proteins. This enables a given extracellular signal, through its action on a plasma-membrane receptor, to influence a large number of intracellular reactions (Fig. 4.4). Examples of the different protein kinases and target proteins present in cells of the brain and liver are shown in Figs 4.5 and 4.6.

The energy required to form the covalent phosphate ester bond with a seryl, threonyl, or tyrosyl residue in a polypeptide chain is comparable in magnitude with that released by hydro-

lysis of the terminal phosphate of ATP. This relatively large energy requirement may be one of the factors which allows selective phosphorylation of target proteins and which prevents indiscriminate phosphorylation of these proteins by other cellular kinase enzymes such as those which phosphorylate metabolites.

The basic elements of the protein kinase network are the protein kinase and phosphoprotein phosphatase enzymes. In this chapter, the properties, regulation, and major natural substrates (target proteins) for each of these enzymes will be described. Whilst a list of natural substrates for each enzyme can readily be drawn up, it should be borne in mind that for the action of each protein kinase in a given cell, the nature,

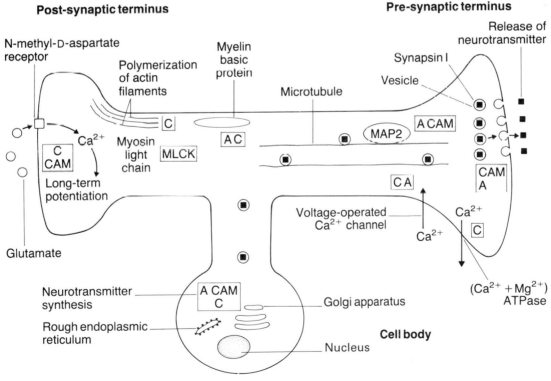

Fig. 4.5 A schematic representation of a nerve cell showing the target proteins for the major protein kinases or the metabolic pathways or processes in which the target protein functions. The protein kinases are represented by the following boxed symbols: A, cyclic AMP-dependent protein kinase; CAM, (Ca^{2+} + calmodulin)-dependent protein kinase; C, protein kinase C; MLCK, myosin light-chain kinase.

priority of phosphorylation, spatial distribution, and mechanism of dephosphorylation of target proteins have not yet been fully described.

4.2　The protein kinases

4.2.1　*The families of protein kinases*

Protein kinases can be broadly classified into two groups. These are kinases which catalyse the phosphorylation of a serine or threonine residue in the polypeptide chain of the target protein, and kinases which catalyse the phosphorylation of tyrosine residues. The majority of target proteins are phosphorylated on serine or threonine residues. Phosphorylation of tyrosine residues represents less than 0.1 per cent of the total phosphorylated protein in a cell. The main protein–serine and –threonine kinases with broad substrate specificity are summarized in

Table 4.1　*The protein–serine and protein–threonine kinases which have a broad specificity for target proteins*

Protein kinase	Regulatory agent(s)
cAMP-dependent protein kinases	cAMP
Cyclic GMP-dependent protein kinase	cGMP
$(Ca^{2+} + calmodulin)$-dependent protein kinase II	Ca^{2+}
Protein kinases C	Diacylglycerol, Ca^{2+}

Table 4.1. There are also many other protein–serine and protein–threonine kinases, such as pyruvate dehydrogenase kinase, with a narrow substrate specificity. These are described later.

There are multiple forms of cyclic AMP-

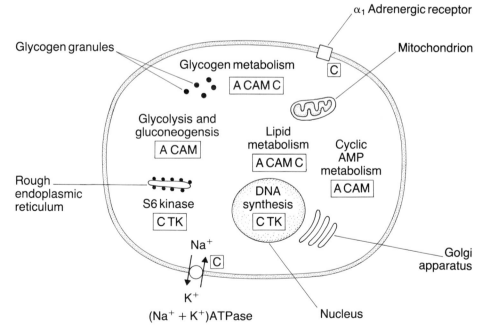

Fig. 4.6　A schematic representation of a hepatocyte showing the target proteins for the major protein kinases or the metabolic pathways in which the target proteins function. The protein kinases are represented by the following boxed symbols: A, cyclic AMP-dependent protein kinase; CAM, $(Ca^{2+} + calmodulin)$-dependent protein kinase; C, protein kinase C; TK, a receptor protein–tyrosine kinase, such as the insulin or EGF receptor kinase.

dependent protein kinase, (Ca^{2+} calmodulin)-dependent protein kinase and protein kinase C. Although the cellular functions of these different species of the same enzyme are not yet fully understood, they may be involved in the delivery of signals to subsets of substrates, may be specific for certain types of cells, and, in the case of protein kinase C, may respond to different activators.

The known protein–tyrosine kinases can be divided into two groups—those that are part of the cytoplasmic domain of the polypeptide chain of plasma-membrane receptors for certain hormones and growth factors, and those which are not components of plasma-membrane receptors. In addition to their specificity for tyrosyl residues, the protein–tyrosine kinases differ from most of the protein–serine and –threonine kinases in that they do not require the presence of mobile intracellular messengers as activators. Mutant forms of a number of the protein–tyrosine kinases are encoded by oncogenes. These oncogenic kinases can have far-reaching effects on cell growth which may lead to cell transformation. The nature of the oncogenic protein–tyrosine kinases is discussed in Chapter 11.

4.2.2   *General structure*

A number of different forms of expression of a general principle which underlies the structures and actions of protein kinases have evolved. These forms are represented by the different types of protein kinases present in animal cells. There are a variety of different protein structures which convert the initial stimulus, such as an increase in the concentration of an intracellular messenger, into activation of the protein kinase.

Cyclic GMP-dependent protein kinase, protein kinase C, and almost all the protein–tyrosine kinases are monomers. Each polypeptide chain contains a catalytic and a regulatory domain. The other protein kinases are oligomers

each of which is composed of a catalytic subunit and one or more regulatory subunits (Table 4.2). The regulatory subunit, for example the R subunit of cyclic AMP-dependent protein kinase, or calmodulin, contains the binding site for an intracellular messenger. The catalytic subunit contains the protein kinase catalytic site and a domain which interacts with the regulatory subunit.

A schematic representation of the primary structures of the major protein kinases, arranged so that the catalytic domains are aligned, is shown in Fig. 4.7. There is considerable homology between the amino-acid sequences in the catalytic domain of the different enzymes. Comparison of the primary amino-acid sequences of the various protein kinases suggests that the catalytic region of each enzyme is derived from a common ancestral gene.

The interaction of substrates with the catalytic site and the release of products takes place in an ordered sequential manner. The binding of $MgATP^{2-}$ is followed by binding of the polypeptide substrate. The phosphate moiety is transferred directly from $MgATP^{2-}$ to the polypeptide. $MgADP^-$ is then released, followed by the phosphorylated polypeptide.

The non-catalytic or regulatory region of the protein kinase enzymes determines how the activity of the kinase is regulated as well as the intracellular location of the kinase. The regulatory domain contains the binding sites for mobile intracellular messengers or, in the case of the receptor protein–tyrosine kinases, the binding sites for hormones or growth factors. The importance of these regulatory sites is illustrated by some oncogenic forms of the receptor protein–tyrosine kinases. These enzymes are constitutively active. This may be because critical amino-acid residues in the regulatory region have been lost.

Each species of protein kinase is inactive in the absence of a regulator molecule. This is pro-

Table 4.2   *Subunit structures of protein–serine and protein–threonine kinases*

Protein kinase	Enzyme molecular weight (kDa)	Subunit structure
Cyclic AMP-dependent		
Type I	178	$R^I_2C_2$
Type II	190	$R^{II}_2C_2$
Cyclic GMP-dependent	175–180	E_2
$(Ca^{2+}$ + calmodulin)-dependent		
Type II (Multifunctional)	650 (forebrain, calmodulin absent)	$\alpha_9(\beta \text{ or } \beta')_3$
	500 (cerebellar, calmodulin absent)	$\alpha_1(\beta \text{ or } \beta')_4$
Type I	42 (calmodulin absent)	C
Glycogen phosphorylase kinase	1300	$(\alpha\beta\gamma\Delta)_4$ (Δ is calmodulin)
Myosin light-chain kinase	130 (smooth muscle, calmodulin absent)	C
	65 (skeletal muscle, calmodulin absent)	
Protein kinases C	77–85	E

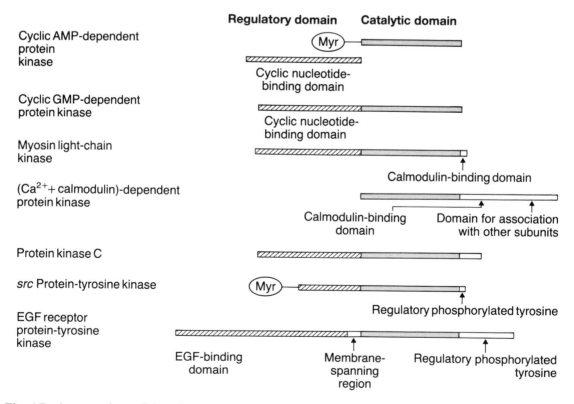

Fig. 4.7   A comparison of the primary structures of the major protein–serine and protein–threonine kinases and two protein–tyrosine kinases. The polypeptide chains have been arranged so that their catalytic domains are aligned. The catalytic domains are the shaded sections and regulatory domains are shown by cross-hatching. 'Myr' represents the site of attachment of a myristyl group.

bably because one of the substrates, ATP, or the protein to be phosphorylated, cannot interact with the catalytic site. Upon binding of the regulator molecule the protein kinase undergoes a conformational change which exposes the catalytic site to the substrates. The regulatory molecule which induces this change may be a cyclic nucleotide, the (Ca^{2+} + calmodulin) complex, diacylglycerol, or, in the case of the receptor protein–tyrosine kinases, an agonist.

There are at least two mechanisms by which the protein kinase catalytic site is autoregulated in the absence of a regulatory molecule. In the absence of Ca^{2+} and calmodulin, the conformation of the catalytic site of (Ca^{2+} + calmodulin)-dependent kinase is such that ATP does not have access to the catalytic site. In myosin light-chain kinase, cyclic AMP-dependent protein kinase, cyclic GMP-dependent protein kinase, and protein kinase C, the catalytic site is masked by its binding to the autoregulatory region of the protein kinase which is called a pseudosubstrate site.

The pseudosubstrate site consists of a sequence of amino acids which mimics the amino-acid sequence of the phosphorylation site in the natural substrate which binds to the active site. However, there is no phosphate transfer to the pseudosubstrate site because there is no ser, thr, or tyr that can be phosphorylated. For example, the amino-acid sequence of the pseudosubstrate site for protein kinase C is arg–phe–ala –arg–lys–gly–ala–leu–arg–gln–lys–asn–val. The consensus sequence of the phosphorylation site in substrates for protein kinase C is ala–lys– ala–lys–thr(P)–thr–lys–lys–arg–pro–gln–arg. The conformational change induced by the binding of a regulatory molecule to its site in the regulatory domain of the protein kinase moves the pseudosubstrate region from close association with the catalytic site and allows the catalytic site access to the natural protein substrate (Fig. 4.8).

4.2.3 *Target proteins*
Most cellular target proteins for protein kinases

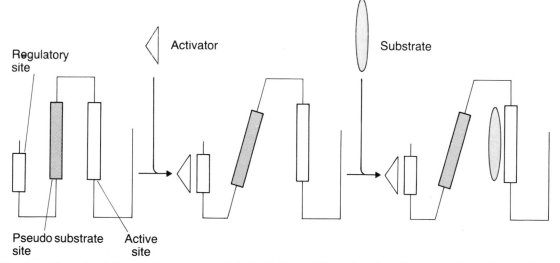

Fig. 4.8 The role of the pseudosubstrate site in inhibition of the active site of a protein kinase in the absence of an activator. The active site of the protein kinase is bound to a region of the polypeptide chain called the pseudosubstrate site in the absence of an activator, such as cyclic AMP, cyclic GMP, (Ca^{2+} + calmodulin), or diacylglycerol. Combination of the activator with the protein kinase alters the conformation of the enzyme and releases the active site so that it can interact with the substrate.

were first identified by observing phosphorylation of the target protein by the protein kinase *in vitro*. Improved techniques of two-dimensional polyacrylamide gel electrophoresis have now enabled extracts of cells labelled with [^{32}P]inorganic phosphate to be scanned systematically. This has permitted the detection of many more target proteins which are phosphorylated in response to the action of a given protein kinase. These include target proteins already detected from studies conducted *in vitro*. Many target proteins are phosphorylated by more than one protein kinase.

The sequence of amino acids around the phosphorylated serine or threonine residue is the predominant factor that determines which proteins are phosphorylated by a given protein–serine or protein–threonine kinase. For the protein-tyrosine kinases, the secondary and tertiary structure of the target protein, as well as the amino-acid sequence around the phosphorylated tyrosine residue, are important in determining the nature of the proteins phosphorylated.

Most protein–serine and protein–threonine kinases recognize a certain configuration of basic amino acids on the amino-terminal side of the phosphorylated serine or threonine in the target protein (Table 4.3). However, one group of protein–serine kinases, the casein kinases, recognize a configuration of acidic residues on the carboxy-terminal side of the phosphorylated serine. The recognition sequence for substrates of the protein–tyrosine kinases are an acidic amino acid at four residues and a basic amino acid at eight residues on the amino-terminal side of the phosphorylated tyrosine (Table 4.3).

Other protein kinases can also be target proteins for the action of protein kinases. For example, protein kinase C phosphorylates the cytoplasmic domain of the EGF receptor. This contributes to regulation of the activity of the EGF receptor through regulation of the activity of the EGF protein–tyrosine kinase (Chapter 3, Section 3.6).

4.2.4 *Multi-site phosphorylation of target proteins*

Many protein targets for protein kinases are phosphorylated at more than one site. This

Table 4.3 *Amino-acid sequences at the phosphorylation sites of target proteins for protein kinases*

Protein kinase	Amino-acid sequence around the phosphorylated serine, threonine, or tyrosine residue
Cyclic AMP-dependent protein kinase	xxx–arg–arg–xxx–*ser*(*P*)–xxx
	arg–xxx–lys–arg–xxx–xxx–*ser*(*P*)–xxx
	xxx–arg–arg–arg–xxx–*thr*(*P*)–xxx
	xxx–arg–lys–xxx–*ser*(*P*)–xxx
Glycogen phosphorylase kinase	xxx–xxx–xxx–*ser*(*P*)–xxx–arg
Myosin light-chain kinase	lys–arg–arg–xxx–xxx–xxx–
	xxx–xxx–*ser*(*P*)–asn–val–phe
Multifunctional (Ca^{2+} + calmodulin)–dependent protein kinase II	xxx–xxx–xxx–arg–xxx–xxx–*ser*(*P*)–xxx–xxx–xxx
Protein kinase C	ala–lys–ala–lys–*thr*(*P*)–thr–lys–lys–arg–pro–gln–arg
Protein–tyrosine kinases	lys–xxx–xxx–asp–xxx–xxx–
	xxx–*tyr*(*P*)–xxx
	arg–xxx–xxx–glu–xxx–xxx–
	xxx–*tyr*(*P*)–xxx

phenomenon is termed multi-site phosphorylation. Different protein kinases may catalyse these phosphorylations. Large numbers of phosphate groups are found associated with some proteins. In the case of microtubule-associated protein-2 (MAP-2) the number is over 20. Glycogen synthetase is one example of a well characterized protein with multiple phosphorylation sites (Fig. 4.9).

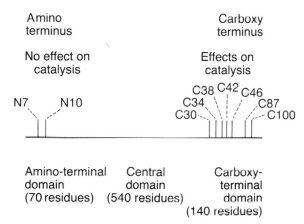

Fig. 4.9 Glycogen synthetase from rabbit skeletal muscle is an example of an enzyme which has multiple phosphorylation sites. The nine phosphorylation sites are designated by the numbers N7, N10, C30, C34, C38, C42, C46, C87, and C100. These numbers refer to the distances from the amino terminus of each of the cyanogen bromide peptides derived from the amino terminus (N) and carboxy terminus (C) of glycogen synthetase. Site N7 is phosphorylated by (Ca^{2+} + calmodulin)-dependent protein kinase II, glycogen phosphorylase kinase, cyclic AMP-dependent protein kinase, and glycogen synthetase kinase-4; site N10 by an unknown protein kinase; site C100 by cyclic AMP-dependent protein kinase and (Ca^{2+} + calmodulin)-dependent protein kinase II; site C87 by cyclic AMP-dependent protein kinase; site C46 by casein kinase II; and sites C42, C38, C34, and C30 by glycogen synthetase kinase-3. Adapted from Cohen (1982) and Poulter *et al.* (1988).

The phosphorylation of at least one of the multiple sites on a target protein leads to an alteration in the activity of that protein. Depending on the nature of the target protein, phosphorylation at other sites may directly alter the

activity of the protein, may modulate the response of the protein to phosphorylation at other sites, or may modify phosphorylation of the protein by other protein kinases. For example, the phosphorylation of glycogen synthase at site C46 by casein kinase II affects the ability of glycogen synthase kinase III to recognize and phosphorylate sites C30, C34, and C38 on the amino-terminal side of site C46.

4.2.5 *Autophosphorylation*

Most protein kinase enzymes themselves contain serine, threonine, or tyrosine residues which can be phosphorylated either by the catalytic site of the same protein kinase or, as described earlier, by another protein kinase. Phosphorylation by the protein kinase itself is an intramolecular reaction and is termed autophosphorylation. This type of phosphorylation is an important mechanism for the control of the activity of the protein kinase. One of the most dramatic examples of the role of autophosphorylation in regulation of the activity of a protein kinase is the autophosphorylation of calmodulin-dependent protein kinase II which renders the enzyme independent of calmodulin. Similarly autophosphorylation of the insulin-receptor kinase leads to an activation of the kinase which is independent of the presence of insulin.

4.2.6 *Intracellular location*

The various protein kinases are located at different intracellular sites. A large proportion of the cyclic nucleotide- and (Ca^{2+} + calmodulin)-dependent protein kinases are found in the cytoplasmic space in a form which is freely dissociable from the intracellular structures present in this space. The receptor protein–tyrosine kinases and a number of other protein–tyrosine kinases without transmembrane regions and extracellular domains are located on the cytoplasmic side of the plasma membrane. When activated, protein kinase C is transiently bound to the cytoplasmic side of the plasma membrane. A number of other protein–serine and –threonine kinases are associated with specific enzyme complexes. While these general conclusions about the intracellular distribution of protein kinases can be made, much is still to be learned about the detailed intracellular distribution of these enzymes. The properties of each type of protein kinase will now be considered in more detail, beginning with the cyclic AMP-dependent protein kinases.

4.3 The cyclic AMP-dependent protein kinases

4.3.1 *Isoenzymes of cyclic AMP-dependent protein kinase*

In 1968, Krebs and his colleagues discovered an enzyme which catalyses the cyclic AMP-dependent phosphorylation of glycogen phosphorylase kinase (Walsh *et al.* 1968). Subse-

quently this enzyme was shown to phosphorylate not only glycogen phosphorylase kinase but also glycogen synthetase and many other substrates. The enzyme was named cyclic AMP-dependent protein kinase.

There are two forms of cyclic AMP-dependent protein kinase present in animal cells. These enzymes, named types I and II by Corbin and his colleagues (1975), have different affinities for DEAE cellulose (Fig. 4.10). It was this property which first indicated the existence of the two isoenzymes. The relative amounts of isoenzymes I and II present in a given type of cell depends on the nature of the cell. For example, heart and testis contain predominantly type I; adipose, stomach mucosa and brain tissues predominantly type II; and liver and skeletal muscle approximately equal amounts of types I and II.

4.3.2 *Activation by cyclic AMP*

In the absence of activator, cyclic AMP-dependent protein kinase exists as a dimer composed of two catalytic (C) and two regulatory (R) subunits (Table 4.2). The catalytic unit is myristylated at the amino terminus. The regulatory subunit contains four functional domains. These are two cyclic AMP binding domains, a dimerization domain, and a domain which interacts with the catalytic unit (Fig. 4.11). The domain which interacts with the catalytic unit contains a pseudosubstrate region. The combination of cyclic AMP with cyclic AMP-dependent protein kinase decreases the affinity of the regulatory subunit for the catalytic subunit by a factor of 10^4. As shown by the following reaction sequence, this causes dissociation of the catalytic and regulatory subunits.

$$R_2C_2 + 4\text{cyclic AMP} \rightleftharpoons R_2C_2 \cdot (\text{cyclic AMP})_4$$
$$\rightleftharpoons 2(\text{cyclic AMP}_2 \cdot R) + 2C.$$

Cyclic AMP combines with both activator binding sites on each regulatory subunit. The association constant for the combination of cyclic AMP

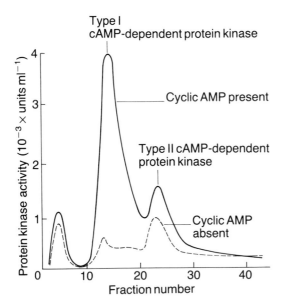

Fig. 4.10 Resolution of heart-muscle type I and type II cyclic AMP-dependent protein kinases by chromatography on DEAE cellulose. The enzymes were eluted with a linear NaCl gradient and assayed in the presence and absence of cyclic AMP. From Corbin *et al.* (1975).

with the regulatory unit is 10 nM. Dissociation of the catalytic subunit is accompanied by a conformational change in the catalytic polypeptide chain. This exposes the active site of the protein kinase and permits the interaction of this site with protein substrates.

The two binding sites for cyclic AMP on each regulatory subunit (Fig. 4.11) differ slightly in structure. Each site has a different affinity for a given analogue of cyclic AMP.

The degree of activation by cyclic AMP of cyclic AMP-dependent protein kinase in cells or tissues can be determined by measuring the activity of the protein kinase in cell extracts incubated in the presence and absence of exogenous cyclic AMP. The ratio of protein kinase activity in the absence of cyclic AMP to that in the presence of the cyclic nucleotide is a measure of the degree of activation of the protein kinase.

Two analogues of cyclic AMP have proved useful in the elucidation of the role of cyclic AMP-dependent protein kinase in intact cells. These are the diastereoisomers of adenosine cyclic 3′,5′ phosphorothioate (cAMPS), S_p-cAMPS and R_p-cAMPS. S_p-cAMPS activates the enzyme whereas R_p-cAMPS inhibits the action

of cyclic AMP. R_p-cAMPS competes with cyclic AMP for the regulatory binding site on the regulatory subunit but does not cause dissociation of the R_2C_2 complex.

The catalytic units of types I and II cyclic AMP-dependent protein kinase have identical amino-acid sequences. The regulatory subunits of the type I and II enzymes differ in primary amino-acid sequence, in their interactions with the catalytic unit and cyclic AMP, and in autophosphorylation by the catalytic unit. Type I cyclic AMP-dependent protein kinase dissociates into catalytic and regulatory units much more readily than the type II enzyme. Some experiments have suggested that cyclic AMP-dependent protein kinases I and II may be selectively activated by different agonists, although the mechanism by which this differential activation might occur has not been elucidated.

4.3.3   *Phosphorylation of target proteins*

Target proteins phosphorylated by cyclic AMP-dependent protein kinases in intact cells include a large number of regulatory enzymes in pathways of intermediary metabolism, enzymes involved in muscle contraction, enzymes which

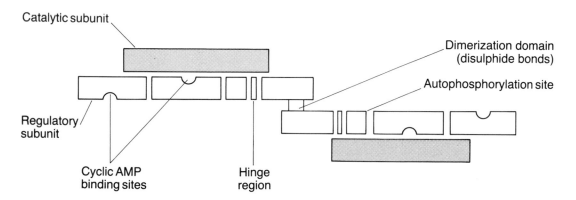

Fig. 4.11   The domains of the primary structures of the regulatory subunits of cyclic AMP-dependent protein kinase. Each regulatory subunit contains two binding sites for cyclic AMP, an autophosphorylation site, a site which interacts with the other regulatory subunit (the dimerization domain), and a region which interacts with the catalytic subunit. From Taylor (1989).

Table 4.4 *Pathways or processes regulated by cyclic AMP-dependent protein kinases, and some protein targets for these kinases*

Metabolic Pathway	Protein target (substrate)
Carbohydrate metabolism	Glycogen phosphorylase kinase Glycogen synthetase Fructose 1,6-bisphosphatase Fructose-6-phosphate-l-kinase Pyruvate kinase (liver)
Lipid metabolism	Hormone-sensitive lipase Hydroxymethylglutanyl-CoA reductase Acetyl-CoA carboxylase
Neurotransmitter synthesis	Tyrosine hydroxylase Phenylalanine hydroxylase
RNA synthesis	RNA polymerase S
Other protein kinases and enzymes of cyclic nucleotide metabolism	*src* protein–tyrosine kinase (Ca^{2+} + calmodulin)-dependent cyclic nucleotide phosphodiesterase Insulin-stimulated low K_M cyclic AMP phosphodiesterase
Muscle contraction	Troponin I regulatory subunit Myosin light-chain kinase

metabolize cyclic nucleotides, and RNA polymerases (Table 4.4). Histones and a number of synthetic peptides are also good substrates for cyclic AMP-dependent protein kinases and have been used in the assay of enzyme activity *in vitro*.

In the target proteins for cyclic AMP-dependent protein kinase there are two types of amino-acid sequence which precede the phosphorylated serine or threonine residues. These are arg(lys)–X–ser(P) and lys–arg–X–X–ser(P) (Table 4.3) where X is any amino acid. The presence of the basic amino acids on the amino-terminal side of the phosphorylated serine, and the distance between these residues and the serine(P), are thought to distinguish target proteins for cyclic AMP-dependent protein kinase from those for other protein kinases.

Serine and threonine residues located in the polypeptide chain of the cyclic AMP-dependent protein kinase enzyme itself can be autophosphorylated. Two residues on the regulatory subunit near the cyclic AMP binding sites (Fig. 4.11) are preferentially phosphorylated in this reaction. In addition, two residues on the catalytic subunit can also be phosphorylated. As described earlier, binding of the active site of the catalytic subunit to an autophosphorylation (pseudosubstrate) site on the regulatory subunit is responsible for inhibition of the activity of the catalytic subunit in the absence of cyclic AMP.

4.4 Cyclic GMP-dependent protein kinase

Although cyclic GMP-dependent protein kinase was discovered soon after the cyclic AMP-dependent kinases (Kuo and Greengard 1970; Hofmann and Sold 1972), the intracellular functions of the cyclic GMP-dependent enzyme are still not well understood some 20 years later. Cyclic GMP-dependent protein kinase is present in many tissues. For example, relatively high concentrations are found in smooth muscle, lung, heart, and in Purkinje cells of the cerebellum. The enzyme appears to be primarily located in the cytoplasmic space.

The substrate specificity of cyclic GMP-dependent protein kinase is more narrow than that of the cyclic AMP-dependent protein kinases. Cyclic GMP-dependent protein kinase phosphorylates a number of proteins *in vitro* (Table 4.5). The enzyme also undergoes autophosphorylation. Only a few of the proteins phosphorylated *in vitro* have clearly been shown to be phosphorylated by cyclic GMP-dependent protein kinase in intact cells. Some of these are discussed in Chapter 5 in connection with the action of cyclic GMP.

Like the cyclic AMP-dependent protein kinases, the nature of the target protein phosphorylated by cyclic GMP-dependent protein kinase is specified by the presence of multiple basic amino-acid residues on the amino-terminal side of the phosphorylated serine residue. In some cases, additional determinants of specificity are the presence of a basic residue immediately on the carboxy-terminal side of the ser(P)

and of a prolyl residue immediately on the amino-terminal side of ser(P).

The catalytic and regulatory domains of cyclic GMP-dependent protein kinase which, as described earlier, are on the same polypeptide chain, can be separated by selective proteolytic cleavage. The polypeptide chain of cyclic GMP-dependent protein kinase normally forms dimers (Table 4.2) with the polypeptide chains arranged in an antiparallel manner. In the absence of cyclic GMP a pseudosubstrate region in the regulatory domain binds to the catalytic site. The interaction of the enzyme (E) with cyclic GMP leads to activation of the catalytic site without dissociation of the dimer, as shown in the following equation:

$$E_2 + 2\text{cyclic GMP} \rightleftharpoons E_2(\text{cyclic GMP})_2.$$

The active dimeric form of the enzyme can then phosphorylate target proteins. The affinity of the kinase for cyclic GMP is about 10^{-8} M.

4.5 The (Ca^{2+} + calmodulin)-dependent protein kinases

4.5.1 *The family of (Ca^{2+} + calmodulin)-dependent protein kinases*

Knowledge of the properties of the (Ca^{2+} + calmodulin)-dependent protein kinases began with the discovery of calmodulin (Cheung 1970) and the detection of protein kinases which are activated by Ca^{2+} and calmodulin but are not affected by cyclic nucleotides (De Lorenzo 1976). The (Ca^{2+} + calmodulin)-dependent protein kinases are activated by Ca^{2+} in the range of Ca^{2+} concentrations through which the intracellular free Ca^{2+} concentration ($[Ca^{2+}]_i$) passes in response to the action of agonists. This group of enzymes consists of glycogen phosphorylase kinase, myosin light-chain kinase, (Ca^{2+} + calmodulin)-dependent protein kinases I and III, each of which has a narrow substrate specificity, and the multifunctional enzyme (Ca^{2+} + calmodulin)-

Table 4.5 *Proteins which are substrates for cyclic GMP-dependent protein kinase* in vitro

Troponin I
Phospholamban
Cyclic AMP-dependent protein kinase
    (R^I subunit)
Phosphorylase kinase
Glycogen synthetase
Phosphatase inhibitor 1
G-substrate (protein-phosphatase inhibitor)

Pyruvate kinase
Fructose 1,6-diphosphatase

Cholesterol esterase
Diglyceride lipase
Hormone-sensitive lipase

S2 ribosomal protein
S10 ribosomal protein
L5 ribosomal protein

Protamine
Histone

Myelin basic protein

Table 4.6 *The (Ca^{2+} + calmodulin)-dependent protein kinases and some of their target proteins*

Kinase	Target proteins
Type I (Ca^{2+} + calmodulin)-dependent protein kinase	Synapsin I (brain) Protein III (brain)
Type II (multifunctional) (Ca^{2+} + calmodulin)-dependent protein kinase	Glycogen synthetase Myosin light chain Tyrosine hydroxylase Tryptophan hydroxylase Myelin basic protein Ribosomal protein S6 (Ca^{2+} + calmodulin)-dependent phosphodiesterase Synapsin I Microtubule-associated protein-2
Type III (Ca^{2+} + calmodulin)-dependent protein kinase	Ef2
Glycogen phosphorylase kinase	Glycogen phosphorylase *b* Glycogen synthetase
Myosin light-chain kinase	Myosin light-chain P (LC_2) Myosin light-chain kinase (autophosphorylation)

dependent protein kinase II which has a broad substrate specificity (Table 4.6). Multifunctional protein kinase II probably mediates the actions of increased $[Ca^{2+}]_i$ on a large number of target proteins, including those involved in the maintenance and modification of the structure of the cytoskeleton. This proposed role of (Ca^{2+} + calmodulin)-dependent protein kinase II is analogous to that of the multifunctional cyclic AMP-dependent protein kinases.

In the absence of calmodulin, some (Ca^{2+} + calmodulin)-dependent protein kinases are monomeric while others are oligomeric. The latter are composed of one or more catalytic subunits and sometimes additional regulatory units (Table 4.2). These monomers and oligomers bind calmodulin in the presence of Ca^{2+}. There is at least one exception to this generalization. This is glycogen phosphorylase kinase in which calmodulin remains as an integral part of the quaternary structure in the absence of Ca^{2+}.

The target proteins phosphorylated by (Ca^{2+} + calmodulin)-dependent protein kinases are specified by the arrangement of one or more basic amino acids located near the phosphorylated serine or threonine residue. For glycogen phosphorylase kinase, an arginine residue on the carboxy-terminal side of the phosphorylated serine (Table 4.3) is a major determinant of the stereochemical features of the site phosphorylated on glycogen phosphorylase. The specificity of myosin light-chain kinase for its substrate is largely determined by the sequence asn–val–phe on the carboxy-terminal side of the phosphorylated seryl residue and by the sequence lys–arg–arg on the amino-terminal side (Table 4.3). For multifunctional (Ca^{2+} + calmodulin)-dependent protein kinase II, an arginine located three residues from the amino-terminal side of the phosphorylated serine or threonine residue specifies the target protein phosphorylated (Table 4.3).

4.5.2 *Glycogen phosphorylase kinase*

Considerably more is known about the properties of glycogen phosphorylase kinase and myosin light-chain kinase than is known about the multifunctional (Ca^{2+} + calmodulin) protein kinases. The main physiological substrate for glycogen phosphorylase kinase is glycogen phosphorylase *b*. However, other substrates, including glycogen synthetase, phospholamban, the $(Na^+ + K^+)$ATPase of the sarcolemma, and the $(Ca^{2+} + Mg^{2+})$ATPase of the sarcoplasmic reticulum, may also be phosphorylated under physiological conditions. Cohen and his colleagues have made extensive studies of the properties of the glycogen phosphorylase kinase enzymes present in muscle and liver (Cohen 1982). Each of these enzymes is composed of four different types of subunit (Table 4.2). These are the catalytic subunit (γ), two regulatory subunits (α and β), and calmodulin (Δ). In contrast to most other $(Ca^{2+}$ + calmodulin)-dependent enzymes, the calmodulin polypeptide (Δ) is tightly bound to the other subunits.

An example of the regulatory function of the α and β subunits of glycogen phosphorylase kinase is the phosphorylation of these peptides by cyclic AMP-dependent protein kinase. This

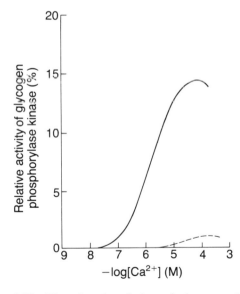

Fig. 4.12 The phosphorylation of glycogen phosphorylase kinase by cyclic AMP-dependent protein kinase markedly increases the sensitivity of the enzyme to activation by Ca^{2+}. Phosphorylated enzyme: full curve. Non-phosphorylated enzyme: broken curve. From Cohen (1980).

decreases the apparent K_M of glycogen phosphorylase kinase for its substrate glycogen phosphorylase *b* and, as shown in Fig. 4.12, increases the affinity of glycogen phosphorylase kinase for Ca^{2+} by about 15-fold. In heart muscle exposed to a β-adrenergic agonist, such as adrenalin, which increases the intracellular concentration of cyclic AMP, the increase in affinity of glycogen phosphorylase kinase for Ca^{2+} enhances the sensitivity of the enzyme to the transient increase in $[Ca^{2+}]_i$ which follows depolarization of the sarcolemma.

4.5.3   *Myosin light-chain kinase*

Myosin light-chain kinase is specific for the P chain of myosin which is phosphorylated on a seryl residue near the amino terminus. This phosphorylation is responsible for the initiation of contraction in smooth-muscle cells, and for the initiation of motility, including movement associated with secretion, in non-muscle cells. In striated muscle, the phosphorylation of myosin modifies the degree of muscle tension. Myosin light-chain kinase is a monomer (Table 4.2). The polypeptide chain contains both a catalytic and a pseudosubstrate site. As described earlier, the binding of calmodulin to the pseudosubstrate site releases the active site and allows this site to bind and phosphorylate substrates.

4.5.4   *(Ca^{2+} + calmodulin)-dependent protein kinases I, II, and III*

Multifunctional $(Ca^{2+}$ + calmodulin)-dependent protein kinase (form II) has been detected in many tissues and is present at high concentrations in brain. The target proteins for this enzyme include synapsin I, tryptophan hydroxylase, glycogen synthetase, and the cytoskeletal proteins tau, tubulin, and MAP-2 (microtubule-associated protein 2). In brain, the enzyme is found both as a membrane-bound form and as a form bound to freely dissociable sites in the cytoplasmic space.

In the absence of Ca^{2+} and calmodulin, $(Ca^{2+}$ + calmodulin)-dependent protein kinase II is an oligomeric protein composed of two types of subunits, α and β. The α subunit has a molecular weight of 50 kDa. There are two forms of the β subunit called β and β'. These have molecular weights of 60 and 58 kDa, respectively. The ratio of α and β (or β') subunits present in $(Ca^{2+}$ + calmodulin)-dependent protein kinase depends on the type of cell in which the enzyme is present (Table 4.2). Each α and β subunit contains a catalytic and a regulatory domain, and a domain involved in interaction with other subunits (Fig. 4.7). The regulatory domain contains the calmodulin binding site. The combination of $(Ca^{2+}$ + calmodulin) with the kinase alters the conformation of the enzyme so that the protein unfolds allowing ATP access to the active site. Under certain conditions, autophosphorylation renders the kinase active in the absence of $(Ca^{2+}$ + calmodulin).

In contrast to the multifunctional $(Ca^{2+}$ + calmodulin)-dependent protein kinase II, $(Ca^{2+}$ + calmodulin)-dependent protein kinases I and III have a very narrow substrate specificity. Type I phosphorylates synapsin I, protein III, and smooth-muscle myosin light chain while Type III phosphorylates a protein called Ef2. In the absence of calmodulin, $(Ca^{2+}$ + calmodulin)-dependent protein kinase I is a monomer with a molecular weight of 42 kDa (Table 4.2).

4.6 Protein kinase C

4.6.1 *The different species of protein kinase C*
In 1977 Nishizuka and his colleagues described a protein kinase, later named protein kinase C, which was activated by proteolytic cleavage (Inoue *et al.* 1977). Subsequently, these workers showed that the enzyme requires phospholipid, Ca^{2+}, and diacylglycerol for maximum activity. Nishizuka proposed that the major physiological activator of protein kinase C is the diacyl-

glycerol which is formed in the plasma membrane by the hydrolysis of phosphoinositides. This idea, and the reactions which form diacylglycerol, are described in Chapter 6.

In 1986 the complete amino-acid sequence of the polypeptide chain of protein kinase C was deduced from the base sequence of the cDNA which encodes this protein (Parker *et al.* 1986; Knopf *et al.* 1986; Ono *et al.* 1986; Makowske *et al.* 1986). The analysis of other cDNA clones has shown that there are at least eight distinct forms of protein kinase C enzymes in mammalian cells. These are designated protein kinase C (PKC) α, βI, βII, γ, δ, ϵ, ζ, and η. Species α, β and γ are encoded by separate genes each located on a separate chromosome. Species βI and βII, which are encoded by the same gene, are synthesized from a single RNA transcript by alternative splicing.

PKC α has been found in all cell types so far examined. By contrast, PKC γ is found solely in the brain and spinal cord and PKC βI and PKC βII are only found in certain cell types. The different species of protein kinase C presumably perform different cellular functions although these functional differences have not yet been clearly defined. Each species of protein kinase C may respond to diacylglycerols which possess a unique fatty-acid composition, or may phosphorylate a specific set of substrates, or may act on target proteins located at a specific site within the cytoplasmic space. For example, in the brain, the intracellular concentration of each of the major species of protein kinase C varies from one location to another. This may reflect a different neuronal function for each isoenzyme of protein kinase C.

4.6.2 *Structures of the protein kinase C enzymes*
Comparison of the amino-acid sequences of the protein kinase C species α, β, and γ has allowed the identification of four conserved and five vari-

able regions in the protein kinase C polypeptide chain (Fig. 4.13). Conserved regions C1 and C2 constitute a domain called the regulatory domain while conserved regions C3 and C4 constitute the catalytic domain (Fig. 4.13). PKCδ, PKCε, and PKCζ are smaller than PKCα, PKCβ, and PKCγ and lack conserved region C2. There are long sequences of the protein kinase C polypeptide chain which are homologous with sequences of the cyclic AMP- and cyclic GMP-dependent protein kinases. In fact, the overall structure of the protein kinase C enzymes is quite similar to that of cyclic GMP-dependent protein kinase.

The region in the protein kinase C molecule which joins the catalytic and regulatory domains is called the hinge region (Fig. 4.13). The regulatory domain probably contains the binding site for Ca^{2+} and the site at which the protein kinase C molecule interacts with the plasma membrane. The latter is thought to be a cysteine-rich sequence near the amino terminus. Within the regulatory domain there are two sequences which resemble the consensus sequence of a structure called the zinc finger which is present in the DNA-binding domain of sequence-specific DNA-binding proteins (Fig. 4.13). (The structures of zinc fingers are described in Chapter 10, Section 10.2.3). Although Zn^{2+} binds to these motifs in protein kinase C, their affinity for Zn^{2+} is lower than the affinity for Zn^{2+} of the zinc fingers of DNA-binding proteins. Sites in both the catalytic and regulatory domains of protein kinase C are autophosphorylated. This results in a decrease in the K_M of the enzyme for its substrates.

4.6.3   *Activation of protein kinase C by diacylglycerol*

In 1980, Nishizuka and his colleagues showed that in the presence of phospholipid, the ability of Ca^{2+} to activate protein kinase C is greatly

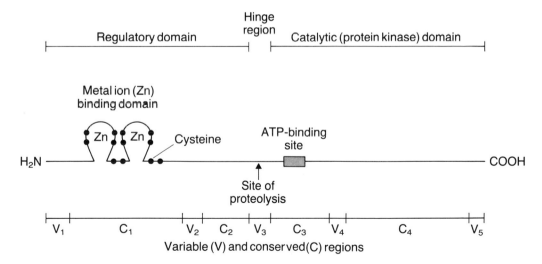

Fig. 4.13 A representation of the primary structures of the α, β, and γ species of protein kinase C. The enzyme is composed of a regulatory and catalytic domain which are joined by the hinge region. This is also the site at which protein kinase C is cleaved by proteolytic enzymes. The regulatory domain includes a region enriched in cysteine residues (indicated by the filled circles) which is the binding site for metal ions such as Zn^{2+} and may be the site of interaction of protein kinase C with the membrane. The distinction between variable (V) and conserved (C) regions of the enzyme is shown in the bottom part of the diagram. These distinctions have been made by comparing the amino-acid sequences of the different species of protein kinase C.

enhanced by diacylglycerols (Kishimoto *et al*, 1980) (Fig. 4.14). Neither phospholipid nor diacylglycerol, when present alone, caused substantial enhancement of the activation of the enzyme by Ca^{2+} (Fig. 4.14). Phosphatidylserine was found to be the most effective phospholipid in co-operating with diacylglycerol and Ca^{2+} in activating the enzyme. These observations led to the conclusion that protein kinase C is activated by diacylglycerol and Ca^{2+} while the enzyme is bound to the cytoplasmic face of the plasma membrane. This process of activation is described in more detail in Chapter 6.

Another important observation made by Nishizuka and his colleagues was that in the presence of phospholipid, purified protein kinase C can be activated by tumour-promoting phorbol esters such as phorbol dibutyrate (Castagna *et al*. 1982; Kikkawa *et al*. 1983). This experiment is shown in Fig. 4.15. Other experiments with purified protein kinase C showed

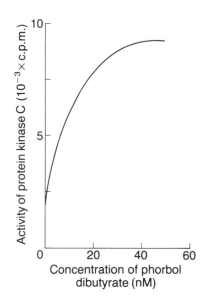

Fig. 4.15 The tumour-promoting phorbol ester, phorbol dibutyrate, activates protein kinase C in the presence of phosphatidylserine. From Kikkawa *et al*. (1983).

that there is a specific binding site for phorbol esters on the protein kinase C molecule (Niedel *et al*. 1983) while experiments conducted with intact cells showed that phorbol esters can replace diacylglycerol in the activation of protein kinase C. There is considerable similarity between the structure of the esterified vicinal carbon atoms 1 and 2 of diacylglycerol and the esterified vicinal carbon atoms 12 and 13 of the phorbol esters (Fig. 4.16).

*Sn*1,2 diacylglycerols in which the fatty acids are unsaturated are more effective activators of isolated protein kinase C than are diacylglycerols in which the fatty acids are saturated. Diacylglycerols with *sn* 1,3 and *sn* 2,3 configurations neither activate nor inhibit protein kinase C. The ester linkage between the glycerol carbon atom and the carbonyl carbon of the fatty acid on each of the vicinal carbon atoms of glycerol, as well as the adjacent 3′ hydroxyl group in 1,2 *sn* diacylglycerol (Fig. 4.16), are essential for the activation of protein kinase C.

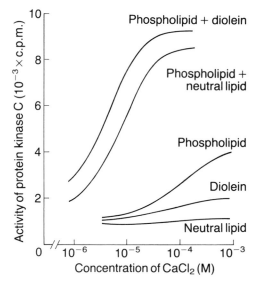

Fig. 4.14 The addition of diacylglycerol, in the form of neutral lipid or diolein, to a mixture of purified protein kinase C and phospholipid markedly enhances the ability of Ca^{2+} to activate the enzyme. The synergistic activation of protein kinase C by diacylglycerol and Ca^{2+} is dependent on the presence of phospholipid. From Kishimoto *et al*. (1980).

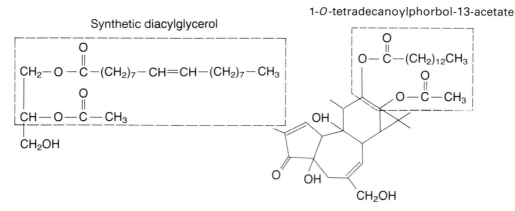

Fig. 4.16 Comparison of the structures of the synthetic diacylglycerol, l-oleolyl-2-acetylglycerol, and the tumour-promoting phorbol ester, 1-*O*-tetradecanoylphorbol-13-acetate. Both compounds are activators of protein kinase C. Ester bonds on vicinal carbon atoms are required for this activation.

The molecular mechanism by which phospholipids, Ca^{2+}, and diacylglycerols activate protein kinase C on the plasma membrane is an interesting, but as yet, incompletely answered question. Activation of the enzyme is probably a two-step process. The first step is the binding of protein kinase C to the plasma membrane in the presence of Ca^{2+} to yield an inactive membrane-bound enzyme. In the second step, diacylglycerol binds to an allosteric site on the enzyme. This site is located in the hydrophobic zinc-finger region of the protein kinase C polypeptide chain and is adjacent to the pseudosubstrate region. The binding site for diacylglycerol is probably also the site to which phorbol esters bind. The binding of diacylglycerol causes a conformational change which leads to a disassociation of the catalytic and pseudosubstrate regions and allows the catalytic site to interact with substrates.

4.6.4   *Proteolytic cleavage of protein kinase C*
The protein kinase C polypeptide chain is readily cleaved at the hinge region by calpain, a Ca^{2+}-activated neutral protease, and by some other proteolytic enzymes. Hydrolysis of protein kinase C occurs at arg 302 in variable region

V_3 (Fig. 4.13) and yields two polypeptide chains, one of molecular weight 50 kDa which contains the carboxy-terminus and the catalytic domain, designated protein kinase M, and one which contains the amino terminus and the regulatory domain. Proteolysis is thought to be initiated by the combination of protein kinase C with Ca^{2+}, diacylglycerol, and the plasma membrane. This sequence of reactions is described in Chapter 6. The carboxy-terminal half of the molecule is catalytically active in the absence of Ca^{2+}, phospholipid, and diacylglycerol. This form of protein kinase C is rapidly further degraded by proteolytic digestion.

The different species of protein kinase C exhibit different susceptibilities to calpain. For example, PKCγ is rapidly degraded whereas PKCα is relatively resistant to degradation. While it has been suggested that the proteolysis of protein kinase C is an alternative mechanism by which the enzyme can be activated, it seems most likely that the role of calpain is to initiate degradation of the enzyme.

4.6.5   *Target proteins for protein kinase C*
Purified protein kinase C phosphorylates a broad range of target proteins on serine or threo-

nine residues. Some of these are listed in Table 4.7. The major categories of target proteins are plasma-membrane receptors, other plasma-membrane proteins, proteins of the cytoskeleton, contractile proteins, regulatory enzymes in metabolic pathways, and sequence-specific DNA-binding proteins involved in the control of gene expression and cell proliferation. Many of the target proteins for protein kinase C are also substrates for cyclic AMP-dependent protein kinase. The phosphorylation by protein kinase C of sequence-specific DNA-binding proteins in the nucleus is the final step in the pathway by which many hormones and growth factors influence cell growth.

In protein targets for protein kinase C, the phosphorylated serine or threonine residue is specified by the presence of a basic amino acid on either the amino- or carboxy-terminal side of the phosphorylated residue. For example, there are two lysine residues on the amino-terminal side and two lysine and two arginine residues on the carboxy-terminal side of the phosphorylated threonine in the smooth-muscle myosin light chain, the substrate for protein kinase C shown in Table 4.3.

4.7   Other protein–serine (threonine) kinases

In the preceding sections, the properties of the major groups of the protein–serine and protein–threonine kinases with broad substrate specificity, and of myosin light-chain kinase and glycogen phosphorylase kinase, were described. In addition to these enzymes, there are a number of other protein–serine and protein–threonine kinases which have a narrow substrate specificity. These are listed in Table 4.8. A number

Table 4.7   *Cellular processes regulated by protein kinases C and target proteins for these protein kinases*

Intracellular process	Substrate
Receptor function	Epidermal growth factor receptor
	Insulin receptor
	Transferrin receptor
Ion transport	$(Ca^{2+} + Mg^{2+})$ATPase Ca^{2+} transporter
	Na^+–H^+ exchange system
	Synaptic B50 (FI) protein
Movement and shape change	Myosin light chain
	Troponins T and I
	Microtubule-associated proteins
	Myosin light-chain kinase
Metabolism	Glycogen phosphorylase kinase
	Glycogen synthetase
	Phosphofructokinase
	Guanylate cyclase
Other processes	Retinal-binding proteins
	Vitamin D-binding protein
	Ribosomal S6 protein
	Middle T antigen
	p60[src]
	p20 and p40 (platelets)
	p87 (brain and other tissues)
DNA transcription	*jun*/Ap-1

of protein kinases phosphorylate only one target protein. The properties and intracellular functions of the two eIF-2α (eukaryotic initiation factor 2α) kinases and of pyruvate dehydrogenase kinase have been most clearly defined. Less is known about the other protein kinases.

Ribosomal S6 kinase plays a key role in the control of protein synthesis by growth factors. Regulation of the activity of ribosomal S6 kinase by growth factors probably involves the phosphorylation of the S6 kinase by other protein kinases. These include protein kinase C and plasma-membrane receptor protein–tyrosine kinases.

Another protein–serine (threonine) kinase with narrow substrate specificity, p34 kinase, plays a major role in control of the cell cycle (Chapter 10, Section 10.4.1). In its active form p34 kinase is the catalytic subunit of a protein factor called maturation promoting factor (MPF), which induces mitosis. The p34 kinase is encoded by the *cdc* 2 (cell division cycle) gene. The regulatory subunit of the maturation promoting factor complex is a cyclin protein. There are various forms of cyclins, such as the A and B forms. Cyclins also play a major role in control of the cell cycle. The substrates for p34 kinase include histone H1, lamins, nucleolin, myosin light chain, and RNA polymerase II. These target proteins may link changes in p34 kinase activity to progression through the cell cycle.

Phosphorylation of RNA polymerase II by p34 kinase is particularly interesting because it involves polyphosphorylation of serine residues in the carboxy terminus of this protein. Within this region of the RNA polymerase II polypeptide chain are multiple repeats of the consensus sequence tyr–ser–pro–thr–ser–pro–ser. p34

Table 4.8 *Other kinases which phosphorylate proteins at serine or threonine residues*

Protein kinase	Regulatory agent(s)	Target proteins
eIF-2α kinase (double stranded RNA-dependent)	Double-stranded RNA	eIF-2 (eukaryotic initiation factor 2)
eIF-2α kinase (haemin dependent)	Haemin	eIF-2
p34 kinase	Proteins encoded by the *wee* 1, *cdc* 25, *suc* 1 genes and cyclins	RNA polymerase II Histone H1
MAP kinase	MAP (microtubule-associated protein) kinases	S6 kinase II
Ribosomal S6 kinase	Other protein kinases	40S ribosomal subunit (S6)
Pyruvate dehydrogenase kinase	Acetyl-CoA, NADH, pyruvate, ADP	Pyruvate dehydrogenase complex
Branched chain α-ketoacid dehydrogenase kinase	Not known	Branched chain α-ketoacid dehydrogenase
Polyamine-dependent protein kinase	Polyamines	Not known
Casein kinases 1 and 2	Not known	Casein, glycogen synthetase
Casein kinase 2 (glycogen synthetase kinase 5)	Not known	Initiation factors
Glycogen synthetase kinases 3 and 4	Not known	Glycogen synthetase
Rhodopsin kinase	Light	Rhodopsin
β-Adrenergic receptor kinase	Not known	β-Adrenergic receptor
AMP-activated kinase	AMP	Acetyl-CoA carboxylase

kinase phosphorylates serine residues in these consensus sequences. Since there are between 25 and 50 copies of the consensus sequence, depending on the species from which the RNA polymerase II is derived, phosphorylation of RNA polymerase II alters its molecular weight.

The activity of p34 kinase is regulated by a complex mechanism which involves the phosphorylation and dephosphorylation of the kinase. These events are part of a cycle in which the p34 kinase exists either as a monomer or as a complex with cyclin. The probable sequence of events for activation of the kinase is as follows.

p34 kinase is prepared for activation by its combination with cyclin. This allows phosphorylation of the p34 kinase first on tyrosine 15 then on threonine 167. These reactions are catalysed by a specific protein–tyrosine kinase and a specific protein–threonine kinase. The p34 kinase becomes active when the cyclin is also phosphorylated and the phosphate moiety on tyrosine 15 of the p34 kinase is removed by a phosphoprotein phosphatase. Inactivation of the p34 kinase is achieved by proteolytic degradation of the cyclin. This occurs very rapidly and is catalysed by a cyclin-specific protease. Removal of the cyclin is followed by dephosphorylation of the threonine 167 on the p34 kinase. In addition to the cyclins, a number of other proteins, including those encoded by the genes *wee* 1, *cdc* 25, and *suc* 1, regulate the phosphorylation and dephosphorylation of p34 kinase.

4.8   The protein–tyrosine kinases

4.8.1   *Classification and discovery of protein–tyrosine kinases*
The protein–tyrosine kinases can be divided into two groups, the receptor protein–tyrosine kinases located in the plasma membrane and the protein–tyrosine kinases without transmembrane regions and extracellular domains. These kinases play a central role in the control of cell growth. In comparison with the protein–serine and protein–threonine kinases, knowledge of the nature and function of the protein–tyrosine kinases is limited and may belie this important role. Not only is the number of different protein–tyrosine kinases large, but relatively little is known about the nature of the target proteins for these enzymes. Thus the division of the protein–tyrosine kinases into two groups is probably an over simplification of a much more complex situation.

The existence of protein–tyrosine kinases was discovered as a result of investigation of the properties of the proteins encoded by the genome of the Rous sarcoma virus. This retrovirus induces solid tumours in chickens and animals. Antisera from rabbits possessing tumours induced by the Rous sarcoma virus was used to precipitate proteins present in extracts of cultured cells transformed by this virus, and also to precipitate the proteins present in cell-free translation products of Rous sarcoma viral RNA. The major protein present in these immunoprecipitates was called polyoma middle T antigen.

Polyoma middle T antigen was found to phosphorylate immunoglobulin heavy chains in the presence of ATP and Mg^{2+} (Collett and Erikson 1978; Levinson *et al.* 1978). Surprisingly, tyrosine rather than serine or threonine residues were phosphorylated (Eckart *et al.* 1979). It was subsequently shown that this protein–tyrosine kinase activity is an intrinsic property of the v-*src* protein (Hunter and Sefton 1980; Collett *et al.* 1980). Since these initial investigations of the *src* protein–tyrosine kinase, a number of different protein–tyrosine kinase enzymes have been discovered. Some of these were initially detected as the products of other retroviral oncogenes while others were found as components of plasma-membrane receptors.

The total protein–tyrosine kinase activity present in a given cell is very much smaller than the total amount of activity of protein–serine and protein–threonine kinases. Elucidation of the function of the protein–tyrosine kinases has been greatly facilitated by the isolation of cDNA molecules which encode the various kinases. This has enabled deduction of the amino-acid sequences from the cDNA base-sequence and the synthesis of relatively large amounts of enzyme by the cloning and expression in bacteria of DNA which encodes the protein kinase.

4.8.2   *The receptor protein–tyrosine kinases*

As described in Chapter 3, the protein–tyrosine catalytic site of the receptor protein–tyrosine kinases is located on the cytoplasmic domain of the receptor protein. The members of this family of protein–tyrosine kinases are listed in Table 4.9. The receptors for unidentified growth factors encoded by the c-*erb*-B-2, c-*kit*, c-*met*,

Table 4.9   *Members of the family of receptor protein–tyrosine kinases*

Receptor
Epidermal growth factor and transforming growth factor-α receptor (the c-*erb*-B protein)
Platelet-derived growth factor receptor
Insulin receptor
Colony-stimulating factor 1 receptor (the c-*fms* protein)
Insulin-like growth factor 1 receptor
Protein encoded by the *sevenless* gene of *Drosophila*
c-*erb*-B-2 protein (receptor similar to the EGF receptor)
c-*kit* protein (receptor for mast cell growth factor)
c-*met* protein (receptor for hepatocyte growth factor)
c-*eph* protein (receptor for unidentified growth factor)
c-*neu* protein (receptor for unidentified growth factor)
c-*trk* protein (receptor for unidentified growth factor)
c-*sea* protein (receptor for unidentified growth factor)
c-*ret* protein (receptor for unidentified growth factor)

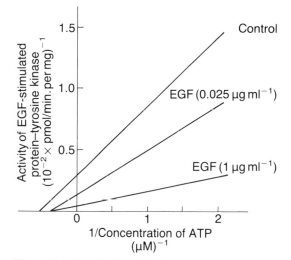

Fig. 4.17   The binding of EGF to the purified EGF receptor leads to an increase in the maximum activity of the receptor protein–tyrosine kinase (intercept on the ordinate) with little change in the apparent K_M for ATP (intercept on the abscissa). From Erneux *et al.* (1983).

and c-*eph* genes were discovered as their oncogenic forms. The properties of the oncogenic forms of a number of these receptor protein–tyrosine kinases are described in Chapter 11.

The protein–tyrosine kinase on the cytoplasmic domain of a plasma-membrane receptor is activated by the binding of the growth factor or hormone to that receptor. In the case of the purified EGF receptor, this leads to an increase in the maximum catalytic activity of the kinase with little change in the apparent K_M of the enzyme for its substrates (Fig. 4.17). A possible mechanism by which hormones and growth factors activate receptor protein–tyrosine kinases in the plasma membranes of cells is described in Chapter 3. This mechanism involves association of the receptors.

The activities of the receptor protein–tyrosine kinases are also regulated by autophosphorylation. As described in Chapter 3, a number of tyrosine residues in the epidermal growth factor and insulin receptor kinase proteins are autophosphorylated. One of these tyrosine residues

Table 4.10. *Substrates for protein–tyrosine kinases*

Protein–tyrosine kinase	Substrate
Receptor protein–tyrosine kinases	*Signal transduction enzymes*
	Phosphatidylinositol-3 kinase
	PtdIns 4,5-P_2-specific phospholipase Cγ
	ras GTP-ase-activating protein
	raf protein–serine (threonine) kinase
	Cytoskeletal proteins and enzymes
	Lipocortin
	Fodrin (β)
	Microtubule-associated protein 2
	Band 3 protein (erythrocytes)
	36 kDa protein
	Tubulin (α)
	Other enzymes
	Glycolytic enzymes
	Ribosomal S6 kinase
Protein–tyrosine kinases without transmembrane regions and extracellular domains	*Signal transduction enzymes*
	Phosphatidylinositol-3 kinase
	PtdIns 4,5-P_2-specific phospholipase Cγ
	ras GTP-ase-activating protein
	raf protein–serine (threonine) kinase
	Cytoskeletal proteins and enzymes
	Vinculin
	Fodrin (2)
	Tubulin
	Band 3 protein (erythrocytes)
	Other proteins and enzymes
	36 kDA protein
	50 kDa protein
	Insulin receptor kinase
	Glycolytic enzymes

in each protein–tyrosine kinase is located near the carboxy terminus and acts as an allosteric regulator of the activity of the kinase. The importance of this control site is emphasized by the consequences which follow its removal. This occurs in the formation of certain oncogenic protein–tyrosine kinases and is described in Chapter 11.

The activity of each of the protein–tyrosine kinases is probably also regulated by phosphorylation at sites other than the autophosphorylation sites. For example certain threonine residues in these proteins are phosphorylated by protein kinase C. Phosphorylation at tyrosine and threonine residues regulates both the activity of the protein–tyrosine kinase and also the rate of endocytosis of the receptor.

Experiments conducted with purified receptors and intact cells have identified a number of proteins phosphorylated by receptor protein–tyrosine kinases (Table 4.10). A number of these phosphoproteins are enzymes involved in signal transduction or proteins which regulate the structure of the cytoskeleton and the interaction of the cytoskeleton with the plasma membrane. It has so far been difficult to obtain conclusive evidence which indicates that the phosphorylation of these putative target proteins is a necessary part of the intracellular mechanism by which responses are induced by growth factors which bind to receptor protein–tyrosine kinases. Attempts to provide this evidence have so far focused on analysis of the effects of antibodies which inhibit receptor–activated protein tyrosine kinase activity, or of mutations at the ATP-binding site which also inhibit the protein–tyrosine kinase activity.

Roth and his colleagues showed that the introduction by microinjection of an antibody, which inhibits the insulin receptor protein–tyrosine kinase activity, into *Xenopus laevis* oocytes, inhibits the ability of insulin to stimulate oocyte maturation (Morgan *et al.* 1986). Ullrich and Rosen and their colleagues have transfected mutant insulin-receptor tyrosine kinase proteins into Chinese hamster ovary cells (Chou *et al.* 1987). Wild-type Chinese hamster ovary cells express relatively few insulin receptors. The actions of normal insulin receptors were compared with those of receptors in which lys 1018 was substituted with ala by site-directed mutage-

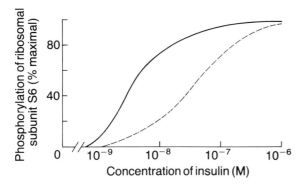

Fig. 4.18 A mutation in the tyrosine kinase domain of the human insulin receptor, in which lysine in position 1018 is replaced by alanine, almost completely inhibits insulin-stimulated protein–tyrosine kinase activity. When this mutant receptor is inserted into the plasma membrane of an intact cell, the sensitivity of ribosomal S6 kinase to activation by insulin is greatly decreased (broken curve) in comparison with cells in which wild-type receptor (full curve) has been inserted. Genes for the normal and mutated human-insulin receptor were introduced into Chinese hamster ovary cells. From Chou *et al.* (1987).

nesis. Although the mutated receptors bind insulin in a normal manner, they have a very low affinity for ATP and hence have a greatly diminished protein–tyrosine kinase activity.

Cells transfected with mutant insulin receptors were found to be far less sensitive to insulin when the ability of the hormone to activate glucose uptake, ribosomal S6 kinase, phosphorylation of the insulin receptor, glycogen synthesis, or thymidine incorporation into DNA was measured. The ability of insulin to activate ribosomal S6 kinase in cells transfected with mutant and wild-type receptors is shown in Fig. 4.18. It has been concluded from these and other similar experiments that activation of the protein–tyrosine kinase is a necessary step in the process by which agonists which bind to plasma-membrane receptors with a cytoplasmic protein–tyrosine kinase domain exert their intracellular effects.

One of the most puzzling aspects of the action of plasma-membrane receptor protein–tyrosine

kinases is the apparent failure to detect many target enzymes or proteins phosphorylated on tyrosine residues in intact cells. Investigation of [^{32}P]-labelled proteins in cells in which protein–tyrosine kinases are activated reveals changes in the phosphorylation of a number of proteins. However, only a few of these changes occur at tyrosine residues.

A further difficulty in explaining the intracellular actions of receptor protein–tyrosine kinase enzymes is the localization of the protein–tyrosine kinase activity at the plasma membrane. This would be expected to prevent the direct interaction of the protein–tyrosine kinase with those target enzymes located within the cytoplasmic space and spatially separated from the plasma membrane. These considerations have led to the idea that receptor protein–tyrosine kinases affect cell function, at least in part, by regulating the activity of a series of protein–serine and protein–threonine kinases, such as ribosomal S6 kinase, which can move within the cytoplasmic compartment (Fig. 4.19).

The receptor protein–tyrosine kinases may also exert their actions by recruiting a series of other signal-transducing enzymes. These include phosphatidylinositol-3 kinase, PtdIns 4,5 P$_2$-specific phospholipase C$_{\gamma-1}$, *ras* GTP-ase-activating protein, and the *raf* protein–serine (threonine) kinase. These are all substrates for a number of receptor protein–tyrosine kinases such as the PDGF receptor kinase. Activation and autophosphorylation of the receptor protein–tyrosine kinase may lead to the interaction of one or more of the signal-transducing enzymes with the protein–tyrosine kinase cytoplasmic domain of the receptor, phosphorylation of the target-signalling enzyme, and generation of an intracellular signal. Association of the signal–transducing enzyme with the receptor protein–tyrosine kinase is aided by the presence of domains in the signalling enzyme called the *src* homology-2 (SH-2) domains. These probably

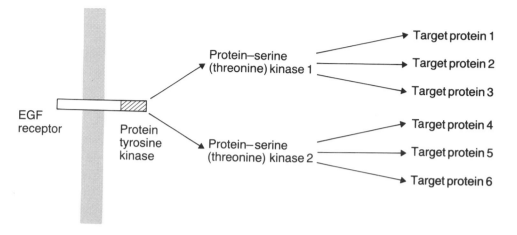

Fig. 4.19 Plasma-membrane receptor protein–tyrosine kinases, such as the EGF receptor kinase, are thought to affect intracellular target proteins by phosphorylating one or more intermediary protein–serine or protein–threonine kinases which, in turn, phosphorylate given target proteins.

form a tight association with the autophosphorylation site on the receptor protein–tyrosine kinase.

4.8.3 *Protein–tyrosine kinases without transmembrane regions and extracellular domains*

There are at least 7 protein–tyrosine kinases which do not possess a transmembrane region and an extracellular domain (Table 4.11). A number of these are members of the *src* family. Many of the protein–tyrosine kinases without transmembrane regions and extracellular domains were initially identified as the products of oncogenes. The properties of these oncogenes and the oncogenic proteins which they encode are described in Chapter 11. Most of the protein–tyrosine kinases without transmembrane regions and extracellular domains are located on the cytoplasmic side of the plasma membrane, but some are found elsewhere in the cytoplasmic space (Table 4.11).

As described earlier, the v-*src* protein–tyrosine kinase was the first protein–tyrosine kinase discovered. The c-*src* protein, the normal counterpart of the v-*src* protein, has a molecular weight of 60 kDa and is composed of 526 amino acids. These include extensive sequences of hydrophobic residues. The mature protein encoded by the c-*src* gene is phosphorylated (Fig. 4.7) and is located on the cytoplasmic face of the plasma membrane. The c-*src* protein consists of three domains, the tyrosine kinase domain, the membrane-binding domain, and a modulatory domain. The tyrosine kinase domain is homologous with the catalytic domains of many other protein–tyrosine kinases and is located in the carboxy half of the molecule.

The membrane-binding domain is small and is composed of amino acids 2 to 14 at the amino terminus. Myristic acid is attached to the amino-terminal glycine residue through a covalent linkage. This fatty acid, together with the hydrophobic amino-acid sequences of the membrane-binding domain, is responsible for attachment of the c-*src* protein to the plasma membrane. Evidence that myristic acid plays an important role in the cellular actions of c-*src* comes from the observation that removal of the fatty-acid moiety from the v-*src* protein destroys the ability of the v-*src* protein to transform cultured cells *in vitro*.

Table 4.11 *Members of the family of protein–tyrosine kinases without transmembrane regions and extracellular domains*

Intracellular location of kinase	Gene encoding kinase
Cytoplasmic side of plasma membrane	c-*src*
	c-*yes*
	c-*lck*
	c-*fgr*
	c-*abl*
	c-*ros*
Internal region of the cytoplasmic space	c-*fps* (c-*fes*)

The modulatory domain lies between the tyrosine kinase and membrane-binding domains. The presence of the modulatory domain has been deduced from studies of the effects of the mutation of amino acids in this domain. Changes in the modulatory domain alter the intrinsic activity of the protein–tyrosine kinase and, in intact cells, alter the phenotypic properties of the cell. The *src* kinase and other protein tyrosine kinases without transmembrane regions and extracellular domains also possess a regulatory autophosphorylation site on a tyrosine residue near the carboxy terminus.

A number of substrates for the c-*src* protein–tyrosine kinase, and for the other protein–tyrosine kinases without transmembrane regions and extracellular domains, have been identified (Table 4.10). The nature of the two or three amino-acid residues which precede the phosphorylated tyrosine residue determines the specific tyrosine, and hence the target protein, which is phosphorylated by the c-*src* kinase. The c-*src* kinase itself can be phosphorylated at ser 17 and tyr 416. As described in Chapter 11, autophosphorylation at tyr 416 probably regulates the catalytic activity of the c-*src* kinase.

The results of experiments conducted by some investigators have been interpreted as indicating that some oncogene protein–tyrosine kinases, including the v-*src* kinase, catalyse the ATP-dependent phosphorylation of phosphatidylinositol and phosphatidylinositol-4-phosphate as well as the phosphorylation of protein substrates. However, subsequent investigation has indicated that the observed phosphorylation of the phosphoinositides by preparations of certain protein–tyrosine kinases is probably due to a very tight association between the protein–tyrosine kinase and a phosphoinositide kinase. Phosphoinositides are not presently considered to be intracellular substrates for the protein–tyrosine kinases.

What signals activate the protein–tyrosine kinases without transmembrane regions and extracellular domains? An answer to this question has been obtained for one member of the *src* family, the *lck* protein–tyrosine kinase. The *lck* protein–tyrosine kinase has so far been found only in T lymphocytes. It is bound to the cytoplasmic face of the lymphocyte plasma membrane and is closely associated with the surface glycoproteins CD4 and CD8. These glycoproteins are involved in the control of T-cell activation by antigens. Interaction of the *lck* protein–tyrosine kinase with the plasma membrane is aided by the presence of a myristic-acid group on gly 2 of the *lck* polypeptide chain.

Each of the CD4 and CD8 glycoproteins is a single polypeptide chain which spans the plasma membrane. Folding of the polypeptide chain leads to a large extracellular domain, a transmembrane segment, and a short cytoplasmic domain or tail. The cytoplasmic tail probably interacts with a region of the *lck* protein–tyrosine kinase.

The combination of an antigen with either CD4 or CD8 leads to activation of the associated *lck* protein–tyrosine kinase, the phosphorylation of a tyrosine residue on the *lck* protein itself, and the phosphorylation of tyrosine residues on other cellular proteins. One of these is the zeta subunit of a protein called the T-cell receptor.

Other members of the *src* family of protein–tyrosine kinases, and possibly other protein–tyrosine kinases without transmembrane regions and extracellular domains, may be activated by interaction of the protein–tyrosine kinase with the cytoplasmic tail of an unknown plasma-membrane receptor in a manner similar to the activation of the *lck* protein–tyrosine kinase.

4.9   The phosphoprotein-serine (threonine) phosphatases

4.9.1   *The family of phosphoprotein–serine (threonine) phosphatases*

There are two main families of phosphoprotein phosphatases. These are the phosphoprotein–serine (threonine) phosphatases which hydrolyse phosphate moieties on serine or threonine residues and the phosphoprotein–tyrosine phosphatases which hydrolyse phosphate moieties on tyrosine residues. A feature of most of the phosphoprotein phosphatases, which is not shared by the protein kinases, is the apparent absence of specific signals, such as intracellular messengers, which activate these enzymes. Although there are some exceptions, most phosphoprotein phosphatases appear to respond to an increase in the concentration of their substrates, that is, specific phosphoproteins.

The properties of the phosphoprotein phosphatases have not been characterized as extensively as those of the protein kinases. This is partly because the phosphoprotein phosphatases have received less attention and partly because studies of this group of enzymes have proved more difficult.

Analysis of purified preparations of many phosphoprotein–serine (threonine) phosphatases indicates that the enzymes are present in multiple molecular forms. A number of different

investigators have isolated the same phospho-protein–serine (threonine) phosphatase enzyme using different substrates for the assay of enzyme activity. Consequently, a variety of different names has been given to each of the major phosphoprotein–serine (threonine) phosphatases (Table 4.12). The detection of multiple forms of these enzymes may be due, in part, to proteolytic degradation of the phosphoprotein phosphatases during their isolation, since a number of phosphoprotein–serine (threonine) phosphatases are susceptible to proteolysis during extraction and purification.

In 1943, Cori and Green (Cori and Green 1943) described the enzyme glycogen phosphorylase *a* phosphatase which was the first phosphoprotein phosphatase discovered. Subsequently, knowledge of the phosphoprotein-serine (threonine) phosphatases, like that of the protein kinases, evolved from studies of the role of phosphoprotein phosphatases in the regulation of glycogen metabolism.

In 1983, Cohen and Ingebritsen (Ingebritsen and Cohen 1983) proposed that most species of phosphoprotein–serine and phosphoprotein–threonine phosphatases identified at that time could be accounted for by the existence of four different principal catalytic subunits with broad and overlapping substrate specificities. These are phosphoprotein phosphatases 1, 2A, 2B, and 2C, designated PP-1, PP-2A, PP-2B, and PP-2C (Table 4.12).

The subdivision of the phosphoprotein–serine (threonine) phosphatases into types I and II was made on the basis of the ability of the enzymes to dephosphorylate subunits of glycogen phosphorylase kinase and their susceptibility to inhibition by two low molecular weight heat- and acid-stable molecules called inhibitor 1 and inhibitor 2. Type 1 phosphoprotein phosphatase (PP-1) preferentially dephosphorylates the β subunit of phosphorylase kinase and is inhibited by inhibitors 1 and 2. Type 2 phosphoprotein phosphatases (PP-2A, PP-2B, and PP-2C) preferentially dephosphorylate the α subunit of phosphorylase kinase and are insensitive to the actions of inhibitors 1 and 2. PP-1, PP-2A, and PP-2B are members of the same gene family whereas PP-2C belongs to a different gene family.

The type 2 phosphoprotein phosphatases have been sub-classified on the basis of their depen-

Table 4.12 *The phosphoprotein–serine (threonine) phosphatases*

Enzyme	Alternative names
Phosphoprotein phosphatase 1 (PP-1)	ATP, Mg-dependent phosphoprotein phosphatase Phosphatase HI and CI
Phosphoprotein phosphatase 2A (PP-2A)	Polycation-stimulated phosphoprotein phosphatase Phosphatase 3 Phosphatase HII and CII
Phosphoprotein phosphatase 2B (PP-2B)	CaM-BP$_{80}$ Calcineurin
Phosphoprotein phosphatase 2C (PP-2C)	Mg^{2+}-dependent phosphoprotein phosphatase Phosphatase 4

dence on divalent cations, activation by calmodulin, and inhibition by okadaic acid, a polyether derivative of a 38-carbon fatty acid. Okadaic acid is a potent tumour promoter which is found in the brown sponge. Unlike the phorbol-ester tumour promoters, it does not activate protein kinase C. Okadaic acid is probably the agent present in those shellfish which cause diarrhetic poisoning in humans. PP-2B and PP-2C each have an absolute requirement for Ca^{2+} and Mg^{2+} whereas PP-2A is active in the absence of these cations. PP-2B is activated by calmodulin. Okadaic acid inhibits PP-2A and PP-2B but not PP-2C.

PP-1, PP-2A, and PP-2C hydrolyse phosphate groups from seryl and threonyl residues and

have a broad substrate specificity. These three phosphatases have been isolated principally from skeletal and heart muscle, and from liver. PP-2B, which hydrolyses phosphorylated tyrosyl residues as well as phosphorylated seryl and threonyl residues, has a narrow substrate specificity. This enzyme is found in large quantities in brain tissue and in smaller quantities in heart muscle, and in liver and many other tissues. Although the isolated PP-2B enzyme can hydrolyse phosphorylated tyrosine residues in purified substrates, it probably only hydrolyses phosphorylated serine or threonine residues under physiological conditions.

4.9.2 *Phosphoprotein phosphatase 1*

Most of the PP-1 present in a given cell is associated with intracellular structures. In skeletal muscle these include glycogen granules, the sarcoplasmic reticulum, and myofibrils. In nerve cells the enzyme associates with post-synaptic densities, and in a number of other types of cell with ribosomes and nuclei. Different forms of PP-1 are associated with glycogen granules (PP-1G), the sarcoplasmic reticulum (PP-1SR), myofibrils (PP-1M), and possibly with other intracellular structures. Each of these forms is a heterodimer composed of a catalytic subunit and a regulatory subunit. The catalytic subunits of each form are identical and have a molecular weight of 37 kDa. The regulatory subunits, which are thought to direct PP-1 to a given target structure, are different. In addition to the bound forms, a soluble form of PP-1 is also present in cells. This form, designated PP-1I, is inactive. As described below, it consists of the PP-1 catalytic subunit and inhibitor protein 2.

The regulatory subunit of the form of PP-1 which binds to glycogen in skeletal muscle, PP-1G, can be phosphorylated by cyclic AMP-dependent protein kinase. This causes the translocation of the catalytic subunit of PP-1G from glycogen granules to the cytoplasmic space, resulting in an inhibition of the dephosphorylation of enzymes involved in glycogen metabolism.

PP-1 has a broad substrate specificity. The substrates include glycogen phosphorylase *a*, the β subunit of glycogen phosphorylase kinase, acetyl-CoA carboxylase, the α subunit of eukaryotic initiation factor 2 (eIF-2), troponin I, hydroxymethylglutaryl (HMG)-CoA reductase, HMG-CoA reductase kinase, and a number of unidentified substrates.

4.9.3 *Inhibition of phosphoprotein phosphatase 1 by heat-stable proteins*

Inhibitor proteins 1 and 2 were discovered by Huang and Glinsman in 1976. Inhibitor protein 2 has also been called modulator protein. These two proteins, which are distributed in a wide variety of tissues, interact with PP-1 but not with other phosphoprotein phosphatases. The inhibitor proteins retain biological activity after being heated at 100°C, precipitated with trichloracetic acid, or treated with sodium dodecyl sulphate. Determination of the complete amino-acid sequences of inhibitor proteins 1 and 2 has shown that these proteins contain no cysteine residues and are very hydrophobic.

Although inhibitors 1 and 2 have interesting chemical properties which suggest that they play an important role in regulation of the activity of PP-1, the biological function of these inhibitors is not yet clear. Inhibitor 1 is phosphorylated by cyclic AMP-dependent protein kinase. The phosphorylated form of the inhibitor protein binds to PP-1 and inactivates it (Fig. 4.20). This may provide a mechanism by which the activity of PP-1 is controlled by cyclic AMP.

The complex formed between PP-1 and inhibitor 2 is the inhibited form of PP-1 (PP-1I) found in the soluble fraction of cells. The interaction of inhibitor 2 with PP-1 depends on the state of phosphorylation of the inhibitor protein. The form of inhibitor 2 which binds to PP-1 has no

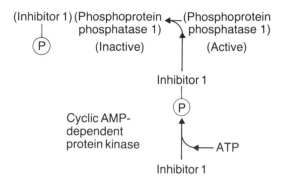

Fig. 4.20 Phosphoprotein phosphatase 1 (PP-1) is inhibited by the phosphorylated form of inhibitor 1, a heat-stable protein. The phosphorylation of inhibitor 1 is catalysed by cyclic AMP-dependent protein kinase.

covalently bound phosphate moieties. Phosphorylation of inhibitor 2 causes dissociation of the inhibitor–phosphatase complex and liberation of the active species of the phosphatase.

4.9.4 *Phosphoprotein phosphatases 2A, 2B, and 2C*

PP-2A is composed of three subunits, one of which is a catalytic unit of molecular weight 36 kDa. Two isoforms of the catalytic subunit have been detected. Each of these shares considerable homology with the catalytic subunit of PP-1. There are a number of different oligomeric forms of PP-2A, each containing one of the two isoforms of the catalytic unit. In contrast to the oligomeric structure of PP-2A, PP-2C is a monomer with a molecular weight of 43 kDa. Two isoforms of this monomer have been detected.

PP-2A and PP-2C have broad substrate specificities which are similar for each enzyme and similar to the substrate specificity for PP-1. Phosphoproteins dephosphorylated by PP-2A and PP-2C include enzymes involved in the regulation of glycogen metabolism, glycolysis and gluconeogenesis, muscle contraction, protein synthesis, cholesterol synthesis, fatty-acid synthesis, aromatic amino-acid degradation, and the degradation of proteins of the cytoskeleton.

As indicated by one of the alternative names for PP-2A, polycation-stimulated phosphoprotein phosphatase (Table 4.12), this phosphoprotein phosphatase is activated by certain cations. These include histone H1, protamine, and polylysine. The activation by these molecules probably reflects the intrinsic properties of the PP-2A protein rather than a regulatory function of the cations. PP-2B is distinguished from the other phosphoprotein–serine and –threonine phosphatases by its interaction with the (Ca^{2+} + calmodulin) complex. PP-2B is a heterodimer composed of subunits designated A and B. These have molecular weights of 61 and 19 kDa, respectively. Subunit A contains the catalytic site and a binding site for calmodulin while subunit B contains a Ca^{2+} binding site.

The substrates for PP-2B are proteins which regulate the activities of protein kinases and other phosphoprotein phosphatases. These include inhibitor 1, regulatory subunit II of cyclic AMP-dependent protein kinase, the α subunit of glycogen phosphorylase kinase, and calmodulin-dependent cyclic-AMP phosphodiesterase. In some cell types, PP-2B may be part of a mechanism by which increases in intracellular free Ca^{2+} inhibit the actions of cyclic AMP.

4.10 The phosphoprotein–tyrosine phosphatases

A large number of different phosphoprotein–tyrosine phosphatases have been detected in animal tissues. For example, seven enzymes have been found in brain. These probably represent different isoenzymes rather than the combination of a common catalytic unit with different regulatory units, or the proteolytic modification of a single type of catalytic unit. The phosphoprotein–tyrosine phosphatases and phosphoprotein–serine (threonine) phosphatases

(described above) are quite clearly different proteins.

The phosphoprotein–tyrosine phosphatases include four enzymes which contain a membrane-spanning region and which are probably plasma-membrane receptors, and two enzymes which do not contain a membrane-spanning region and are probably located in the cytoplasmic space. The receptor phosphoprotein–tyrosine phosphatases are called CD45 (a human leucocyte surface protein called leucocyte common antigen), LAR (leucocyte common antigen related protein), DPTP (a phosphoprotein–tyrosine phosphatase from *Drosophila melanogaster*), and DLAR (LAR from *Drosophila*). The cytoplasmic phosphoprotein–tyrosine phosphatases are phosphoprotein–tyrosine phosphatase 1B, which was first isolated from human placenta, and T-cell phosphoprotein–tyrosine phosphatase which was first isolated from human T cells.

The amino-acid sequence of phosphoprotein–tyrosine phosphatase 1B was determined by Charbonneau *et al.* in 1988. Comparison of this amino-acid sequence with the amino-acid sequence of protein CD45, which was not then known to be a phosphoprotein–tyrosine phosphatase, suggested that the CD45 protein may contain a phosphoprotein–tyrosine phosphatase catalytic site. This was subsequently confirmed by expression of the DNA encoding the suspected catalytic site of CD45 in a non-mammalian cell.

Cytoplasmic phosphoprotein–tyrosine phosphatase 1B has a molecular weight of 35 kDa. Like T-cell phosphoprotein–tyrosine phosphatase, which is of a similar size, phosphoprotein–tyrosine phosphatase 1B has a very high intrinsic catalytic activity. Although little is known about the substrates for the cytoplasmic phosphoprotein–tyrosine phosphatases, it is probable that these enzymes dephosphorylate phosphotyrosine residues in proteins following the phosphorylation of these residues by protein–tyrosine kinases. An experimental reflection of this action of phosphoprotein–tyrosine phosphatase 1B is the delay in the ability of insulin to induce the maturation of *Xenopus* oocytes when pure phosphoprotein–tyrosine phosphatase 1B has been introduced into the oocytes by microinjection.

The receptor phosphoprotein–tyrosine phosphatases each consist of a large amino-terminal extracellular domain, a single membrane-spanning region, and a large carboxy-terminal cytoplasmic domain. The extracellular domain is *O*- and *N*-glycosylated, and contains a number of cysteine residues. The cytoplasmic domain contains a tandem repeat of the phosphoprotein–tyrosine phosphatase catalytic site. This contrasts with the cytoplasmic phosphoprotein–tyrosine phosphatases which contain only one copy of this catalytic site.

The catalytic activity of the receptor phosphoprotein–tyrosine phosphatase may be controlled by the binding of an agonist or ligand to the extracellular domain. In the case of LAR this may be part of the system by which molecules on the surface of one cell transmit information to the surface of an adjacent cell through cell–cell contact. A large portion of the extracellular domain of LAR is homologous with amino-acid sequences of neural cell-adhesion molecules (N-CAMs). CD45 may play a role in the normal response of leucocytes to antigens through the dephosphorylation of the *lck* protein–tyrosine kinase and the cytoskeletal protein, fodrin.

4.11 Summary

The protein kinases catalyse the phosphorylation of target proteins using ATP as the phosphate donor. The resulting change in conformation of the phosphorylated target protein leads to a change in the catalytic activity or in the regulation of the activity of the phosphoprotein. The process of phosphorylation is reversed by the action of a phosphoprotein phosphatase. Protein kinases catalyse the phosphorylation of serine or threonine residues (protein–serine or protein–threonine kinases), or tyrosine residues (protein–tyrosine kinases).

The major multi-substrate protein–serine and –threonine kinases are the cyclic nucleotide-dependent protein kinases, the (Ca^{2+} + calmodulin)-dependent protein kinases, and the protein kinases C. There are multiple forms of each of these kinases. The different forms of each of these protein kinases may play a role in the delivery of extracellular signals to subsets of proteins within the cell. The protein–tyrosine kinases can be divided into two groups: receptor protein–tyrosine kinases and protein–tyrosine kinases without transmembrane regions and extracellular domains.

Activation of the cyclic nucleotide and (Ca^{2+} + calmodulin)-dependent protein kinases involves diffusion of the cyclic nucleotide or Ca^{2+} from the site of formation or release to the site at which the protein kinase is located. The active protein kinase is then available to phosphorylate target proteins in that region of the cytoplasmic space. The activation of protein kinase C takes place at the plasma membrane and requires increases in both the concentration of diacylglycerol in the membrane and Ca^{2+} in the cytoplasmic space. Activated protein kinase C may move through the cytoplasmic space to phosphorylate target proteins, or may phosphorylate intermediary kinases which, in turn, phosphorylate the ultimate target proteins. The receptor protein–tyrosine kinases are activated by the binding of an agonist to the receptor in the plasma membrane. The active protein–tyrosine kinase may phosphorylate some target proteins directly and others through intermediary protein–serine or –threonine kinases.

Each protein kinase enzyme contains a catalytic and a regulatory domain. In addition to exerting control on the catalytic domain and providing a site with which mobile intracellular messengers, calmodulin, or extracellular agonists can interact, the regulatory domain contains information which specifies the intracellular location of the kinase. A number of the protein kinases have an oligomeric subunit structure. However, in all kinases except the cyclic AMP-dependent protein kinases, the catalytic and regulatory domains are on the same subunit.

The nature of the target proteins phosphorylated by a given protein kinase is determined chiefly by the number and location of basic amino-acid residues near the phosphorylated serine, threonine, or tyrosine residue on the polypeptide chain of the target protein. The cyclic nucleotide-dependent protein kinases, $(Ca^{2+}$ + calmodulin)-dependent kinase II, protein kinase C, the receptor protein–tyrosine kinases, and some other protein–tyrosine kinases have a broad substrate specificity. Other protein kinases such as $(Ca^{2+}$ + calmodulin)-dependent kinases I and III and a number of other protein–serine and –threonine kinases have a narrow substrate specificity.

Target proteins for protein–serine and –threonine kinases include enzymes which catalyse steps in pathways of intermediary metabolism and protein synthesis, and enzymes and proteins responsible for regulation of the structure of the cytoskeleton, receptor function, and the concentration of mobile intracellular messengers. Target proteins for protein–tyrosine kinases are predominantly enzymes and proteins involved in the regulation of the structure of the cytoskeleton. The nature of the target proteins varies from one cell type to another. Most protein kinases also undergo autophosphorylation in an intramolecular reaction. In some cases, autophosphorylation may play a role in regulation of the activity of the protein kinase.

The properties of the phosphoprotein phosphatases are less well defined than those of the protein kinases. The phosphoprotein phosphatase which have been isolated by different workers have been classified into groups on the basis of substrate specificity, susceptibility to inhibition by two low molecular weight heat-stable inhibitor proteins, and to activation or inhibition by divalent cations and brown-sponge tumour promoter, okadaic acid. The major phosphoprotein phosphatases are types 1, 2A, and 2C, which principally hydrolyse phosphorylated serine and threonine residues, type 2B which hydrolyses phosphorylated tyrosine residues as well as phosphorylated serine and threonine residues, and the protein–phosphotyrosine phosphatases. Phosphoprotein phosphatase 1 is bound to glycogen and other intracellular structures, has a broad substrate specificity and is inhibited by the low molecular-weight heat-stable inhibitor proteins, inhibitors 1 and 2. Phosphoprotein phosphatases 2A and 2C also have broad substrate specificities whereas type 2B, which is activated by $(Ca^{2+}$ + calmodulin), has a more restricted substrate specificity.

Studies of the protein kinases and phosphoprotein phosphatases conducted so far have provided a good understanding of the nature, mechanism of activation, and catalytic function of the protein kinases. Future research is likely to be directed towards studies of the mechanism of activation of the protein–tyrosine kinases, determination of a complete description of the nature and location of the physiological intracellular substrates for each protein kinase, especially the protein–tyrosine kinases, and elucidation of the nature of the phosphoprotein phosphatases and their mechanisms of action and regulation.

References

Castagna, M., Takai, Y., Kaibuchi, K., Sano, K., Kikkawa, U., and Nishizuka, Y. (1982). Direct activation of calcium-activated, phospholipid-dependent protein kinase by tumour-promoting phorbol esters. *J. Biol. Chem.*, **257**, 7847–51.

Charbonneau, H., Tonks, N. K., Walsh, D. A., and Fischer, E. H. (1988). The leukocyte common antigen (CD45): a putative receptor-linked protein tyrosine phosphatase. *Proc. Natl Acad. Sci. USA*, **85**, 7182–6.

Cheung, W. Y. (1970). Cyclic 3′,5′-nucleotide phosphodiesterase. Demonstration of an activator. *Biochem. Biophys. Res. Commun.*, **38**, 533–8.

Chou, C. K., Dull, T. J., Russell, D. S., Gherzi, R., Lebwohl, D., Ullrich, A., and Rosen, O. (1987). Human insulin receptors mutated at the ATP-binding site lack protein tyrosine kinase activity and fail to mediate post-receptor effects of insulin. *J. Biol. Chem.*, **262**, 1842–7.

Cohen, P. (1980). The role of calcium ions, calmodulin and troponin in the regulation of phosphorylase kinase from rabbit skeletal muscle. *Eur. J. Biochem.*, **111**, 563–74.

Cohen, P. (1982). The role of protein phosphorylation in neural and hormonal control of cellular activity. *Nature*, **296**, 613–20.

Collett, M. S. and Erikson, R. L. (1978). Protein kinase activity associated with the avian sarcoma virus *src* gene product. *Proc. Natl Acad. Sci. USA*, **75**, 2021–4.

Collett, M. S., Purchio, A. F., and Erikson, R. L. (1980). Avian sarcoma virus-transforming protein, pp60^{src} shows protein kinase activity specific for tyrosine. *Nature*, **285**, 167–9.

Corbin, J. D., Keely, S. L., and Park, C. R. (1975). The distribution and dissociation of cyclic adenosine 3′,5′-monophosphate-dependent protein kinases in adipose, cardiac, and other tissues. *J. Biol. Chem.*, **250**, 218–25.

Cori, G. T. and Green, A. A. (1943). Crystalline muscle phosphorylase. II Prosthetic group. *J. Biol. Chem.*, **151**, 31–8.

Davies, S. P., Sim, A. T. R., and Hardie, D. G. (1990). Location and function of three sites phosphorylated on rat acetyl-CoA carboxylase by the AMP-activated protein kinase. *Eur. J. Biochem.*, **187**, 183–90.

De Lorenzo, R. J. (1976). Calcium-dependent phosphorylation of specific synaptosomal fraction proteins: possible role of phosphoproteins in mediating neurotransmitter release. *Biochem. Biophys. Res. Commun.*, **71**, 590–7.

Eckhart, W., Hutchinson, M. A., and Hunter, T. (1979). An activity phosphorylating tyrosine in polyoma T antigen immunoprecipitates. *Cell*, **18**, 925–33.

Erneux, C., Cohen, S., and Garbers, D. L. (1983). The kinetics of tyrosine phosphorylation by the purified epidermal growth factor receptor kinase of A-431 cells. *J. Biol. Chem.*, **258**, 4137–42.

Fischer, E. H. and Krebs, E. G. (1955). Conversion of phosphorylase *b* to phosphorylase *a* in muscle extracts. *J. Biol. Chem.*, **216**, 121–32.

Hoffman, F. and Sold, G. (1972). A protein kinase activity from rat cerebellum stimulated by guanosine-3′,5′-monophosphate. *Biochem. Biophys. Res. Commun.*, **49**, 1100–7.

Huang, F. L. and Glinsman, W. H. (1976). Separation and characterization of two phosphorylase phosphatase inhibitors from rabbit skeletal muscle. *Eur. J. Biochem.*, **70**, 419–26.

Huijing, F. and Larner, J. (1966). On the mechanism of action of adenosine 3′,5′-cyclophosphate. *Proc. Natl Acad. Sci. USA*, **56**, 647–53.

Hunter, T. and Sefton, B. M. (1980). Transforming gene product of Rous sarcoma virus phosphorylates tyrosine. *Proc. Natl Acad. Sci. USA*, **77**, 1311–15.

Ingebritsen, T. S. and Cohen, P. (1983). The protein phosphatases involved in cellular regulation. 1. Classification and substrate specificities. *Eur. J. Biochem.*, **132**, 255–61.

Inoue, M., Kishimoto, A., Takai, Y., and Nishizuka, Y. (1977). Studies on a cyclic nucleotide-independent protein kinase and its proenzyme in mammalian tissues. *J. Biol. Chem.*, **252**, 7610–16.

Kikkawa, U., Takai, Y., Tanaka, Y., Miyake, R., and Nishizuka, Y. (1983). Protein kinase C as a possible receptor protein of tumour-promoting phorbol esters. *J. Biol. Chem.*, **258**, 11442–5.

Kishimoto, A., Takai, Y., Mori, T., Kikkawa, U., and Nishizuka, Y. (1980). Activation of calcium and phospholipid-dependent protein kinase by diacylglycerol, its possible relation to phosphatidylinositol turnover. *J. Biol. Chem.*, **255**, 2273–6.

Knopf, J. L., Lee, M-H., Sultzman, L. A., Kriz, R. W., Loomis, C. R., Hewick, R. M., and Bell, R. M. (1986). Cloning and expression of multiple protein kinase C cDNAs. *Cell*, **46**, 491–502.

Kuo, J. F. and Greengard, P. (1970). Cyclic nucleotide-dependent protein kinases. VI. Isolation and partial purification of a protein kinase activated by guanosine 3′,5′-monophosphate. *J. Biol. Chem.*, **245**, 2493–8.

Levinson, A. D., Oppermann, H., Levintow, L., Varmus, H. E., and Bishop, J. M. (1978). Evidence that the transforming gene of avian sarcoma virus encodes a protein kinase associated with a phosphoprotein. *Cell*, **15**, 561–72.

Makowske, M., Birnbaum, M. J., Ballester, R., and Rosen, O. M. (1986). A cDNA encoding protein kinase C identifies two species of mRNA in brain and GH$_3$ cells. *J. Biol. Chem.*, **261**, 13389–92.

Morgan, D. O., Ho, L., Korn, L. J., and Roth, R. A. (1986). Insulin action is blocked by a monoclonal antibody that inhibits the insulin receptor kinase. *Proc. Natl Acad. Sci. USA*, **83**, 328–32.

Niedel, J. E., Kuhn, L. J., and Vandenbark, G. R. (1983). Phorbol diester receptor copurifies with protein kinase C. *Proc. Natl Acad. Sci. USA*, **80**, 36–40.

Ono, Y., Kurokawa, T., Kawahara, K., Nishimura, O., Marumoto, R., Igarashi, K., *et al.* (1986). Cloning of rat brain protein kinase C complementary DNA. *FEBS Lett.*, **203**, 111–15.

Parker, P. J., Coussens, L., Totty, N., Rhee, L., Young, S., Chen, E., *et al.* (1986). The complete primary structure of protein kinase C—the major phorbol ester receptor. *Science*, **233**, 853–9.

Poulter, L., Ang, S.-G., Gibson, B. W., Williams, D. H., Holmes, C. F. B., Caudwell, F. B. *et al.* (1988). Analysis of the *in vivo* phosphorylation state of rabbit skeletal muscle glycogen synthase by fast-atom bombardment mass spectrometry. *Eur. J. Biochem.*, **175**, 497–510.

Rall, T. W., Sutherland, E. W., and Berthet, J. (1957). The relationship of epinephrine and glucagon to liver phosphorylase. IV Effect of epinephrine and glucogen on the reactivation of phosphorylase in liver homogenates. *J. Biol. Chem.*, **224**, 463–75.

Taylor, S. S. (1989). cAMP-dependent protein kinase: model for an enzyme family. *J. Biol. Chem.*, **264**, 8443–6.

Walsh, D. A., Perkins, J. P., and Krebs, E. G. (1968). An adenosine 3′,5′-monophosphate-dependent protein kinase from rabbit skeletal muscle. *J. Biol. Chem.*, **243**, 3763–5.

Further reading

Cohen, P. (1980). *Recently discovered systems of enzyme regulation by reversible phosphorylation.* Elsevier, Amsterdam.

Cohen, P. (1989). The structure and regulation of protein phosphatases. *Ann. Rev. Biochem.*, **58**, 453–508.

Cohen, P., Holmes, C. F. B., and Tsukitani, Y. (1990). Okadaic acid: a new probe for the study of cellular regulation. *Trends in Biochemical Sciences*, **15**, 98–102.

Freeman, R. S. and Donoghue, D. J. (1991). Protein kinases and protooncogenes: biochemical regulators of the eukaryotic cell cycle. *Biochemistry*, **30**, 2293–302.

Glass, D. B. and Krebs, E. G. (1980). Protein phosphorylation catalysed by cyclic AMP-dependent and cyclic GMP-dependent protein kinases. *Ann. Rev. Pharmacol. Toxicol.*, **20**, 363–88.

Hunter, T. (1989). Protein-tyrosine phosphatases: the other side of the coin. *Cell*, **58**, 1013–16.

Hunter, T. and Cooper, J. A. (1985). Protein–tyrosine kinases. *Ann. Rev. Biochem.*, **54**, 897–930.

Kikkawa, U., Kishimoto, A., and Nishizuka, Y. (1989). The protein kinase C family: heterogeneity and its implications. *Ann. Rev. Biochem.*, **58**, 31–44.

Krebs, E. G. and Beavo, J. A. (1979). Phosphorylation–dephosphorylation of enzymes. *Ann. Rev. Biochem.*, **48**, 923–59.

Krebs, E. G. (1983). Historical perspectives on protein phosphorylation and a classification system for protein kinases. *Phil. Trans. Roy. Soc. London*, **B 302**, 3–11.

Lau, K-H. W., Farley, J. R., and Baylink, D. J. (1989). Phosphotyrosyl protein phosphatases. *Biochem. J.*, **257**, 23–36.

Merlevede, W. (1985). Protein phosphates and the protein phosphatases. Landmarks in an eventful century. In *Advances in protein phosphatases* (ed. W. Merlevede and J. Di Salvo), Vol. 1, pp. 1–18. Leuven University Press, Belgium.

Soderling, T. R. (1990). Protein kinases. Regulation by autoinhibitory domains. *J. Biol. Chem.* **265**, 1823–6.

Taylor, S. S. (1987). Protein kinases: a diverse family of related proteins. *BioEssays*, **7**, 24–9.

Taylor, S. S., Buechler, J. A., and Yonemoto, W. (1990). cAMP-dependent protein kinase: framework for a diverse family of regulatory enzymes. *Ann. Rev. Biochem.*, **59**, 971–1005.

Weller, M. (1979). *Protein phosphorylation. The nature, function and metabolism of proteins which contain covalently bound phosphorus.* Pion Limited, London.

5 *The cyclic nucleotides*

5.1 Cyclic nucleotides as intracellular messengers in animal cells

Adenosine 3',5'-monophosphate (cyclic AMP) and guanosine 3',5'-monophosphate (cyclic GMP) (Fig. 5.1) have evolved as intracellular messengers in animal cells. The intracellular concentration of each of these cyclic nucleotides is controlled by the relative rates of synthesis, catalysed by adenylate or guanylate cyclase, and degradation, catalysed by cyclic nucleotide phosphodiesterases (Fig. 5.2). This is illustrated by the action of glucagon in the liver. Fig. 5.3 shows how the prolonged infusion of glucagon, which activates adenylate cyclase, induces an increase in cyclic AMP over a corresponding period of time. This is due to the greater activity of adenylate cyclase in relation to cyclic AMP phosphodiesterase in the presence of glucagon. An agonist can alter the intracellular concentration of cyclic AMP or cyclic GMP by increasing the rate of synthesis or changing the rate of degradation of the cyclic nucleotide.

Cyclic AMP acts as an intracellular messenger in almost all types of animal cell. Some of the major categories of response to cyclic AMP are shown in Table 5.1. In animal cells all the known actions of cyclic AMP except one are mediated through binding of the cyclic nucleotide to cyclic AMP-dependent protein kinases. This role is shown schematically in Fig. 5.4(a). The known exception is in the olfactory cell, in which cyclic

Table 5.1 *Examples of the role of cyclic AMP as an intracellular messenger*

Response	Cell	Agonist
Modulation of muscle contraction	Heart muscle	Adrenalin (β)
	Smooth muscle	Adrenalin (β)
		Acetylcholine (M)
Glucose synthesis and glycogenolysis	Liver, kidney, heart muscle	Glucagon (G_1)
		Adrenalin (β_1)
Secretion of hormones and proteins	Pancreatic β cell	Glucagon
		Glucose
		Acetylcholine
	Pancreatic acinar cell	Acetylcholine
	Adrenal medulla	Adrenalin (β)
Secretion of ions and fluid	Parotid gland	Adrenalin (β)
	Salivary gland	5-Hydroxytryptamine
	Kidney	Vasopressin
Mitogenesis	Fibroblasts	Growth factors
Shape change and secretion	Blood platelet	ADP

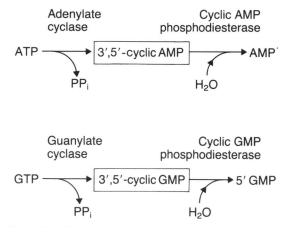

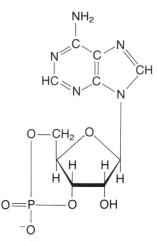

Adenosine 3′,5′-monophosphate (cyclic AMP)

Fig. 5.2 The reactions involved in the synthesis and degradation of cyclic AMP and cyclic GMP. The concentration of the cyclic nucleotide which is present in a given region of the cytoplasmic space at any given time is determined by the balance of the biosynthetic and degradative reactions.

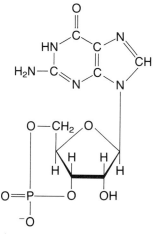

Guanosine 3′,5′-monophosphate (cyclic GMP)

Fig. 5.1 The two cyclic nucleotides with intracellular messenger function in animal cells, 3′,5′-cyclic adenosine monophosphate and 3′,5′-cyclic guanosine monophosphate.

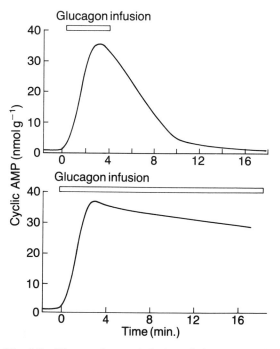

Fig. 5.3 The continuous infusion of glucagon to the perfused liver induces an increase in the concentration of cyclic AMP which is maintained while the concentration of the hormone is raised. The upper panel shows that switching off the glucagon infusion results in a decrease in the concentration of cyclic AMP. From Exton *et al.* (1971).

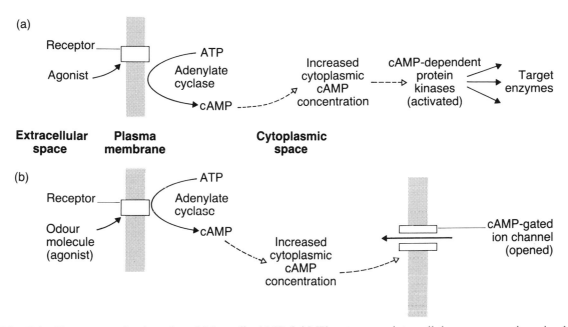

Fig. 5.4 The two mechanisms by which cyclic AMP (cAMP) acts as an intracellular messenger in animal cells. (a) Almost all effects of this cyclic nucleotide on target proteins are mediated by cyclic AMP-dependent protein kinases. (b) In olfactory cells, cyclic AMP activates a cyclic AMP-gated ion channel without the requirement for a protein kinase.

AMP binds to a cyclic AMP-gated cation channel and increases the movement of ions through the channel. This function is shown schematically in Fig. 5.4(b). This action of cyclic AMP does not involve a cyclic AMP-dependent protein kinase.

Cyclic GMP has been detected in most animal cells. In many of these the concentration of this cyclic nucleotide has been shown to increase in response to the action of an agonist. However, a clear role for cyclic GMP as an intracellular messenger has so far only been defined in a few cell types (Table 5.2)

There are two known mechanisms by which the intracellular actions of cyclic GMP are exerted. These are the activation of cyclic GMP-dependent protein kinase (Fig. 5.5(a)) and the binding of cyclic GMP to an allosteric site on an ion channel (Fig. 5.5(b)). Although many cells contain cyclic GMP-dependent protein kinase, a physiological function for this protein

kinase has so far only been clearly defined for the actions of atrial natriuretic peptide, sperm-activating peptides, and endothelium-derived relaxing factor (EDRF) which is probably nitric oxide or S-nitrosocysteine. The action of cyclic GMP in rod and cone cells of the retina involves the binding of the nucleotide to a stereospecific site on a cyclic GMP-gated cation channel. This alters the conformation of the protein and the rate of Na^+ transport as shown schematically in Fig. 5.5(b). This action of cyclic GMP does not require cyclic GMP-dependent protein kinase.

The cyclic nucleotides not only transfer information from the plasma membrane to intracellular sites but also amplify the initial signal received by the cell. In the pathway that has evolved for the function of cyclic AMP as an intracellular messenger, there are at least four catalytic steps at which the information conveyed by the extracellular agonist is amplified

Table 5.2 *Examples of the role of cyclic GMP as an intracellular messenger*

Response	Cell	Agonist
Light-induced nerve impulse	Rod and cone cells of the retina	Light
Excretion of Na$^+$ and water	Kidney	Atrial natriuretic peptide
Muscle relaxation	Smooth muscle	Atrial natriuretic peptide
Modification of function of spermatozoa	Spermatozoa	Speract and other sperm-activating peptides secreted by egg cells
Increased Ca^{2+} inflow	Nerve cells	5-Hydroxytryptamine
Muscle relaxation	Smooth muscle	Endothelial-derived relaxing factor (EDRF)

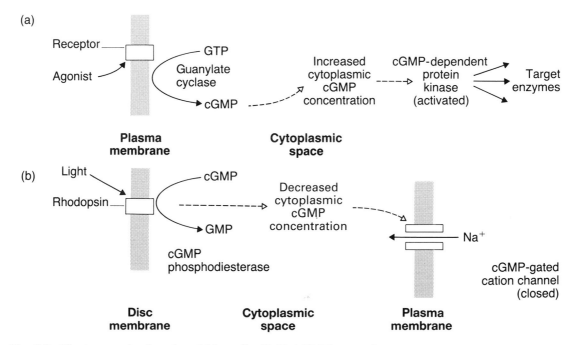

Fig. 5.5 The two mechanisms by which cyclic GMP (cGMP) exerts its action as an intracellular messenger in animal cells. (a) In some cell types agonist-receptor complexes activate guanylate cyclase and increase the concentration of cyclic GMP. The effects of increased cyclic GMP on target proteins are mediated by the activation of cyclic GMP-dependent protein kinase. A variation of this mechanism (not shown) is the activation of a cytoplasmic guanylate cyclase. (b) In photoreceptor cells, the interaction of light with rhodopsin activates cyclic GMP phosphodiesterase which leads to a decrease in the concentration of cyclic GMP and closure of a cation channel. In these cells cyclic GMP acts as an allosteric activator of a cyclic GMP-gated cation channel.

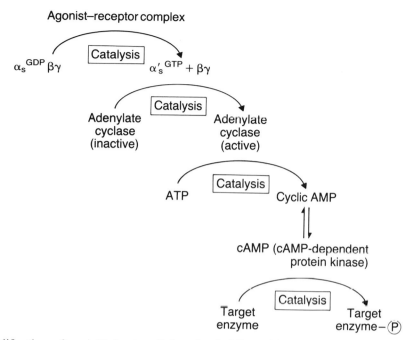

Fig. 5.6 Amplification of an initial extracellular signal delivered by a hormone or other agonist through the components of the cyclic AMP intracellular messenger system. Amplification is achieved by the catalytic activities of the agonist–receptor complex which activates G_s ($\alpha_s^{GDP}\beta\gamma$); the active form of G_s (α'_s^{GTP}), which activates adenylate cyclase; adenylate cyclase, which converts ATP to cyclic AMP; and the cyclic AMP-dependent protein kinases which phosphorylate target enzymes.

(Fig. 5.6). The amplification at each step has been estimated to be at least 10-fold so that the total amplification of the initial signal is greater than 10^4. Another example of the role of a cyclic nucleotide in the amplification of an extracellular signal is the action of cyclic GMP in photoreceptor cells (Section 5.8.4)

The abilities of cyclic AMP and cyclic GMP to act as intracellular messengers in animal cells depend on the unique chemical structures of these molecules. The sole function of cyclic AMP and cyclic GMP is to act as intracellular messengers. Likewise, the reactions which form and degrade each cyclic nucleotide have no function other than to regulate the concentration of these intracellular messengers. By contrast, the non-cyclic adenosine and guanosine nucleotides are intermediates in many pathways of intermediary metabolism.

The function of each of the cyclic nucleotides as an intracellular messenger will now be considered in more detail. The scope of the actions of the cyclic nucleotide in different cell types will be indicated, the enzymatic reactions responsible for its synthesis and degradation described, and the regulation of these reactions discussed. Since the role of cyclic AMP as a messenger in prokaryotes and lower eukaryotes and knowledge of the discovery of cyclic AMP and cyclic GMP helps in understanding the roles of the cyclic nucleotides as intracellular messengers in animal cells, these topics will be considered first.

5.2 Cyclic AMP as an inter- and intracellular messenger in prokaryotes and lower eukaryotes

The function of cyclic AMP in animal cells is

thought to have evolved from the role of this cyclic nucleotide as an inter- and intracellular messenger in prokaryotes and in lower eukaryotes. In *Escherichia coli* and in some other bacteria, cyclic AMP is synthesized and secreted when high concentrations of carbon sources other than glucose are present in the growth medium. In the presence of extracellular glucose, cyclic AMP concentrations are decreased. In these bacteria, the mechanism of action of cyclic AMP is to bind to a cyclic AMP receptor protein in the nucleus. This, in turn, stimulates the synthesis of enzymes required for the metabolism of non-glucose sugars. Bacteria do not possess a cyclic AMP-dependent protein kinase. How-

ever, there are substantial regions of homology between regulatory subunit R_{II} of cyclic AMP-dependent protein kinase in animal cells and the cyclic-AMP-receptor protein in bacteria.

In the cellular slime mould *Dictyostelium discordeum* the function of cyclic AMP is more complex than in *E. coli*. In *Dictyostelium discordeum* cyclic AMP acts both at receptors on the cell membrane and at intracellular sites (Fig. 5.7). In the absence of nutrients, the amoeba of *Dictyostelium discordeum* secretes cyclic AMP. This acts as an attractant for nearby cells and induces large numbers of cells to aggregate and form multicellular structures. The extracellular concentration of the cyclic nucleotide is

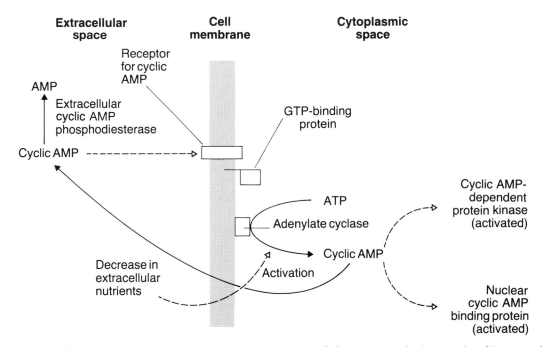

Fig. 5.7 Cyclic AMP acts as both an intracellular and an extracellular messenger in the amoeba of *Dictyostelium discoideum*. The synthesis of cyclic AMP is stimulated by a decrease in the concentration of extracellular nutrients. Cyclic AMP is formed by the action of adenylate cyclase attached to the cytoplasmic side of the plasma membrane. Intracellular actions of the cyclic nucleotide are mediated by binding of the nucleotide to a nuclear cyclic-AMP-binding protein (stimulation of protein synthesis) and by cyclic AMP-dependent protein kinase. Cyclic AMP formed in the cytoplasmic space is also secreted into the extracellular medium. Extracellular cyclic AMP acts as a chemical attractant for nearby amoebae by binding to a receptor on the external face of the plasma membrane of these cells. This activates adenylate cyclase through a GTP-binding protein and is the chief signal responsible for stimulation of the formation of cyclic AMP in the cytoplasmic space. An extracellular cyclic AMP phosphodiesterase degrades cyclic AMP present in the extracellular medium.

determined by the activities of an intracellular adenylate cyclase and an extracellular cyclic AMP phosphodiesterase (Fig. 5.7). The adenylate cyclase is activated by the binding of cyclic AMP to a receptor on the cell surface. The intracellular effects of cyclic AMP are exerted through both a nuclear cyclic AMP receptor protein and a cyclic AMP-dependent protein kinase (Fig. 5.7).

Since prokaryotes and some eukaryotes possess a nuclear cyclic-AMP-binding protein, it has been suggested that such a protein may be present in animal cells. However, no evidence for this has yet been obtained.

5.3 The discovery of cyclic AMP and cyclic GMP

5.3.1 *Cyclic AMP*

The discovery of cyclic AMP as an intracellular messenger arose from the studies of Sutherland and his colleagues during the period between 1955 and 1960. They were investigating the mechanism by which adrenalin and glucagon increase the activity of glycogen phosphorylase in liver slices. C. and G. Cori (1945) had previously isolated two forms (*a* and *b*) of glycogen phosphorylase from skeletal muscle. Form *b* was shown to require AMP as an activator (Cori and Cori 1945). Sutherland and Rall and their colleagues showed that ATP and Mg^{2+} were required for the conversion of isolated liver glycogen phosphorylase *b* (inactive in the absence of AMP) to phosphorylase *a* (Rall *et al.* 1956). This enabled Rall *et al.* (1957) to develop a cell-free system in which the addition of adrenalin or glucagon to a liver homogenate in the presence of ATP and Mg^{2+} caused an increase in phosphorylase activity. After searching for a compound which might be formed as a result of the action of the hormones, a heat-stable factor was isolated from liver slices treated with hormone. This factor was shown to activate glycogen phosphor-

ylase in liver homogenates incubated in the absence of hormones (Fig. 5.8).

At the time Sutherland and his colleagues were studying the activation of glycogen phosphorylase, Lipkin was investigating the chemistry of compounds formed when ATP was treated with $Ba(OH)_2$ (Lipkin *et al.* 1959). One of the products of this reaction was found to be similar in biological properties to the heat-stable activator of phosphorylase. The two groups collaborated in the elucidation of the structure of the activator which was subsequently identified as 3',5'-cyclic AMP (Suther-

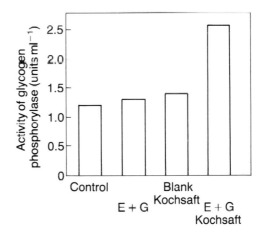

Fig. 5.8 The activation by a heat-stable factor, subsequently shown to be cyclic AMP, of glycogen phosphorylase in the experiments described in 1957 by Rall and his colleagues. The heat-stable factor was prepared by the incubation of a liver-membrane fraction with adrenalin and glucagon. The mixture was boiled and the soluble heat-stable factor separated by centrifugation. Control extracts were prepared in a similar manner by incubation of liver membranes in the absence of hormones. The activity of glycogen phosphorylase was measured in a supernatant fraction prepared from a liver homogenate and incubated in the presence of ATP, Mg^{2+}, and the following additions: control, no further additions; E + G, addition of adrenalin and glucagon directly to the supernatant fraction; blank Kochsaft (boiled extract prepared from membranes incubated in the absence of hormones); E + G Kochsaft (boiled extract prepared from membranes incubated with hormones). From Rall *et al.* (1957).

land and Rall 1958; Lipkin *et al.* 1959). Shortly after this, the enzymes adenylate cyclase (Sutherland and Rall 1958), cyclic AMP phosphodiesterase (Butcher and Sutherland 1962), and cyclic AMP-dependent protein kinase (Walsh *et al.* 1968) were identified and isolated.

Once cyclic AMP was discovered as the intracellular mediator required for the activation by adrenalin and glucagon of glycogen phosphorylase in liver, the possibility that this cyclic nucleotide plays a similar role in the actions of hormones on other cells was investigated. The criteria used to determine whether cyclic AMP acts as an intracellular messenger in a given cell are listed in Table 5.3. One of the important tests was the ability of derivatives of cyclic AMP to mimic the action of the cyclic nucleotide in intact cells. Cyclic AMP itself does not readily diffuse across the plasma membrane. However, a number of derivatives of cyclic AMP with increased lipid solubility, for example $N^6, O^{2'}$-

Table 5.3 *Criteria used to establish that cyclic AMP acts as an intracellular messenger in the process by which a given agonist induces a specific response in a target cell (Robison* et al. *1971)*

1. The response induced by the given agonist is associated with an increase in the activity of adenylate cyclase. This effect is specific for all other agonists which induce the same response.

2. The given agonist increases the concentration of cyclic AMP in the cell. Changes in cyclic AMP concentration measured as a function of (a) the time elapsed after addition of the agonist and (b) the concentration of the agonist correlate with the time-course and the dose-response curves for the response induced by the agonist.

3. Inhibitors of cyclic AMP phosphodiesterase, for example theophylline and caffeine, act synergistically with the given agonist in inducing the response.

4. A response similar to that elicited by the given agonist is induced by dibutyryl cyclic AMP and other less polar derivatives of cyclic AMP.

dibutyryl cyclic AMP, move across the plasma membrane much faster than cyclic AMP itself. These derivatives bind to cyclic AMP-dependent protein kinase with an affinity similar to that of cyclic AMP itself. One difficulty with these experiments is that some derivatives like $N^6, O^{2'}$-dibutyryl cyclic AMP are rapidly metabolized within the cell. The resulting metabolites may, themselves, influence cell metabolism, and hence complicate interpretation of the results of these experiments.

The importance of the discovery of cyclic AMP by Sutherland and his colleagues lies not only in its contribution to knowledge of the existence and function of cyclic AMP, but also in its role in the development of the concept of the nature of an intracellular messenger and in the principles which underlie experimental tests of this concept. The work of Sutherland and his colleagues set a pattern which could be followed in future searches for other intracellular messengers such as Ca^{2+}, inositol 1,4,5-trisphosphate, and diacylglycerol.

5.3.2 *Cyclic GMP*

Studies of the distribution of cyclic AMP in extracellular fluids in animals led to the discovery, in mammalian urine, of another cyclic nucleotide, cyclic GMP (Ashman *et al.* 1963). The subsequent detection of cyclic GMP in many cells, and of cyclic GMP-dependent protein kinase, suggested that this cyclic nucleotide may have a role as an intracellular messenger similar to that of cyclic AMP. The discovery of the activation by light of cyclic nucleotide phosphodiesterase in photoreceptor cells (Miki *et al.* 1973; Chader *et al.* 1974) led to the elucidation of the role of cyclic GMP in the transfer of light-induced signals in photoreceptor cells. This was the first description of a clearly defined function of cyclic GMP as an intracellular messenger.

In 1973, Goldberg and his colleagues proposed that cyclic GMP acts by opposing the effects of cyclic AMP on intracellular enzymes (Goldberg *et al.* 1973). It was proposed that in some cells, for example smooth-muscle cells, cyclic AMP activates and cyclic GMP inhibits common target enzymes. In other cells, for example heart muscle cells, cyclic GMP was proposed to activate and cyclic AMP to inhibit target enzymes. Subsequent experiments have shown that this simple hypothesis, known as the 'Yin Yang' hypothesis, is not correct.

It was not until 1984 that definitive evidence for an intracellular messenger function for cyclic GMP in a system other than the photoreceptor cell was obtained. This was the observation that atrial natriuretic peptide stimulates guanylate cyclase and the formation of cyclic GMP in smooth-muscle cells (Winquist *et al.* 1984). It is likely that cyclic GMP has a more widespread role as an intracellular messenger than present knowledge indicates. Experimental difficulties may have prevented elucidation of this role in many cells.

5.4 Adenylate cyclase and the formation of cyclic AMP

5.4.1 *The adenylate cyclase enzymes*
The products of the reaction catalysed by adenylate cyclase are cyclic AMP and inorganic pyrophosphate (Fig. 5.9). The adenylate cyclase catalytic centre is located on the cytoplasmic side

$$MgATP^{2-} \longrightarrow Cyclic\ AMP^- + MgPP_i^{2-} + H^+$$

Adenylate cyclase

Fig. 5.9 The formation of 3′,5′-cyclic adenosine monophosphate from ATP is catalysed by adenylate cyclase.

of the plasma membrane. Many cells possess more than one form of adenylate cyclase. Two of the main isoenzymes are the calmodulin-activated and the calmodulin-independent ade-

nylate cyclases. Some of the other forms of adenylate cyclase detected in cell extracts may be artefacts that are a result of proteolytic degradation which has occurred after homogenization of the cells.

The relative amounts of calmodulin-activated and calmodulin-independent adenylate cyclase present in a given tissue can be determined by the use of an antibody which is specific for calmodulin-activated adenylate cyclase. Figure 5.10 shows the relative proportions of these enzymes present in a number of tissues. Significant quantities of the calmodulin-activated enzyme are present in brain, heart, kidney, and lung whereas practically none of this form of the enzyme is present in liver and testis.

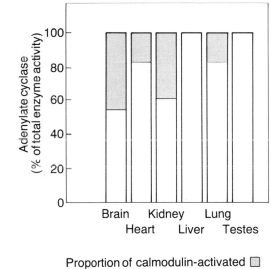

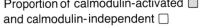

Proportion of calmodulin-activated ▨ and calmodulin-independent ☐

Fig. 5.10 The relative proportions of calmodulin-independent and calmodulin-activated adenylate cyclase in tissues. A membrane fraction from each tissue was treated with detergent in order to release membrane-bound adenylate cyclase. Calmodulin-activated (shaded bars) and calmodulin-independent (open bars) adenylate cyclases were distinguished by treatment of the solubilized enzymes with an antibody to calmodulin-activated adenylate cyclase. From Rosenberg and Storm (1987).

Most adenylate cyclase enzymes are activated by pharmacological concentrations of the compound forskolin. One exception is sperm-cell adenylate cyclase which is not affected by this agent. Forskolin is a diterpene (Fig. 5.11) isolated from the plant *Coleus forskohlii*. The interaction of forskolin with adenylate cyclase

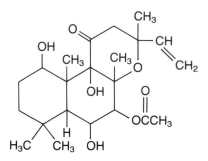

Fig. 5.11 The structure of the diterpene forskolin. This compound activates adenylate cyclase by a mechanism which does not involve GTP-binding regulatory proteins.

requires the presence of another protein, the nature of which has not been elucidated although it is known that it is not the alpha subunit (α_s) of the stimulatory GTP-binding regula-

tory protein, G_s. Forskolin has been used to activate adenylate cyclase in the absence of the normal requirements for α_s in studies of the physiological roles of adenylate cyclase and cyclic AMP.

5.4.2 *Structure of adenylate cyclase*

The adenylate cyclase enzymes from brain and heart have been purified to homogeneity using affinity chromatography columns in which calmodulin or forskolin are bound to a solid support such as Sepharose. Adenylate cyclase is composed of a single glycosylated polypeptide chain with a molecular weight of about 120 kDa. In highly purified preparations of adenylate cyclase from some cells, α_s is found to be tightly associated with the enzyme.

In 1989 Gilman and his colleagues obtained a cDNA clone which encodes bovine brain adenylate cyclase and determined the predicted amino-acid sequence of this enzyme (Krupinski *et al.* 1989). The predicted tertiary structure of the enzyme shows surprising complexity (Fig. 5.12). A region of six membrane-spanning sequences near the amino terminus is joined to

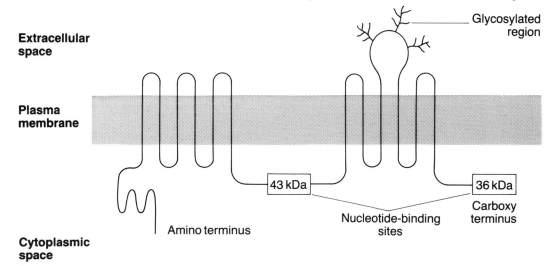

Fig. 5.12 The predicted tertiary structure of adenylate cyclase from bovine brain. This molecule is a single polypeptide chain which contains two hydrophobic domains separated by a large hydrophilic domain located in the cytoplasmic space. A second large hydrophilic domain is located at the carboxylic end of the molecule.

a second region of six membrane-spanning sequences by a large 43 kDa cytoplasmic hydrophilic sequence. At the carboxy terminus there is a second large cytoplasmic hydrophilic sequence. The two cytoplasmic hydrophilic sequences contain nucleotide binding sites and may represent the catalytic site of the enzyme. Glycosylation sites are present on a large extracellular sequence which lies between two of the membrane-spanning sequences. With the exception of the two large hydrophilic intracellular domains, the membrane-spanning regions have some similarities to the structures of plasma-membrane ion channels.

5.4.3   *Regulation of adenylate cyclase activity*

The activity of adenylate cyclase is principally controlled by extracellular agonists. These act through a plasma-membrane receptor and either G_s or the inhibitory GTP-binding regulatory protein, G_i. The component of G_s which interacts with adenylate cyclase and induces a conformational change in the enzyme is $\alpha_s'^{GTP}$. This allows the active site of adenylate cyclase to bind ATP. The inhibition of adenylate cyclase through the actions of G_i is mediated indirectly by released $\beta_i\gamma_i$ subunits and directly by the interaction of α_i with adenylate cyclase. These processes are discussed in more detail in Chapter 3 (Section 3.4.5).

Adenylate cyclase is also controlled by intracellular signals through the phosphorylation of the plasma-membrane receptors or α_s and, in cells which possess calmodulin-activated adenylate cyclase, through changes in $[Ca^{2+}]_i$. Phosphorylation of receptors or α_s inhibits the activation of adenylate cyclase by agonists. These phosphorylation reactions are discussed in Chapter 3 (Section 3.6). The control of the actions of receptors and α_s by phosphorylation may be a negative-feedback system which limits the agonist-induced increase in cyclic AMP. The activation by Ca^{2+} of calmodulin-activated ade-

nylate cyclase provides a mechanism by which cyclic AMP can be increased in the absence of an external agonist in association with an increase in $[Ca^{2+}]_i$ in cells which possess calmodulin-activated adenylate cyclase.

5.5   The cyclic AMP phosphodiesterases

5.5.1   *Multiple forms of cyclic AMP phosphodiesterase*

Hydrolysis of the 3′ ester bond of 3′,5′-cyclic AMP to form 5′ cyclic AMP is catalysed by cyclic AMP phosphodiesterase (Fig. 5.13). Regulation of the activity of this enzyme is considerably more complex than the regulation of adenylate cyclase. In contrast to adenylate cyclase, which is confined to the cytoplasmic face of the plasma membrane, cyclic AMP phosphodiesterase is distributed in a number of different intracellular compartments.

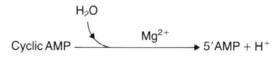
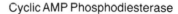
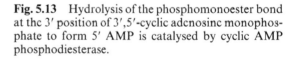

Cyclic AMP Phosphodiesterase

Fig. 5.13   Hydrolysis of the phosphomonoester bond at the 3′ position of 3′,5′-cyclic adenosine monophosphate to form 5′ AMP is catalysed by cyclic AMP phosphodiesterase.

A general feature of intracellular communication seems to be that regulation of the enzymes which catalyse the hydrolysis of phosphate ester groups on cyclic nucleotides, inositol 1,4,5-trisphosphate and phosphorylated proteins, is considerably more complex than regulation of the enzymes which catalyse addition of the phosphate group. Consequently, it has been much more difficult to elucidate the nature of the pathways involved in hydrolysis of the phosphate ester groups on these metabolites and proteins.

Cells contain multiple forms of cyclic AMP phosphodiesterase. For example, up to eight dif-

Table 5.4 *Multiple forms of cyclic AMP phosphodiesterase detected in homogenates of heart, liver, brain, and platelets*

Tissue	Association with membrane	Distinguishing features
Heart	Membrane-bound form	Not characterized
	Soluble form 1	Calmodulin-activated
	Soluble form 2	High K_M for cyclic AMP, activated by cyclic GMP
	Soluble form 3	Low K_M for cyclic AMP
	Soluble form 4	Low K_M for cyclic AMP
Liver	Membrane-bound form 1	Peripheral plasma membrane, low K_M for cyclic AMP, simulated by insulin
	Membrane-bound form 2	Dense vesicle, low K_M for cyclic AMP, stimulated by insulin and glucagon
	Membrane-bound form 3	Calmodulin-activated
	Membrane-bound form 4	Cyclic GMP-activated
	Soluble form 1	Insulin-sensitive
	Soluble form 2	Cyclic GMP-activated
Brain	Membrane-bound form	Not characterized
	Soluble form 1	Calmodulin-activated
	Soluble form 2	Calmodulin-activated
	Soluble form 3	Calmodulin-activated
	Soluble form 4	Cyclic GMP-activated
Platelets	Membrane-bound form	Not characterized
	Soluble form 1	Low K_M for cyclic AMP
	Soluble form 2	K_M for cyclic GMP lower than K_M for cyclic AMP
	Soluble form 3	Calmodulin-activated

ferent forms have been detected in liver. Some of the different forms of cyclic AMP phosphodiesterases which have been detected in heart, liver, brain, and platelets are listed in Table 5.4. In most cells, less that 10 per cent of the total detectable phosphodiesterase activity is associated with the particulate fraction of cell extracts. However, in brain, 50 per cent of the total enzyme activity is found in the particulate fraction.

The physical and chemical properties which characterize a given form of cyclic nucleotide phosphodiesterase include the affinity with which the enzyme is bound to intracellular membranes or proteins, the apparent K_M values for cyclic AMP and cyclic GMP, and the mechanisms by which the activity of the enzyme is regulated. The terms 'low K_M' and 'high K_M' are sometimes used to designate cyclic AMP phosphodiesterases with different affinities for cyclic AMP. A difference in the physical properties of four forms of cyclic AMP phosphodiesterase present in the soluble fraction of homogenates of heart tissue is illustrated by separation of the enzymes by DEAE-Sepharose chromatography as shown in Fig. 5.14. Some forms of cyclic AMP phosphodiesterase may be responsible for the degradation of cyclic GMP as well as cyclic AMP.

Cyclic nucleotide phosphodiesterase enzymes, especially the membrane-bound forms, have been difficult to purify. More is known about the nature of the soluble enzymes than about the membrane-bound forms. Cyclic AMP phosphodiesterase enzymes are composed of either a single polypeptide chain or a dimer of the same or different polypeptides. The molecular weights of the polypeptides range between 45 and 60 kDa.

The apparent K_M values of the low K_M phosphodiesterases for cyclic AMP are in the range 0.1 to 5 μM. For a number of purified cyclic AMP phosphodiesterases, kinetic plots of reaction velocity as a function of cyclic AMP concentration obtained under steady-state conditions are non-hyperbolic and the double reciprocal plots are non-linear. An example of the latter plot, obtained for the dense vesicle cyclic AMP phosphodiesterase from liver, is shown in Fig. 5.15. Plots of the type shown in Fig. 5.15 have generally been interpreted as indicating the presence on the enzyme of at least two types of interactive binding sites for cyclic AMP in which the binding of cyclic AMP to one site on a molecule

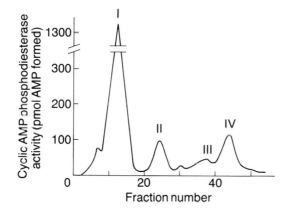

Fig. 5.14 Four forms of cyclic AMP phosphodiesterase, designated I, II, III, and IV, are present in homogenates of heart muscle. These can be separated by chromatography on DEAE-Sepharose. Enzyme activity has been measured in the presence of 25 μM cyclic AMP. From Reeves *et al.* (1987).

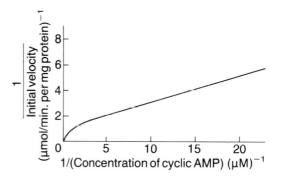

Fig. 5.15 A double reciprocal plot of initial reaction velocity as a function of cyclic AMP concentration for the reaction catalysed by purified dense-vesicle low K_M cyclic AMP phosphodiesterase from liver. The non-linearity of the plot has been interpreted as indicating apparent negative co-operativity between two interacting active sites. Limiting apparent K_M values for cyclic AMP of 0.3 and 30 μM can be obtained from these data. From Pyne *et al.* (1987).

Table 5.5 *Derivatives of cyclic AMP which inhibit cyclic AMP phosphodiesterase and activate cyclic AMP-dependent protein kinase. From Beebe et al.* (1984)

Derivative of cyclic AMP	Substituent	Concentration which gives half-maximal effect (μM)	
		Inhibition of phosphodiesterase	Activation of protein kinase
2-Trifluoromethyl cyclic AMP	2-CF$_3$	0.005	1.6
Cyclic AMP		–	0.2
Cyclic IMP		0.6	6.9
8-Bromo cyclic AMP	8-Br	14	0.2
8-Amino cyclic AMP	8-NH$_2$	40	0.2
8-Thiomethyl cyclic AMP	8-S–CH$_3$	46	0.3
N^6-Benzoyl cyclic AMP	N^6-CO$_2$-C$_6$H$_5$	90	2.1
N^6-Butyryl cyclic AMP	N^6-CO$_2$-C$_3$H$_7$	600	3.0

of phosphodiesterase decreases the affinity for cyclic AMP of the second site on the same enzyme molecule. This is called a negative co-operative interaction. Kinetic plots of the type shown in Fig. 5.15 may also arise when a mixture

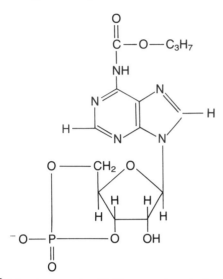

N⁶Butyryl adenosine 3',5'-monophosphate

Fig. 5.16 N⁶-butyryl adenosine 3',5'-monophosphate, a derivative of cyclic AMP which inhibits cyclic AMP phosphodiesterase.

of different phosphodiesterases with different K_M values for cyclic AMP is present in preparations of partially purified cyclic AMP phosphodiesterases.

5.5.2 *Pharmacological inhibitors of cyclic AMP phosphodiesterases*

Inhibitors of cyclic AMP phosphodiesterases have proved valuable in the elucidation of the role of cyclic AMP as an intracellular messenger in intact cells (Beavo *et al.* 1970). Cyclic AMP phosphodiesterases are inhibited by derivatives of cyclic AMP and by a variety of other cyclic organic molecules. The first inhibitors discovered were xanthine and its derivatives (Sutherland and Rall 1958). Many inhibitors of cyclic AMP phosphodiesterase preferentially inhibit certain forms of the enzyme.

Some of the derivatives of cyclic AMP which act as inhibitors are listed in Table 5.5. The structure of one of these, N⁶-butyryl adenosine 3', 5'-monophosphate, is shown in Fig. 5.16. The concentrations of the cyclic AMP derivatives which give half-maximal inhibition of cyclic AMP hydrolysis range from 5nM for 2-trifluoro-

Table 5.6 *Inhibitors of cyclic AMP phosphodiesterase enzymes*

Family of inhibitors	Examples of specific inhibitors
Methylxanthine derivatives	1,3,7-trimethylxanthine (caffeine) 1,3-dimethylxanthine (theophylline) 1-methyl-3-isobutylxanthine
Papaverine and related compounds	Papaverine
Oxo-quinoline derivatives	6,7-dimethoxy-4-ethylquinazoline
Imidazolidinones	4-(3,4-dimethoxybenzyl)-2-imidazolidone 4-(3-butoxy-4-methoxybenzyl)-2-imidazolidine
Pyrrolidone derivatives	4-(3-cyclopentyloxy-4-methoxyphenyl)-2-pyrrolidone
Pyrazine derivatives	5-(4-acetamidophenyl)pyrazine-2[1H]-one
Pyrazolopyridines	1-ethyl-4-(isopropylidene hydrazine)-1H-pyrazolo-(3,4-*b*)-pyridine-5-carboxylic acid, ethyl ester, HCl
Benzodiazepines	Chlordiazepoxide

methyl cyclic AMP to 600 μM for N^6-butyryl cyclic AMP (Table 5.5). A number of derivatives of cyclic AMP are also substrates for cyclic AMP phosphodiesterase and are hydrolysed at a slow rate. Most derivatives of cyclic AMP which bind to cyclic AMP phosphodiesterase also bind to each of the cyclic AMP-binding sites on the regulatory subunit of cyclic AMP-dependent protein kinase (Chapter 4, Section 4.3.2) and are effective activators of the purified enzyme. The concentrations which give half-maximal activation of cyclic AMP-dependent protein kinase are also listed in Table 5.5.

When added to intact cells, derivatives of cyclic AMP activate cyclic AMP-dependent protein kinase by two mechanisms—the direct interaction of the cyclic AMP derivative with the regulatory subunit of cyclic AMP-dependent protein kinase and the indirect effect of the increase in

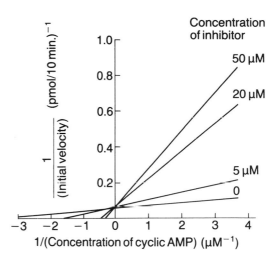

Fig. 5.18   The inhibition of purified soluble cyclic AMP phosphodiesterase from heart muscle cells by 5-(4-acetamidophenyl)-pyrazin-2[1H]-one (SK and F 94120) is competitive with respect to cyclic AMP. From Reeves *et al.* (1987).

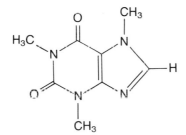

1,3,7-Trimethylxanthine (Caffeine)

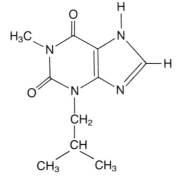

1-Methyl-3-isobutylxanthine

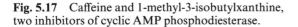

Fig. 5.17   Caffeine and 1-methyl-3-isobutylxanthine, two inhibitors of cyclic AMP phosphodiesterase.

the concentration of cyclic AMP caused by inhibition of cyclic AMP phosphodiesterase. The effect of a given derivative of cyclic AMP on the activity of cyclic AMP-dependent protein kinase in intact cells is also influenced by the ability of the derivative to permeate the plasma membrane.

Some of the cyclic organic molecules which inhibit cyclic AMP phosphodiesterases are listed in Table 5.6. The structures of caffeine and 1-methyl-3-isobutylxanthine are shown in Fig. 5.17. Many of the inhibitors listed in Table 5.6 are competitive inhibitors with respect to cyclic AMP. This is shown by the observation that double reciprocal plots of reaction rate as a function of cyclic AMP concentration obtained in the presence of different concentrations of a given inhibitor consist of a series of straight lines which intersect at the ordinate (Fig. 5.18). However, the xanthine derivatives are an exception and bind at a site which is separate from the catalytic site. Methylisobutylxanthine and other xanthine derivatives have been invaluable in the artificial manipulation of the concentration of cyclic AMP in intact cells and tissues.

5.5.3 *Regulation of the activity of the cyclic AMP phosphodiesterases*

The activities of cyclic AMP phosphodiesterases are regulated by several different mechanisms. The main ones are activation by cyclic AMP-dependent protein kinases, Ca^{2+} and insulin. The activation of cyclic AMP phosphodiesterase by cyclic AMP-dependent protein kinase appears to be a widespread mechanism which regulates the activity of many forms of phosphodiesterase. The other regulatory mechanisms control the activity of specific forms of the enzyme. The nature of the regulatory mechanism for a given cyclic AMP phosphodiesterase depends on the type of cell, the isoenzyme of cyclic AMP phosphodiesterase, and the intracellular location of the phosphodiesterase.

In many cells the activity of at least one form of cyclic AMP phosphodiesterase is increased by phosphorylation of the enzyme catalysed by cyclic AMP-dependent protein kinase. In the liver, this form is the dense vesicle phosphodiesterase. The phosphorylation of cyclic AMP phosphodiesterase by cyclic AMP-dependent protein kinase is probably a negative-feedback mechanism by which the increase in cyclic AMP induced by an agonist is tightly controlled. This is shown schematically in Fig. 5.19. Some forms of cyclic AMP phosphodiesterase are activated by cyclic GMP which binds to an allosteric site on the phosphodiesterase.

The activation by calmodulin of purified calmodulin-activated cyclic nucleotide phosphodiesterase from brain is shown in Fig. 5.20. In cells or cytoplasmic compartments in which calmodulin-activated cyclic AMP phosphodiesterase is present, an increase in $[Ca^{2+}]_i$ above the

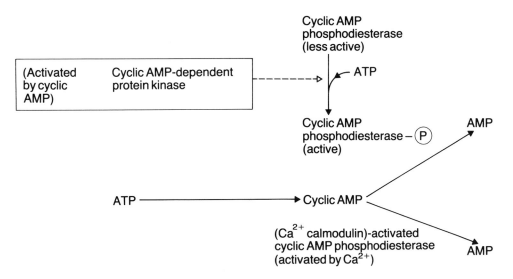

Fig. 5.19 In many cells, the activation of different forms of cyclic AMP phosphodiesterase by cyclic AMP and Ca^{2+} contributes to regulation of the intracellular concentration of cyclic AMP. Ca^{2+} acts through (Ca^{2+} + calmodulin)-activated isoenzymes of cyclic AMP phosphodiesterase. The activation by cyclic AMP involves another form of the phosphodiesterase which is phosphorylated by cyclic AMP-dependent protein kinase. The stimulation by cyclic AMP of the activity of cyclic AMP phosphodiesterase is thought to be a negative-feedback system which limits the increase in cyclic AMP induced by the activation of adenylate cyclase.

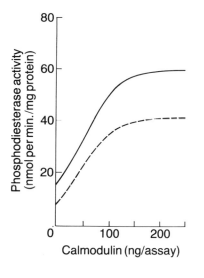

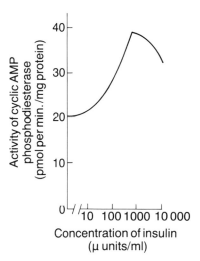

Fig. 5.20   The activation by calmodulin of partially purified soluble cyclic nucleotide phosphodiesterase from brain. The activity of the enzyme was measured in the presence of a fixed concentration of Ca^{2+}, increasing concentrations of calmodulin, and either cyclic AMP (broken curve) or cyclic GMP (full curve) as the substrate. From Strada *et al.* (1984).

Fig. 5.21   The activation by insulin of membrane-bound cyclic AMP phosphodiesterase in rat hepatocytes. Isolated hepatocytes were incubated with a given concentration of insulin, the cells homogenized, cyclic AMP phosphodiesterase extracted from the particulate fraction, and the activity of the enzyme measured. From Loten *et al.* (1978).

basal value stimulates the degradation of cyclic AMP. This regulatory pathway is shown schematically in Fig. 5.19.

In cells of the liver and adipose tissue, insulin activates one or more forms of cyclic AMP phosphodiesterase. This effect was first observed in liver cells by Loten and Sneyd (1970). The change induced by insulin can be observed in partially purified preparations of the phosphodiesterase isolated from the homogenates of cells previously exposed to insulin (Fig. 5.21). In liver cells, both the peripheral plasma-membrane enzyme and the dense-vesicle enzyme are activated by insulin. A soluble cyclic AMP phosphodiesterase in liver is also activated by this hormone. Activation of the two membrane-bound enzymes is associated with phosphorylation of the phosphodiesterases. A GTP-binding protein, G_{ins}, is involved in the mechanism by which insulin activates the peripheral plasma-membrane enzyme. The activation of cyclic

AMP phosphodiesterase by insulin and the subsequent decrease in the intracellular concentration of cyclic AMP may be one of several pathways by which insulin induces responses in cells. This pathway is shown schematically in Fig. 5.22.

5.6   The binding of cyclic AMP to cytoplasmic proteins and its diffusion through the cytoplasmic space

The effect of cyclic AMP on cyclic AMP-dependent protein kinase at any given location in the cytoplasmic space is determined by the concentration of cyclic AMP at that particular intracellular location. In addition to the relative rates of synthesis and degradation of cyclic AMP, the concentration of the cyclic nucleotide is also governed by its binding to cytoplasmic proteins and by its rate of diffusion between adenylate cyclase and cyclic AMP phosphodiesterase.

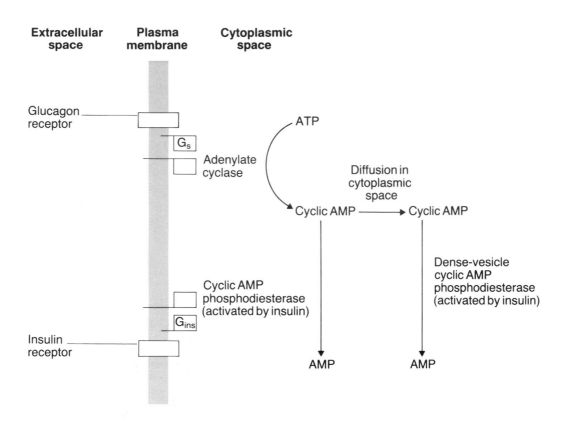

Fig. 5.22 A schematic representation of the role of insulin in the stimulation of cyclic AMP degradation in hepatocytes. Insulin activates a plasma-membrane cyclic AMP phosphodiesterase, possibly through a GTP-binding regulatory protein called G_{ins}, and a cyclic AMP phosphodiesterase called the dense-vesicle phosphodiesterase which is located elsewhere in the cytoplasmic space. The mechanism by which insulin activates the dense-vesicle phosphodiesterase is not known.

In the unstimulated cell, the concentration of total cyclic AMP present in the cytoplasmic space is about 1 μM. This is comparable with the concentration of cyclic AMP which gives half-maximal activation of isolated cyclic AMP-dependent protein kinase. However, in the cell, the protein kinase is not active in the unstimulated state. This is probably because a large portion of the total cyclic AMP is bound to cyclic AMP phosphodiesterases and to non-specific sites on other proteins in the cytoplasmic space. This means that in the unstimulated cell, although the concentration of total cyclic AMP would be sufficient to activate cyclic AMP-dependent protein kinase, the enzyme is not acti-

vated because the concentration of free cyclic AMP is substantially lower than that of the total cyclic nucleotide. When adenylate cyclase is activated, the concentration of free cyclic nucleotide increases within the range which activates the cyclic AMP-dependent protein kinases.

In many cells the cyclic AMP-dependent protein kinases are located some distance from the plasma membrane. For example, in the liver cell, significant quantities of these enzymes are associated with glycogen granules and the smooth endoplasmic reticulum. This means that cyclic AMP formed by adenylate cyclase at the plasma membrane must diffuse through the cytoplasmic space in order to bind to the protein kinase.

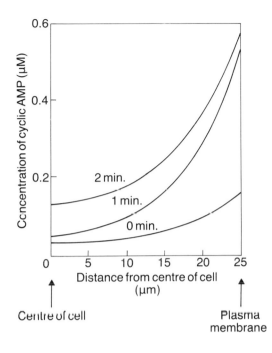

Fig. 5.23 Calculated concentrations of free (unbound) cyclic AMP at various points between the centre of a hypothetical cell and the plasma membrane following the onset of a three-fold increase in the activity of adenylate cyclase at the plasma membrane. The model employed assumes that the cell is a sphere with a radius of 25 μm. It has been assumed that adenylate cyclase and a low K_M cyclic AMP phosphodiesterase are uniformly distributed on the inner surface of the plasma membrane, and a high K_M phosphodiesterase is uniformly distributed in the cytoplasmic space. The value employed for the diffusion coefficient for cyclic AMP is $4 \times 10^{-11}\,\mathrm{m^2\,s^{-1}}$. The curves shown represent the concentrations of cyclic AMP before the three-fold increase in adenylate cyclase activity (0 min), and at 1 min and 2 min after the onset of the increase in enzyme activity. From Fell (1980).

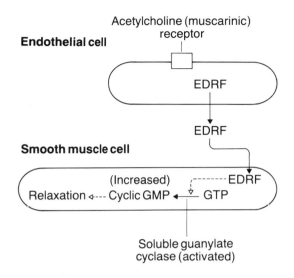

Fig. 5.24 Cyclic GMP acts as an intracellular messenger in the action of endothelial-derived relaxing factor (EDRF) on smooth-muscle cells. EDRF, which is probably nitric oxide or S-nitrosocysteine, is synthesized by endothelial cells in response to acetylcholine and other agonists. EDRF diffuses from the endothelial cells to the cytoplasmic space of smooth muscle cells where it stimulates the soluble form of guanylate cyclase. This leads to an increase in the concentration of cyclic GMP in the region of the cytoplasmic space which surrounds guanylate cyclase. This, in turn, causes a decrease in $[\mathrm{Ca^{2+}}]_i$ and relaxation of the myofibrils.

Calculations made using a theoretical model show that, following the stimulation of adenylate cyclase at the plasma membrane, the increase in cyclic AMP near the plasma membrane is more rapid in onset and much larger than the increase near the centre of the cell (Fig. 5.23). The model employs an estimate of the diffusion coefficient for cyclic AMP, and assumes that adenylate cyclase is located only at the plasma membrane, and cyclic AMP phosphodiesterase at both the plasma membrane and at intracellular sites. Another reason for predicting that the concentration of cyclic AMP varies between different regions of the cytoplasmic space is the observation that within a given cell, the multiple forms of cyclic AMP phosphodiesterase are present in different intracellular locations and would be likely to lead to different rates of degradation of the cyclic nucleotide in these locations.

5.7 Increases in cyclic GMP as intracellular signals

5.7.1 *Systems in which agonists induce an increase in cyclic GMP*

There are three systems in which it has clearly been shown that an increase in cyclic GMP plays a role in the transmission of extracellular signals to intracellular target proteins. These are the actions of atrial natriuretic peptide (ANP) on mammalian cells, the actions of sperm-stimulating peptides on invertebrate sperm cells, the actions of endothelium-derived relaxing factor (EDRF), which is probably nitric oxide (NO) or *S*-nitrocysteine, on smooth-muscle cells and the actions of nitric oxide as both an extracellular and intracellular messenger in other tissues such as the brain. Whilst many agonists which bind to receptors on the plasma membranes of other types of cell increase the concentration of cyclic GMP in those cells, it has been difficult to show that this increase results from the stimulation of guanylate cyclase by the agonist–receptor complex.

The major target cells for ANP are those of the kidney, smooth muscle and the adrenal glomerulosa, and lung fibroblasts. EDRF is released by endothelial cells, diffuses through the interstitial fluid, and across the plasma membrane to the cytoplasmic space of smooth-muscle cells, where it binds to a cytoplasmic form of guanylate cyclase and activates this enzyme (Fig. 5.24). The resulting increase in cyclic GMP induces a decrease in $[Ca^{2+}]_i$ and relaxation of the muscle cell. Cytoplasmic guanylate cyclase is also activated by other nitrovasodilators, prostaglandins, and free radicals.

Peptides which stimulate invertebrate sperm cells include speract, resact, alloresact, and mosact. These peptides are produced by egg cells, bind to receptors on the sperm cell membrane, and induce an increase in the intracellular concentration of cyclic GMP. The increase in

cyclic GMP may mediate the stimulation by the peptides of sperm metabolism and motility.

5.7.2 *The guanylate cyclases*

There are three forms of guanylate cyclase. These are plasma-membrane guanylate cyclase, which possesses a membrane-spanning domain, a cytoplasmic form of the enzyme, which is activated by EDRF, and a Ca^{2+}-activated form, which is found associated with the cytoskeleton and plasma membrane. Thus, in contrast to adenylate cyclase which is located only at the plasma membrane, there are both membrane-bound and soluble forms of guanylate cyclase.

Knowledge of the structures of the plasma-membrane guanylate cyclases which are activated by ANP and sperm-activating peptides has been derived using conventional biochemical techniques and knowledge of the amino-acid sequence of the proteins obtained by Garbers and his colleagues (Singh *et al.* 1988). These proteins were also considered in Chapter 3 (Section 3.1) as one of the families of plasma-membrane receptors.

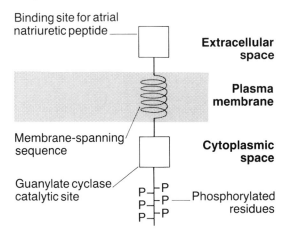

Fig. 5.25 The structure of the plasma-membrane form of guanylate cyclase. This molecule is a single polypeptide chain which contains a single membrane-spanning sequence. The extracellular domain contains the agonist binding site and the cytoplasmic domain the guanylate cyclase catalytic site. The cytoplasmic domain is phosphorylated at multiple sites.

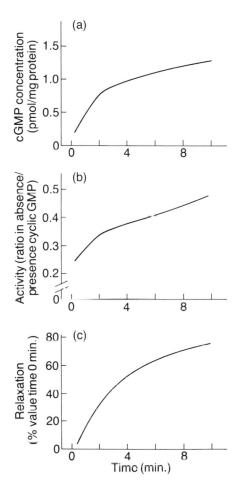

Fig. 5.26 Correlation of the time-courses for the effects of atrial natriuretic peptide (ANP) on (a) cyclic GMP (cGMP) concentration, (b) the activity of cyclic GMP-dependent protein kinase, and (c) the degree of relaxation in smooth-muscle cells isolated from rat thoracic aorta. The activity of cyclic GMP-dependent protein kinase is expressed as the ratio of the activities measured in cell extracts in the absence and presence of exogenous cyclic GMP. From Fiscus *et al.* (1985).

The plasma-membrane guanylate cyclases are each composed of a single polypeptide chain with a molecular weight between 120 and 180 kDa. The polypeptides possess an extracellular domain which binds ANP or a sperm-activating peptide, a single membrane-spanning sequence, and a guanylate cyclase catalytic domain on the cytoplasmic side of the membrane (Fig. 5.25).

A region of the polypeptide chain in the cytoplasmic domain is phosphorylated at multiple sites. Within the cytoplasmic domain there are regions with considerable homology to a region of the cytoplasmic form of guanylate cyclase and regions of the cytoplasmic domains of the receptor for platelet-derived growth factor and adenylate cyclase.

The binding of an agonist to the extracellular domain of the plasma-membrane guanylate cyclase induces a conformational change in the polypeptide chain which, in turn, stimulates the activity of guanylate cyclase. For sperm-cell guanylate cyclase this conformational change also induces a dephosphorylation of the cytoplasmic domain and a subsequent decrease in guanylate cyclase activity even though the agonist remains bound to the extracellular domain of the guanylate cyclase.

The cytoplasmic form of guanylate cyclase which is activated by EDRF is composed of two subunits with molecular weights of 82 and 70 kDa. One of these contains haem as a prosthetic group. Activation of the enzyme by EDRF involves combination of this molecule with the haem group resulting in a conformational change in the guanylate cyclase.

The third form of guanylate cyclase is activated or inhibited by Ca^{2+}. These actions of Ca^{2+} are probably exerted through an intermediary binding protein.

5.7.3   *The role of cyclic GMP-dependent protein kinase in the actions of cyclic GMP*

The best evidence for a role of cyclic GMP-dependent protein kinase in the action of cyclic GMP has come from investigation of the action of ANP on target cells. For this peptide there is a good correlation between increased cytoplasmic cyclic GMP concentration, the activation of cyclic GMP-dependent protein kinase, and myofibril relaxation in smooth-muscle cells (Fig. 5.26). This role of cyclic GMP-dependent

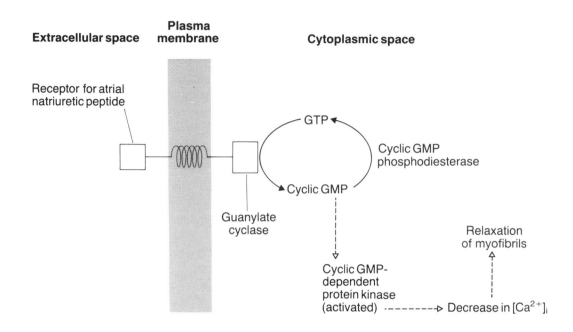

Fig. 5.27 The role of cyclic GMP as an intracellular messenger in the actions of atrial natriuretic peptide (ANP) on smooth-muscle cells. The binding of ANP to the receptor activates guanylate cyclase and increases the concentration of cyclic GMP in the cytoplasmic space. This, in turn, leads to a decrease in $[Ca^{2+}]_i$ and relaxation of myofibrils. The actions of cyclic GMP are mediated by cyclic GMP-dependent protein kinase. Cyclic GMP is degraded by a cyclic GMP phosphodiesterase.

protein kinase is shown schematically in Fig. 5.27. Myofibril relaxation is caused by a decrease in the cytoplasmic free Ca^{2+} concentration which, in turn, is probably due to the activation by cyclic GMP-dependent protein kinase, of the plasma-membrane $(Ca^{2+} + Mg^{2+})$ATPase.

5.8 A system in which a decrease in cyclic GMP acts as an intracellular signal: the photoreceptor cell

5.8.1 *Cyclic GMP and the dark Na⁺ current*
Before considering details of the role of cyclic GMP as an intracellular messenger in photoreceptor cells, it is necessary to consider the structure of these cells and the link between the absorption of light by rhodopsin and transmission of a signal to the brain. The two main types of photoreceptor cell in animals are the

rod and cone cells. These are elongated cells arranged in the retina so that one end is located to receive incident light and the other to release a neurotransmitter. The neurotransmitter initiates a nerve impulse to the brain.

Rod cells are composed of an outer and an inner segment (Fig. 5.28). The outer segment contains the machinery by which light is absorbed while neurotransmitters are released from the inner segment. Within the cytoplasmic space of the outer segment are a large number of discs. The composition of the disc membranes differs greatly from that of the plasma membrane. The disc membranes contain approximately equal amounts of lipid and protein, which is chiefly rhodopsin. The phospholipids contain a high percentage of unsaturated fatty acids so that the membrane is relatively fluid.

In the dark, Na⁺ ions and smaller amounts

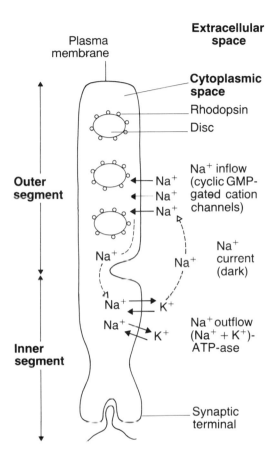

of Ca^{2+} and Mg^{2+} ions flow from the extracellular space to the cytoplasmic space of the outer segment of the rod through cyclic GMP-gated cation channels located in the plasma membrane adjacent to the discs (Fig. 5.28). The cyclic GMP-gated cation channels were discovered in 1985 by Fesenko *et al.* using the patch-clamp technique. The Na^+ ions then flow from the cytoplasmic space in the outer segment of the rod to the adjacent inner segment where they are transported out of the cell by an $(Na^+ + K^+)$ATPase (Fig. 5.28). This creates a current which cycles between the outer and inner segments. Upon the absorption of light by rhodopsin, Na^+ inflow through the rod's outer-segment cation channels is inhibited, the ion current decreases, and the state of polarization of the membrane is altered. The membranes of vertebrate rod cells become hyperpolarized and those of invertebrate cells become depolarized. These changes, in turn, induce the release of neurotransmitter by the inner segment of the rod cell.

Whilst cyclic GMP is the major intracellular messenger in the action of light on photoreceptor cells, a number of experiments indicate that Ca^{2+} also plays a role. These experiments include the observation that Ins 1, 4, 5 P_3 releases Ca^{2+} from intracellular stores in invertebrate rod cells (Chapter 6, Section 6.1) and the detection of cyclic GMP-gated Ca^{2+} channels in rod cells.

Fig. 5.28 The outer and inner segments of a rod cell from the retina of a vertebrate. Rhodopsin is associated with the disc membrane. Cyclic GMP-gated cation channels are located in the plasma membrane adjacent to the discs. In the dark, the concentration of cyclic GMP in the cytoplasmic space is maintained at a relatively high value. This causes the cyclic GMP-gated cation channels in the plasma membrane to remain open and allows Na^+ ions and smaller amounts of Ca^{2+} and Mg^{2+} ions to flow from the extracellular space to the cytoplasmic space in the outer segment. Na^+ ions are transported back to the extracellular space by $(Na^+ + K^+)$ATPases located in the inner segment. This creates a current which flows in a cycle between the outer and inner segments. The absorption of light by rhodopsin leads to a rapid decrease in the concentration of cyclic GMP, closure of the cation channels, hyperpolarization of the membrane, and release of a neurotransmitter.

5.8.2   *Activation of cyclic GMP phosphodiesterase in response to light*

Each molecule of rhodopsin spans the disc membrane (Fig. 5.29). On the cytoplasmic surface, rhodopsin can interact with cyclic GMP phosphodiesterase through the GTP-binding regulatory protein, transducin (G_t) (Chapter 3, Section 3.4.2). Cyclic GMP phosphodiesterase and transducin are attached to the cytoplasmic face of the disc membrane (Fig. 5.29). In the dark, the concentration of cyclic GMP present in the

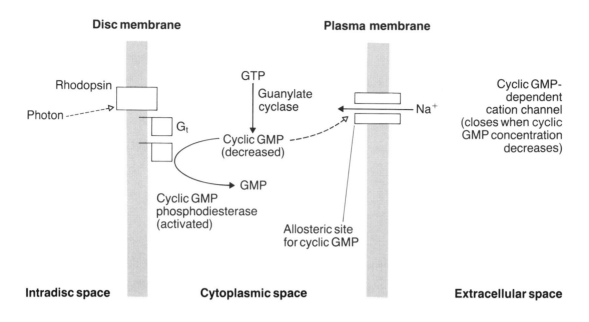

Fig. 5.29 The role of cyclic GMP phosphodiesterase in the mechanism by which light induces the closure of cyclic GMP-gated cation channels in the rod outer segment. Rhodopsin molecules span the disc membranes whereas transducin (G_t) and cyclic GMP phosphodiesterase are bound to the cytoplasmic face of this membrane. The cyclic GMP-gated cation channels are located in the plasma membrane. The absorption of a photon of light by rhodopsin leads to a stimulation of cyclic GMP phosphodiesterase, a decrease in the concentration of cyclic GMP in this region of the cell, dissociation of cyclic GMP from cyclic GMP-gated channels, and inhibition of the inflow of cations (principally Na^+ with smaller quantities of Ca^{2+} and Mg^{2+}) across the plasma membrane.

cytoplasmic space of the rod's outer segment is about 100 μM. (This is much higher than the concentration of cyclic GMP present in the inner segment, and the concentration present in most other animal cells.) Cyclic GMP binds to cyclic GMP-gated cation channels in the plasma membrane and maintains these in the open state.

The absorption of a photon of light by 11-*cis* retinal at the active site of rhodopsin changes the conformation of this molecule to the *trans* retinal form. This, in turn, induces changes in the conformations of rhodopsin, G_t, and cyclic GMP phosphodiesterase. This leads to activation of the phosphodiesterase and to a very rapid decline in the concentration of cyclic GMP in the cytoplasmic space of the rod's outer segment (Fig. 5.30). Subsequent dissociation of cyclic

GMP from the cyclic GMP-gated cation channels closes the channels and decreases the inflow of Na^+. Thus the main consequence of the rapid decrease in the concentration of cyclic GMP is a decrease in the rate of Na^+ inflow. It is interesting to note that there is a similarity between the decrease in cyclic GMP induced by light in the photoreceptor cell and the decrease in cyclic AMP induced by insulin in the liver cell (Section 5.5.3).

The cyclic GMP phosphodiesterase enzyme is composed of three subunits, α, β, and γ (Fig. 5.31). These have molecular weights of 88, 84, and 13 kDa, respectively. Enzyme activity resides in the α and β subunits while the γ subunit acts as an inhibitory regulatory subunit. Activation of the phosphodiesterase by $\alpha_t{'}^{GTP}$,

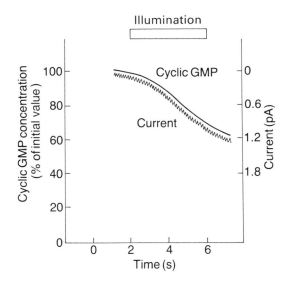

Fig. 5.30 Illumination causes a rapid decrease in the concentration of cyclic GMP in rod outer segments purified from the retina of the frog. At the low intensity of illumination employed in this experiment, the decrease in cyclic GMP concentration correlates well with the decrease in current across the plasma membrane. Illumination was applied during the times indicated by the open bar. From Cote *et al.* (1986).

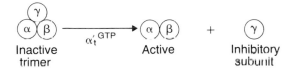

Fig. 5.31 The activation of cyclic GMP phosphodiesterase in rod outer segments by the active form of transducin, $\alpha'_t{}^{GTP}$, involves dissociation of the $\alpha\beta\gamma$ phosphodiesterase oligomer. In the absence of the inhibitory subunit, γ, the active site of the $\alpha\beta$ complex can bind and hydrolyse cyclic GMP.

the active form of the GTP-binding protein, causes dissociation of the γ subunit from the oligomer (Fig. 5.31).

5.8.3   *The cyclic GMP-gated cation channel*
The cyclic GMP-gated cation channel protein in the plasma membrane is composed of several subunits each with an estimated molecular

weight of about 65 kDa. The channel has a broad specificity for cations. In addition to Na$^+$, other monovalent cations, Ca^{2+} and some other divalent cations are admitted. In contrast to the voltage-dependent Na$^+$ and Ca^{2+} channels present in other cell types, the light-sensitive current in rod outer segments carried by Na$^+$ is not influenced by changes in membrane potential.

Cyclic GMP is an allosteric activator of the cation channels. Half-maximal activation is given by a concentration of 5–50 μM cyclic GMP. Each channel molecule possess two binding sites for the cyclic nucleotide. The binding of cyclic GMP to one site increases the affinity of the other site for the cyclic nucleotide so that the observed binding curve exhibits positive cooperativity.

Inactivation of the photoreceptor system requires inactivation of the activated rhodopsin molecule, inactivation of $\alpha_t{}'^{GTP}$ and the regeneration of cyclic GMP. After the absorption of a photon, the conformation of the rhodopsin molecule returns to the inactive state and the *trans* form of retinal is replaced by the 11-*cis* form. Under some conditions, rhodopsin is also inactivated by phosphorylation, catalysed by rhodopsin kinase. The active form of transducin, $\alpha_t{}'^{GTP}$, is inactivated by the hydrolysis of GTP. This is a relatively slow process which may take about a minute to reach completion. Cyclic GMP is regenerated by guanylate cyclase (Fig. 5.29). During the recovery period, the activity of guanylate cyclase is stimulated by the decrease in $[Ca^{2+}]_i$. The effect of Ca^{2+} is mediated by a 23 kDa Ca^{2+} binding protein called recoverin, which activates guanylate cyclase when $[Ca^{2+}]_i$ is low.

5.8.4   *Amplification of the cyclic GMP signal*
The rhodopsin–cyclic GMP system achieves a very large amplification of the initial signal. There are about 10^7 molecules of rhodopsin in one rod outer segment. It has been estimated

Cumulated
amplification

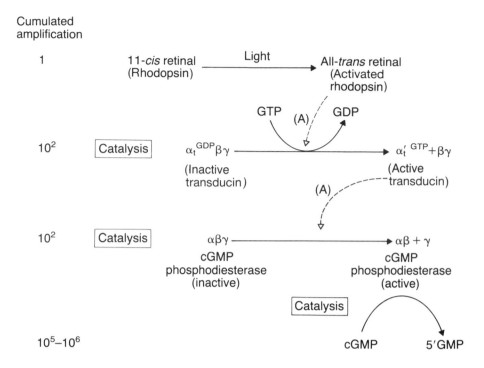

Fig. 5.32 The signal initiated by the interaction of one photon with 11-*cis* retinal in rhodopsin is magnified by a factor of between 10^5 and 10^6-fold by the steps which lie between rhodopsin and the hydrolysis of cyclic GMP (cGMP). This is due to the catalytic activities of activated rhodopsin, activated transducin ($\alpha_t'^{GTP}$), and activated cyclic GMP phosphodiesterase.

that the absorption of one photon by just one of these rhodopsin molecules reduces the permeability of the plasma membrane to Na^+ by about 3 per cent. This is equivalent to inhibition of the movement of about 10^7 Na^+ ions. This large amplification of the initial signal is achieved by the catalytic activities of activated rhodopsin and cyclic GMP phosphodiesterase (Fig. 5.32).

In one animal retina, about $10^3–10^4$ molecules of cyclic GMP are synthesized and hyrolysed per minute. This requires the consumption of milli-equivalents of ATP. The presence of this very large flux through the reactions catalysed by cyclic GMP phosphodiesterase and guanylate cyclase led Goldberg and his colleagues to propose that it is the change in the magnitude of this flux between cyclic GMP and 5' GMP, rather than the absolute concentration of cyclic GMP in the cytoplasmic space, which correlates with the change in current across the rod outer segment (Goldberg and Haddox 1977). However, there has been no further experimental support for this idea.

5.9 Summary

Two cyclic nucleotides, adenosine 3',5'-monophosphate (cyclic AMP) and guanosine 3',5'-monophosphate (cyclic GMP) act as intracellular messengers in animal cells. These molecules are unique in that unlike most other intracellular messengers, they play no other known role in biological systems apart from their function as intracellular messengers. Cyclic AMP has a widespread role as an intracellular messenger whereas the role of cyclic GMP is more restricted. The action of these intracellular cyclic nucleotides allows considerable amplification of extracellular signals.

Cyclic AMP is formed from ATP in the reaction catalysed by adenylate cyclase, and is degraded by cyclic AMP phosphodiesterase. Adenylate cyclase is inserted in the plasma membrane with its hydrophilic catalytic site on the cytoplasmic face of this membrane. There are at least two forms of adenylate cyclase, the (Ca^{2+} + calmodulin)-activated and (Ca^{2+} + calmodulin)-independent enzymes. The activities of both enzymes are regulated through receptors and GTP-binding regulatory proteins which stimulate or inhibit enzyme activity. The (Ca^{2+} + calmodulin)-activated enzyme is also regulated by changes in the intracellular free Ca^{2+} concentration ($[Ca^{2+}]_i$).

Regulation of the enzymes involved in the degradation of cyclic AMP is less well understood than the processes by which cyclic AMP is formed. Most cells possess a number of different forms of the enzyme cyclic AMP phosphodiesterase. These forms can be distinguished on the basis of differences in their ability to bind to the plasma membrane or other intracellular membranes, their affinities for cyclic AMP and cyclic GMP, their interaction with calmodulin, and their susceptibility to activation by insulin. Most types of cell possess at least one form of cyclic AMP phosphodiesterase which is bound to the plasma membrane and one form which is located elsewhere in the cytoplasmic space. The activities of different forms of cyclic AMP phosphodiesterase are regulated by the intracellular concentrations of cyclic AMP (through phosphorylation by cyclic AMP-dependent protein kinase), by $[Ca^{2+}]_i$, and by insulin. A number of organic compounds, including synthetic derivatives of cyclic AMP, caffeine, and other

xanthines, inhibit cyclic AMP phosphodiesterase. These inhibitors have proved invaluable in the elucidation of the role of cyclic AMP as an intracellular messenger.

Almost all the intracellular effects of cyclic AMP are mediated through the activation of cyclic AMP-dependent protein kinases. One exception is the action of cyclic AMP in olfactory cells in which the cyclic nucleotide binds to an allosteric site on a cation channel.

An increase in the concentration of cyclic GMP serves as an intracellular signal in the actions of atrial natriuretic peptide on smooth muscle, kidney, and other cells, sperm-activating peptides on sperm cells, endothelium-derived relaxing factor (EDRF) on smooth-muscle cells, and light on photoreceptor cells. In target cells for atrial natriuretic peptide and in the action of sperm-activating peptides, the concentration of cyclic GMP is controlled by a plasma-membrane guanylate cyclase. This enzyme is composed of a single polypeptide which possesses an extracellular domain which binds the agonist, a single membrane-spanning sequence, and an intracellular domain which possesses guanylate cyclase activity.

In smooth-muscle cells, EDRF binds to a cytoplasmic form of guanylate cyclase through a haem prosthetic group. In the cells which are targets for atrial natriuretic peptide, sperm-activating peptides, and EDRF, cyclic GMP exerts its effects through cyclic GMP-dependent protein kinase. In smooth-muscle cells this results in a decrease in $[Ca^{2+}]_i$ and relaxation of the muscle.

In photoreceptor cells a decrease in cyclic GMP acts as an intracellular signal. In these cells the interaction of light with rhodopsin in the disc membrane causes an activation of cyclic GMP phosphodiesterase through the agency of the GTP-binding regulatory protein, transducin. The resulting decrease in cyclic GMP causes a closure of cyclic GMP-activated Na^+ channels in the plasma membrane, a decrease in Na^+ inflow across the plasma membrane, and a depolarization of this membrane.

References

Ashman, D. F., Lipton, R., Melicow, M. M., and Price, T. D. (1963). Isolation of adenosine 3′,5′ monophosphate and guanosine 3′,5′-monophosphate from rat urine. *Biochem. Biophys. Res. Commun.*, **11**, 330–4.

Beavo, J. A., Rogers, N. L., Crofford, O. B., Hardman, J. G., Sutherland, E. W., and Newman, E. V. (1970). Effects of xanthine derivatives on lipolysis and on adenosine 3′,5′-monophosphate phosphodiesterase activity. *Mol. Pharmacol.*, **6**, 597–603.

Beebe, S. J., Holloway, R., Rannels, S. R., and Corbin, J. D. (1984). Two classes of cAMP analogs which are selective for the two different cAMP-binding sites of type II protein kinase demonstrate synergism when added together to intact adipocytes. *J. Biol. Chem.*, **259**, 3539–47.

Butcher, R. W. and Sutherland, E. W. (1962). Adenosine 3′,5′-phosphate in biological materials. 1. Purification and properties of cyclic 3′-5′-nucleotide phosphodiesterase and use of this enzyme to characterise adenosine 3′,5′-phosphate in human urine. *J. Biol. Chem.*, **237**, 1244–50.

Chader, G., Fletcher, R., Johnson, M., and Bensinger, R. (1974). Rod outer segment phosphodiesterase: factors affecting the hydrolysis of cyclic-AMP and cyclic-GMP. *Exp. Eye Res.*, **18**, 509–15.

Cori, G. T. and Cori, C. F. (1945). The enzymatic conversion of phosphorylase *a* to *b*. *J. Biol. Chem.*, **158**, 321–32.

Cote, R. H., Nicol, G. D., Burke, S. A., and Bownds, M. D. (1986). Changes in cGMP concentration correlate with some, but not all, aspects of the light-regulated conductance of frog rod photoreceptors. *J. Biol. Chem.*, **261**, 12965–75.

Exton, J. H., Robison, G. A., Sutherland, E. W., and Park, C. R. (1971). Studies on the role of adenosine 3′,5′-monophosphate in the hepatic actions of glucagon and catecholamines. *J. Biol. Chem.*, **246**, 6166–77.

Fell, D. A. (1980). Theoretical analyses of the functioning of the high- and low-K_M cyclic nucleotide phosphodiesterases in the regulation of the concentration of adenosine 3′,5′-cyclic monophosphate in animal cells. *J. Theor. Biol.*, **84**, 361–85.

Fesenko, E. E., Kolesnikov, S. S., and Lyubarsky, A. L. (1985). Induction by cyclic GMP of cationic conductance in plasma membrane of retinal rod outer segment. *Nature*, **313**, 310–13.

Fiscus, R. R., Rapoport, R. M., Waldman, S. A., and Murad, F. (1985). Atriopeptin II elevates cyclic GMP, activates cyclic GMP-dependent protein kinase and causes relaxation in rat thoracic aorta. *Biochim. Biophys. Acta*, **846**, 179–84.

Goldberg, N. D. and Haddox, M. K. (1977). Cyclic GMP metabolism and involvement in biological regulation. *Ann. Rev. Biochem.*, **46**, 823–96.

Goldberg, N. D., O'Dea, R. F., and Haddox, M. K. (1973). Cyclic GMP. *Adv. Cyclic Nucleotide Res.*, **3**, 155–223.

Krupinski, J., Coussen, F., Bakalyar, H. A., Tang, W-J., Feinstein, P. G., Orth, K., *et al.* (1989). Adenyl cyclase amino acid sequence: possible channel- or transporter-like structure. *Science*, **244**, 1558–64.

Lipkin, D., Markham, R., and Cook, W. H. (1959). The degradation of adenosine-5′-triphosphoric acid (ATP) by means of aqueous barium hydroxide. *J. Am. Chem. Soc.*, **81**, 6075–80.

Loten, E. G. and Sneyd, J. G. T. (1970). An effect of insulin on adipose-tissue adenosine 3′,5′-cyclic monophospate phosphodiesterase. *Biochem. J.*, **120**, 187–93.

Loten, E. G., Assimacopoulos-Jeannet, F. D., Exton, J. H., and Park, C. R. (1978). Stimulation of a low K_M phosphodiesterase from liver by insulin and glucagon. *J. Biol. Chem.*, **253**, 746–57.

Miki, N., Keirns, J. J., Marcus, F. R., Freeman, J., and Bitensky, M. W. (1973). Regulation of cyclic nucleotide concentrations in photoreceptors: an ATP-dependent stimulation of cyclic nucleotide phosphodiesterase by light. *Proc. Natl Acad. Sci. USA*, **70**, 3820–4.

Pyne, N. J., Cooper, M. E., and Houslay, M. D. (1987). The insulin- and glucagon-stimulated 'dense-vesicle' high-affinity cyclic AMP phosphodiesterase from rat liver. *Biochem. J.*, **242**, 33–42.

Rall, T. W., Sutherland, E. W., and Wosilait, W. D. (1956). The relationship of epinephrine and glucagon to liver phosphorylase III. Reactivation of liver phosphorylase in slices and in extracts. *J. Biol. Chem.*, **218**, 483–95.

Rall, T. W., Sutherland, E. W., and Berthet, J. (1957). The relationship of epinephrine and glucagon to liver phosphorylase. IV. Effects of epinephrine and glucagon on the reactivation of phosphorylase in liver homogenates. *J. Biol. Chem.*, **224**, 463–75.

Reeves, M. L., Leigh, B. K., and England, P. J. (1987). The identification of a new cyclic nucleotide phosphodiesterase activity in human and guinea-pig cardiac ventricle. *Biochem. J.*, **241**, 535–41.

Rosenberg, G. B. and Storm, D. R. (1987). Immunological distinction between calmodulin-sensitive and calmodulin-insensitive adenylate cyclases. *J. Biol. Chem.*, **262**, 7623–8.

Singh, S., Lowe, D. G., Thorpe, D. S., Rodriguez, H., Kuang, W-J., Dangott, L. J., *et al.* (1988). Membrane guanylate cyclase is a cell surface receptor with homology to protein kinases. *Nature*, **334**, 708–12.

Strada, S. J., Martin, M. W., and Thompson, W. J. (1984). General properties of multiple molecular forms of cyclic nucleotide phosphodiesterase in the nervous system. *Adv. Cyclic Nucleotide Prot. Phosphory. Res.*, **16**, 13–29.

Sutherland, E. W. and Rall, T. W. (1958). Fractionation and characterisation of a cyclic adenine ribonucleotide formed by tissue particles. *J. Biol. Chem.*, **232**, 1077–91.

Walsh, D. A., Perkins, J. P., and Krebs, E. G. (1968). An adenosine 3′,5′-monophosphate–dependent protein kinase from rabbit skeletal muscle. *J. Biol. Chem.*, **243**, 3763–5.

Winquist, R. J., Faison, E. P., Waldman, S. A., Schwartz, K., Murad, F., and Rapoport, R. M. (1984). Atrial natriuretic factor elicits an endothelium-independent relaxation and activates particulate guanylate cyclase in vascular smooth muscle. *Proc. Natl Acad. Sci. USA*, **81**, 7661–4.

Further reading

Casperson, G. F. and Bourne, H. R. (1987). Biochemical and molecular genetic analysis of hormone-sensitive adenylyl cyclase. *Ann. Rev. Pharmacol. Toxicol.*, **27**, 371–84.

Hurley, J. B. (1987). Molecular properties of the cGMP cascade of vertebrate photoreceptors. *Ann. Rev. Physiol.*, **49**, 793–812.

Ignarro, L. J. and Kadowitz, P. J. (1985). The pharmacological and physiological role of cyclic GMP in vascular smooth muscle relaxation. *Ann. Rev. Pharmacol. Toxicol.*, **25**, 171–91.

Owen, W. G. (1987). Ionic conductances in rod photoreceptors. *Ann. Rev. Physiol.*, **49**, 743–64.

Robison, G. A., Butcher, R. W., and Sutherland, E. W. (1971). *Cyclic AMP*. Academic Press, New York.

Ross, E. M. and Gilman, A. G. (1980). Biochemical properties of hormone-sensitive adenylate cyclase. *Ann. Rev. Biochem.*, **49**, 533–64.

Schnapf, J. L. and Baylor, D. A. (1987). How photoreceptor cells respond to light. *Sci. Am.*, **256**, 32–9.

Schulz, S., Chinkers, M., and Garbers, D. L. (1989). The guanylate cyclase/receptor family of proteins. *FASEB J.*, **3**, 2026–35.

Yau, K.-W. and Baylor, D. A. (1989). Cyclic GMP-activated conductance of retinal photoreceptor cells. *Ann. Rev. Neurosci.*, **12**, 289–327.

6 *The inositol polyphosphates and diacylglycerols*

6.1 Inositol 1,4,5-trisphosphate and *sn*-1,2-diacylglycerols as intracellular messengers in animal cells

The roles of *myo* inositol 1,4,5-trisphosphate (Ins 1,4,5 P_3) and *sn*-1,2-diacylglycerols (Fig. 6.1) as intracellular messengers in animal cells have been elucidated only during the past seven years. Although the mechanisms of action of these two intracellular messengers differ considerably, they are considered together for two reasons. Firstly, for a number of plasma membrane receptors, increases in Ins 1,4,5 P_3 and diacylglycerol are both required in the process by which the receptor induces an intracellular response. Secondly, the same enzyme, phosphatidylinositol 4,5-bisphosphate (PtdIns 4,5 P_2)-specific phospholipase C, often catalyses the for-

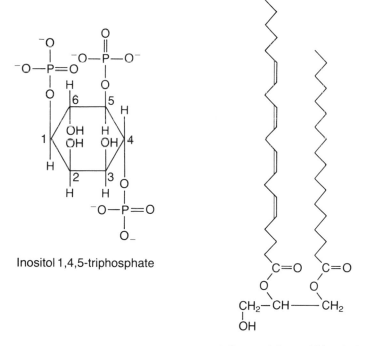

Inositol 1,4,5-triphosphate

sn-1-Stearoyl-2-arachidonyl glycerol

Fig. 6.1 The water-soluble intracellular messenger inositol 1,4,5-trisphosphate (Ins 1,4,5 P_3) and the lipid-soluble messenger *sn*-1-stearoyl-2-arachidonyl glycerol, one of a number of *sn*-1,2-diacylglycerols with intracellular messenger function. The numbers refer to the position of the carbon atoms in the inositol ring.

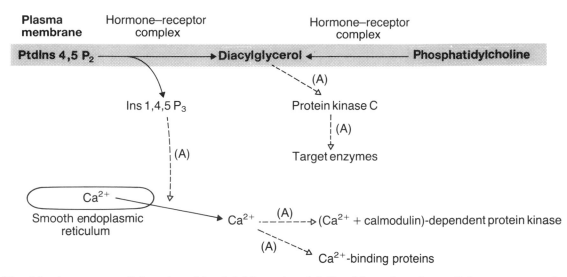

Fig. 6.2 A summary of the roles of Ins 1,4,5 P_3 and *sn*-1,2-diacylglycerols as intracellular messengers. Ins 1,4,5 P_3 is formed by the hydrolysis of PtdIns 4,5 P_2 located in the cytoplasmic leaflet of the phospholipid bilayer of the plasma membrane. Diacylglycerols are formed by the hydrolysis of PtdIns 1,4 P_2, phosphatidylcholine, and other non-inositol phospholipids also located in the cytoplasmic leaflet of the phospholipid bilayer. Ins 1,4,5 P_3 binds to the endoplasmic reticulum and induces the release of Ca^{2+} from this organelle. Diacylglycerol activates protein kinase C at the cytoplasmic face of the plasma membrane. The symbol (A) represents the activation of an enzyme or Ca^{2+} channel.

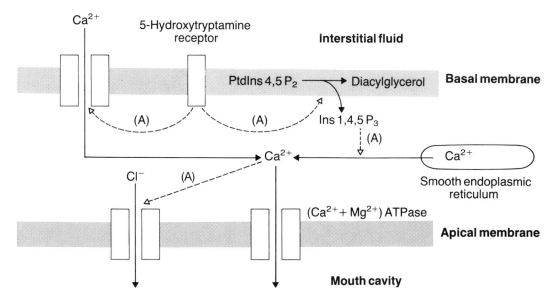

Fig. 6.3 Stimulation of fluid secretion by 5-hydroxytryptamine in the blowfly salivary gland. Ins 1,4,5 P_3, formed as a result of the combination of 5-hydroxytryptamine with plasma-membrane receptors, increases the $[Ca^{2+}]_i$ which, in turn, stimulates the movement of Cl^- out of the cell across the apical membrane. This anion, together with water and other ions, constitutes the fluid secreted by the salivary gland in response to 5-hydroxytryptamine. Some of the Ca^{2+} which enters the cytoplasmic space is transported across the apical membrane by a $(Ca^{2+} + Mg^{2+})$ATPase. The symbol (A) represents the activation of an enzyme or ion channel.

mation of both Ins 1,4,5 P_3 and diacylglycerol.

The role of Ins 1,4,5 P_3 as an intracellular messenger can be briefly summarized as follows. Ins 1,4,5 P_3 is released into the cytoplasmic space following hydrolysis within the plasma membrane of PtdIns 4,5 P_2 (Fig. 6.2). Ins 1,4,5 P_3 releases Ca^{2+} from the endoplasmic reticulum resulting in a transient increase in the cytoplasmic free Ca^{2+} concentration ($[Ca^{2+}_i]$) which, through the combination of Ca^{2+} with Ca^{2+}-binding proteins, induces a cellular response (Fig. 6.2). For example, in the salivary gland of the blowfly the Ca^{2+} released from the endop-lasmic reticulum by Ins 1,4,5 P_3 stimulates Cl^- outflow across the apical membrane (Fig. 6.3). The movements of Cl^-, other ions, and water contribute to fluid secretion from the apical membrane. Agonists which induce Ins 1,4,5 P_3 formation in the salivary gland also enhance Ca^{2+} inflow across the plasma membrane (Chapter 7, Section 7.7.1).

Diacylglycerols are formed in the inner leaflet of the plasma membrane by the hydrolysis of phospholipids, of which PtdIns 4,5 P_2 and phosphatidylcholine are the most important (Fig. 6.2). In the presence of increased $[Ca^{2+}]_i$, the affi-

Table 6.1 *Cellular responses which require the action of inositol 1,4,5-trisphosphate as an intracellular messenger*

Cellular response	Stimulus	Cell
Secretion		
Amylase	Cholecystokinin Acetylcholine	Pancreatic acinar
Fluid	5-Hydroxytryptamine	Insect salivary gland
Prolactin	Thyrotropin-releasing hormone	Pituitary
Insulin	Glucose	Pancreatic β-cell
Neurotransmitter release	Membrane depolarization	Nerve cells
Shape change and aggregation	Thrombin Collagen Thromboxane A_2 5-Hydroxytryptamine (5-HT_1)	Platelets
Defence actions of white blood cells		
Phagocytosis, degranulation, respiratory burst	Chemotactic peptides	Neutrophils (polymorphonuclear leucocytes)
Prostaglandin synthesis	Zymogens	Macrophages
Regulation of metabolism		
Glycogenolysis	Adrenalin (α_1-adrenergic) Vasopressin (V_1) Angiotensin II	Liver
Muscle contraction	Noradrenalin	Smooth muscle
Cell growth and proliferation		
Synthesis of DNA and proteins	Fibroblast-derived growth factor Platelet-derived growth factor	Fibroblasts (e.g. cultured Swiss 3T3 cells)
Detection of light		
Membrane depolarization	Absorption of light by rhodopsin	Photoreceptor
Fertilization		
Cortical granule exocytosis	Interaction with sperm cell	Unfertilized egg

Table 6.2 *Intracellular processes which require the action of diacylglycerol as an intracellular messenger*

Intracellular process	Examples of target proteins for diacylglycerol-activated protein kinase C
Regulation of receptor function	
Protein–tyrosine kinase receptors	Receptors for EGF, insulin
Receptors linked to GTP-binding proteins	β-adrenergic receptors
Regulation of concentration of intracellular messengers	
Ca^{2+}	Voltage-operated Ca^{2+} channels
	$(Ca^{2+} + Mg^{2+})$ATPase Ca^{2+} transporters
Cyclic GMP	Guanylate cyclase
Plasma-membrane ion transport	$Na^{+} - H^{+}$ exchange system
	$(Na^{+} + K^{+})$ATPase
	Nicotinic acetylcholine receptor (Na^{+} movement)
Muscle contraction and movement of cytoskeleton	Myosin light chains
	Myosin light-chain kinase
	Cytoskeletal proteins
Protein syntheses	Ribosomal S6 protein
	DNA methylase
	Initiation factor 2
RNA synthesis	Phorbol ester-responsive-sequence-specific DNA-binding protein
Metabolic pathways	Regulatory enzymes of glycogenolysis and glycolysis
	Glucose transport
	Tyrosine hydroxylase (neurotransmitter release)

nity of the cytoplasmic face of the plasma membrane for protein kinase C is increased. Upon binding to phospholipids and diacylglycerol in the plasma membrane the protein kinase undergoes a conformational change so that the active site becomes available to interact with target proteins.

In comparison with the cyclic nucleotides, Ca^{2+} and Ins 1,4,5 P_3, there are a number of unusual features in the role of diacylglycerols as intracellular messengers. The presence of these features has complicated elucidation of the role of diacylglycerols as intracellular messengers and their mechanism of action.

Whereas almost all other known intracellular messengers are water soluble, the hydrophobic diacylglycerols are confined to the lipid environ-

ment of membranes. Like other lipids, the only ways in which diacylglycerols can move from one region of a cell to another are by diffusion within the plane of the plasma membrane or by transport through the cytoplasmic space as a complex with a lipid transfer protein, or as a component of a lipoprotein vesicle, a secretory vesicle, or an endocytotic vesicle. This means that the movement of diacylglycerol as an intracellular messenger in cells is far more restricted than that of cyclic nucleotides, Ca^{2+}, and Ins 1,4,5 P_3.

In contrast to the cyclic nucleotides and Ins 1,4,5 P_3, the only cellular functions of which are to act as intracellular messengers, the *sn*-1,2-diacylglycerols function as intermediates in the synthesis of phospholipids and triacylglycerols as well as being intracellular messengers. The differences between diacylglycerol and the other intracellular messengers are also reflected in the range of structures which effectively act as intracellular messengers. Variations in the structures of the cyclic nucleotides and Ins 1,4,5 P₃ lead to molecules with markedly reduced effectiveness as intracellular messengers. On the other hand, it seems that many species of diacylglycerols, which differ in the nature of their fatty acid chains, can act as intracellular messengers.

Ins 1,4,5 P₃ is employed as an intracellular messenger in a large number of cellular responses induced by agonists. Some examples of these are shown in Table 6.1. Some of the consequences of the action of Ins 1,4,5 P₃, such as the provision of Ca^{2+} which activates vesicle secretion, are common to different types of cells whilst others are observed in only one or a few cell types. Ins 1,4,5 P₃ conveys information for cell responses which are chiefly rapid in onset and involve changes in the structure of the cytoskeleton and its interaction with cellular membranes.

In contrast to Ins 1,4,5 P₃, diacylglycerol and protein kinase C chiefly convey information for cell responses which are slow in onset and involve longer-term changes in cell growth, proliferation, differentiation, and in movement of the cytoskeleton. Some examples of the roles of protein kinase C in these processes are shown in Table 6.2. Diacylglycerol also plays a major role in the regulation of other pathways of intracellular communication (Table 6.2).

This chapter will be concerned with more details of the reactions involved in the formation and removal of Ins 1,4,5 P₃ and the diacylglycerols, and the mechanisms by which these intracellular messengers act. Since the discovery of the intracellular messenger roles of Ins 1,4,5 P₃ and diacylglycerol in animal cells represents an interesting episode in the development of knowledge of cell biology, this will be considered first.

6.2 Discovery of the roles of inositol trisphosphate and diacylglycerol as intracellular messengers

The first indication that inositol phospholipids are involved in intracellular signal transduction in animal cells came from the observations of L. and M. Hokin in 1953. They showed that acetylcholine stimulates the incorporation of [³²P]HPO₄⁻ into phospholipids in pancreatic acinar cells (Fig. 6.4). This result was interpreted as a stimulation by acetylcholine of the synthesis of phospholipid. Further experiments showed that phosphatidylinositol (PtdIns) was the major phospholipid involved.

The significance and implications of the results obtained by the Hokins, and of the observations by others of similar phenomena in other

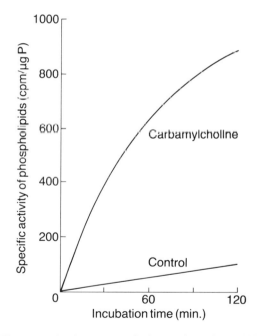

Fig. 6.4 The first reported observation of the ability of certain agonists to increase the turnover of PtdIns in animal cells. The addition of acetylcholine to pancreatic acinar cells labelled with [³²P]HPO₄⁻ causes a large increase in the rate of [³²P] incorporation into phospholipids, chiefly phosphatidylinositol. From Hokin and Hokin (1953).

cell types, were not realized until many years later. This was partly because it was thought by many investigators that cyclic AMP and cyclic GMP were the main, and possibly only, intracellular messengers in animal cells. These cyclic nucleotides were discovered at about the same time as the Hokins first observed agonist-induced phosphoinositide turnover. During the period 1970 to 1975, it became apparent that for many agonists which bind to receptors on the plasma membrane, cyclic AMP is not responsible for conveying information from the plasma membrane to intracellular sites. At the same time, indirect evidence which indicated that changes in intracellular Ca^{2+} concentration are essential for the actions of many of these agonists was obtained.

In the period between 1970 and 1975, Durell, De Robertis and Michell and their colleagues performed a series of experiments which led to the idea that agonist-stimulated PtdIns hydrolysis causes an increase in plasma membrane Ca^{2+} inflow which, in turn, increases $[Ca^{2+}]_i$ (Durell; *et al.* 1969; De Robertis 1971; Lapetina and Michell 1973; Michell 1975). Experiments to test this proposal directly were difficult to perform and were not conducted immediately.

Consequently the nature of the proposed link between phosphoinositides and Ca^{2+} movement remained obscure for several more years. The question being investigated became more complex when it was shown that many agonists cause not only an increase in plasma-membrane Ca^{2+} inflow but also induce the release of Ca^{2+} from intracellular stores.

An important but less widely recognized step in the development of ideas about the role of inositol lipids in intracellular communication came from the experiments of Fain and Berridge in Cambridge. They showed that the ability of 5-hydroxytryptamine to stimulate Ca^{2+} movement across the plasma membrane of blowfly salivary glands was greatly diminished by prior

depletion of the inositol content of the glands (Fain and Berridge 1979). Responses to 5-hydroxytryptamine could be restored by addition of exogenous inositol. This suggested that inositol metabolites play an essential role in the action of 5-hydroxytryptamine. At about that time, Abdel-Latif and his colleagues, and Michell and Kirk, working with iris smooth muscle and liver, respectively, showed that agonists which use Ca^{2+} as an intracellular messenger induce the rapid hydrolysis of PtdIns 4,5 P_2 and phosphatidylinositol 4-phosphate (PtdIns 4 P) as well as the hyrolysis of PtdIns (Abdel-Latif *et al.* 1977; Michell *et al.* 1981).

The observation that a number of agonists stimulate PtdIns 4,5 P_2 hydrolysis helped to focus attention on the unique chemistry of the inositol polyphosphate head-group. In pursuing this further, Berridge (1983) observed that in the blowfly salivary gland, 5-hydroxytryptamine increases the intracellular concentration of inositol trisphosphates together with the concentrations of inositol bis- and monophosphates. Streb, Berridge, Irvine, and Shultz then showed that in permeabilized pancreatic acinar cells, Ins 1,4,5 P_3 facilitates the outflow of Ca^{2+} from an intracellular store (Streb *et al.* 1983). This observation has now been repeated with many other cell types, and the site of Ca^{2+} release shown to be most likely a component of the endoplasmic reticulum.

While early ideas on the roles of Ca^{2+} and phosphoinositides in intracellular communication were developing, Nishizuka and his colleagues discovered a protein kinase that requires Ca^{2+} and phospholipid for activity (Inoue *et al.* 1977). This was originally called Ca^{2+} and phospholipid-dependent protein kinase and is now called protein kinase C. Nishizuka's group observed that diacylglycerols and tumour-promoting phorbol esters are potent activators of this protein kinase (Kishimoto *et al.* 1980; Kikkawa *et al.* 1983). They proposed that diacylglycerols, formed from the hydrolysis of PtdIns 4,5 P_2 as a result of agonist action, activate protein kinase C (Kishimoto *et al.* 1980).

6.3   The formation of inositol trisphosphate

6.3.1   *The polyphosphoinositides*
The species of phosphoinositides which have been identified in animal cells are PtdIns, PtdIns 4 P, PtdIns 4,5 P_2 and very small amounts of PtdIns 3 P, PtdIns 3,4 P_2 and PtdIns 3,4,5 P_3. The structure of PtdIns 4,5 P_2 is shown in Fig. 6.5. PtdIns 3,4 P_2 and PtdIns 3,4,5 P_3 are only detected in cells stimulated by a growth factor, for example PDGF, insulin, or CSF-1, or in cells, such as cultured mouse 3T3 fibroblasts, transformed with the *src* oncogene which, as described in Chapter 4 (Section 4.8), encodes a protein–tyrosine kinase. The *src* oncogene is present in polyoma virus and in the Rous sarcoma virus.

Accurate values for the amounts of PtdIns 4 P and PtdIns 4,5 P_2 present in cells and tissues have been difficult to obtain. This is chiefly due to the acidic nature of these phospholipids, which has made quantitative extraction difficult, and to the rapid hydrolysis of phospho–ester bonds during the initial stages of extraction. In brain, the amount of PtdIns is about 3 per cent of total lipid phosphorus while the amounts of PtdIns 4 P and PtdIns 4,5 P_2 are about 0.6 and 2.6 per cent of total lipid phosphorus, respectively. Similar values have been obtained for other cell types. The amount of PtdIns 3 P present in unstimulated cells is about 3 per cent of the amount of PtdIns 4 P.

The precise intracellular location of the phosphoinositides has also been difficult to determine in an unequivocal manner. Nevertheless, it seems that the phosphoinositides are principally located in the plasma membrane although they have also been detected in other membranes such as the nuclear membrane and the membranes of secretory vesicles.

Some investigators have proposed that PtdIns 4,5 P_2 located in the inner leaflet of the phospholipid bilayer of the plasma membrane may bind Ca^{2+} and provide a store of Ca^{2+} which could be released upon agonist-stimulated hydrolysis of the polyphosphoinositide. At the pH of the cytoplasmic space (about pH 7.2) there are approximately four negative charges on the hydrophilic domain of PtdIns 4,5 P_2. These would allow this phosphoinositide to bind Ca^{2+}, Mg^{2+} or other divalent cations. However, the proposal that PtdIns 4,5 P_2 binds significant amounts of Ca^{2+} in an intact cell is considered unlikely since the concentration of free Mg^{2+} in the cytoplasmic space (1.0 mM) is approximately 10 000 times that of free Ca^{2+} (0.1 μM). This means that in the ionic milieux of the cytoplasmic space the predominant divalent cation bound to PtdIns 4,5 P_2 is likely to be Mg^{2+}.

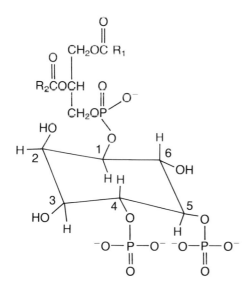

Fig. 6.5   The structure of phosphatidylinositol 4,5-bisphosphate (PtdIns 4,5 P_2). The fatty-acid moiety at position 1 (R_1) is predominantly stearic acid whilst that at position 2 (R_2) is predominantly arachidonic acid. The numbers refer to the position of the carbon atoms in the inositol ring.

6.3.2 *The hydrolysis of polyphosphoinositides*

Ins 1,4,5 P_3 is formed from PtdIns 4,5 P_2 in the reaction catalysed by PtdIns 4,5 P_2-specific phospholipase C (Fig. 6.2). This reaction occurs on the cytoplasmic face of the plasma membrane. Changes in the concentrations of PtdIns 4,5 P_2 and Ins 1,4,5 P_3 have been measured using cells in which the phospholipids have been labelled with either $[^{32}P]HPO_4^-$ or $[^3H]$inositol. Agonist-induced increases in Ins 1,4,5 P_3 are accompanied by increases in inositol bis- and monophosphates (Fig. 6.6). In many cell types, agonists induce a substantial decrease in PtdIns 4,5 P_2, PtdIns 4 P and PtdIns (Fig. 6.7). In some cell types, two functionally distinct pools of each phosphoinositide have been detected. Phosphoinositides in only one of these pools are hydrolysed as a result of the action of agonists.

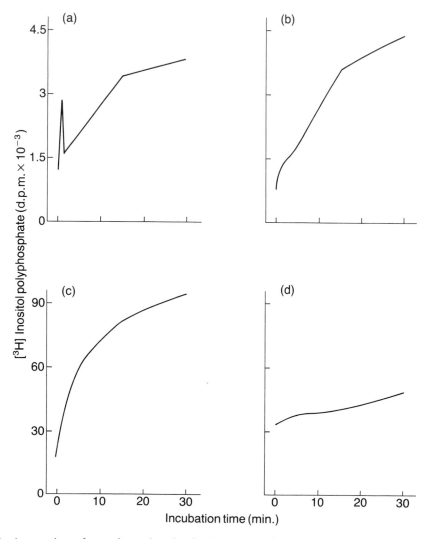

Fig. 6.6 The interaction of gonadotropin-releasing hormone with cultured pituitary ganadotrophs increases the intracellular concentrations of (a) Ins 1,4,5 P_3, (b) Ins 1,4 P_2, (c) Ins 4 P, and (d) Ins 1 P. The inositol polyphosphates have been detected using cells labelled with $[^3H]$inositol. From Morgan *et al.* (1987).

The decreases in PtdIns 4 P and PtdIns which are observed following the binding of an agonist to a receptor coupled to phosphoinositide hydrolysis are caused by the phosphorylation of PtdIns and PtdIns 4 P and probably also by the hydrolysis of PtdIns and PtdIns 4 P. The

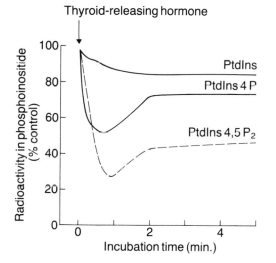

Fig. 6.7   The addition of thyroid-releasing hormone to cultures of GH_3 pituitary cells labelled with [³H]inositol decreases the concentrations of [³H]-labelled PtdIns 4, 5 P_2, PtdIns 4 P and PtdIns. From Rebecchi and Gershengorn (1983).

phosphorylation reactions are described later in Section 6.5.1. The hydrolytic reactions, which are shown in Fig. 6.8, are catalysed by phosphoinositide-specific phospholipases C and yield Ins 1 P and Ins 1,4 P_2 as well as diacylglycerols.

In many cells, increases in inositol 1,4,5-trisphosphate and inositol bis- and monophosphates are accompanied by increases in cyclic forms of the inositol polyphosphates. The major cyclic species are inositol 1,2-(cyclic) 4,5-trisphosphate (Ins 1,2-(cyclic)4,5 P_3), the structure of which is shown in Fig. 6.9, inositol 1,2-(cyclic) 4-bisphosphate (Ins 1,2-(cyclic)4 P_2) and inositol 1,2-(cyclic) phosphate (Ins 1,2-(cyclic)P). Ins 1,2-(cyclic)4,5 P_3 is formed from PtdIns 4,5 P_2 in the reaction catalysed by the same PtdIns 4,5 P_2-specified phospholipase C which generates non-cyclic Ins 1,4,5 P_3 (Fig. 6.10). About 5 per cent of the PtdIns 4,5 P_2 hydrolysed yields Ins 1,2-(cyclic)4,5 P_3 while about 95 per cent yields Ins 1,4,5 P_3. Ins 1,2-(cyclic)4 P_2 and Ins 1,2-(cyclic)P are formed by dephosphorylation of Ins 1,2-(cyclic)4,5 P_3 as described later, and can also be formed in association with the generation of Ins 1,4 P_2 and Ins 1 P in the actions of phospholipases C on PtdIns 4 P and PtdIns. With the

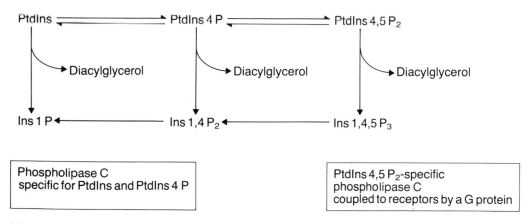

Fig. 6.8   In platelets and in some other types of cells, agonists which increase Ins 1,4,5 P_3 and $[Ca^{2+}]_i$ induce the hydrolysis of PtdIns and PtdIns 4 P as well as the hydrolysis of PtdIns 4,5 P_2. Some experiments indicate that the phospholipase C which hydrolyses PtdIns and PtdIns 4 P differs from PtdIns 4,5 P_2-specific phospholipase C in that it is probably activated by an increase in $[Ca^{2+}]_i$ rather than by a GTP-binding regulatory protein coupled to a receptor.

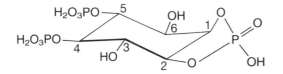

Fig. 6.9 Inositol 1,2-(cyclic)4,5 P_3, a minor product of the hydrolysis of PtdIns 4,5 P_2. The numbers refer to the position of the carbon atoms in the inositol ring.

possible exception of Ins 1,2-(cyclic)4,5 P_3, which, as described below, can release Ca^{2+} from the endoplasmic reticulum, the cyclic inositol polyphosphates probably do not have a physiological function.

6.3.3　*Phosphatidylinositol 4,5 P_2-specific phospholipase C*

Several phosphoinositol-specific phospholipases C which can hydrolyse PtdIns 4,5 P_2 have been detected in most types of cell. Many of the forms of this enzyme which have been purified so far are soluble proteins but there are also a number of membrane-bound phosphoinositide-specific phospholipases C. There are several different species of soluble PtdIns 4,5 P_2-specific phospholipases C. These have been designated as the α, β, γ, Δ, Σ, and ζ species. As described below, phospholipase $C_{γ-1}$ is activated by certain receptor protein–tyrosine kinases and probably by some protein–tyrosine kinases which do not

possess an extracellular or membrane spanning domain. The different species can be distinguished by differences in their molecular weight, isoelectric point, pH optimum, and dependence on Ca^{2+}. Some purified soluble PtdIns 4,5 P_2-specific phospholipases C have molecular weights in the range of 150 kDa while others have molecular weights in the range of 80 kDa. The difference in molecular weights may reflect differences in cell type from which the enzymes are derived, or modifications to the enzyme which occur during purification.

Regions of the amino-acid sequence of some PtdIns 4,5 P_2-specific phospholipases C are homologous with amino-acid sequences in some of the protein–tyrosine kinases encoded by oncogenes. These homologous regions may represent membrane binding sites. The purified soluble phosphoinositide-specific phospholipases C hydrolyse PtdIns 4,5 P_2, PtdIns 4 P and PtdIns. The rate of hydrolysis of PtdIns 4,5 P is often faster than that of PtdIns 4 P and PtdIns.

PtdIns 4,5 P_2-specific phospholipase C is probably bound to the cytoplasmic face of the plasma membrane. There are three mechanisms by which this enzyme is activated. These involve a GTP-binding-regulatory protein (G protein), phosphorylation by a protein–tyrosine kinase, or Ca^{2+} ions. G proteins which activate PtdIns 4,5 P_2-specific phospholipase C include the per-

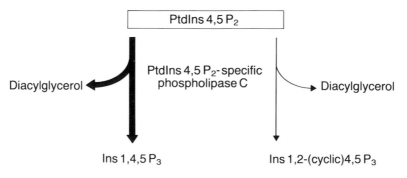

Fig. 6.10 Inositol 1,2-(cyclic)4,5 P_3 is formed in small amounts in association with the formation of Ins 1,4,5 P_3 during the hydrolysis of PtdIns 4,5 P_2 catalysed by PtdIns 4,5 P_2-specific phospholipase C.

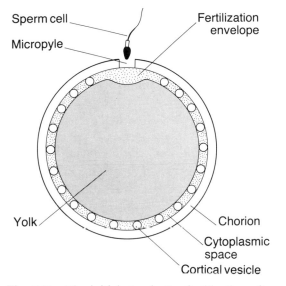

Sperm cell

Micropyle

Fertilization envelope

Yolk

Chorion

Cytoplasmic space

Cortical vesicle

Fig. 6.11 The initial step in the fertilization of an invertebrate egg. When the sperm cell crosses the chorion through the micropyle and enters the cytoplasmic space, a wave of cortical vesicle secretion is initiated. From Gilkey *et al.* (1978).

tussis toxin-sensitive protein G_o and the pertussis toxin-insensitive proteins G_z, G_q, and a novel pertussis toxin-insensitive G protein from liver. Presumably the interaction between G protein and phospholipase causes a conformational change in the phospholipase C which changes the orientation of the active site so that it can interact with PtdIns 4,5 P_2 in the inner leaflet of the plasma membrane. The role of G proteins in the activation of PtdIns 4,5 P_2-specific phospholipase C was described in Chapter 3 (Section 3.4).

The second mechanism involves the phosphorylation of PtdIns 4,5 P_2-specific phospholipase $C_{\gamma-1}$ by the protein–tyrosine kinase catalytic site of an activated receptor such as the PDGF and EGF receptors. Phosphorylation of the phospholipase $C_{\gamma-1}$ on a tyrosine residue leads to a change in the conformation of the protein

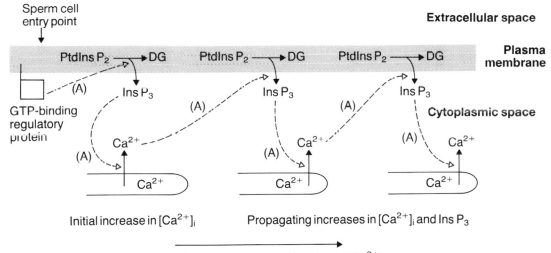

Sperm cell entry point

Extracellular space

PtdIns P_2 ⟶ DG   PtdIns P_2 ⟶ DG   PtdIns P_2 ⟶ DG

Plasma membrane

(A)   Ins P_3 Ins P_3 Ins P_3

GTP-binding regulatory protein

(A)   (A)

Cytoplasmic space

Ca^{2+} (A) Ca^{2+} (A) Ca^{2+}

(A)

Ca^{2+} Ca^{2+} Ca^{2+}

Initial increase in $[Ca^{2+}]_i$ Propagating increases in $[Ca^{2+}]_i$ and Ins P_3

Direction of propagated wave of Ins P_3 and $[Ca^{2+}]_i$

Fig. 6.12 A Ca^{2+}-induced increase in the concentration of Ins 1,4,5 P_3 (Ins P_3) is probably responsible for propagating the wave of increased $[Ca^{2+}]_i$ which travels through the cytoplasmic space of an invertebrate egg cell after fertilization. It is thought that the entry of the sperm cell activates a G protein which, in turn, activates a G protein-activated PtdIns 4,5 P_2-specific phospholipase C and induces the hydrolysis of PtdIns 4,5 P_2 to form an initial quantity of Ins 1,4,5 P_3. The resulting release of Ca^{2+} from nearby endoplasmic reticulum may increase $[Ca^{2+}]_i$ which, in turn, may activate a Ca^{2+}-activated phospholipase C which induces the hydrolysis of further PtdIns 4,5 P_2, the formation of Ins 1,4,5 P_3, and the release of further Ca^{2+}. This generates a wave of increased Ins 1,4,5 P_3 concentration and a wave of increased $[Ca^{2+}]_i$ which move through the cytoplasmic space. Only hydrolysis of PtdIns 4,5 P_2 at the point of entry of the sperm cell is thought to be dependent on a G protein. The symbol (A) represents the activation of an enzyme or Ca^{2+} channel and DG represents diacylglycerol.

and activation of the catalytic site. Regulation of PtdIns 4,5 P_2 hydrolysis by phospholipase $C_{\gamma\text{-}1}$ may also involve profilin, an actin-binding protein which binds PtdIns 4,5 P_2.

The agonist-stimulated phospholipase C which hydrolyses PtdIns 4,5 P_2 in cells requires Ca^{2+} as a cofactor. However, most forms of the enzyme are maximally active at the $[Ca^{2+}]_i$ present in the unstimulated cell (about 0.1 μM) so that the activation by an agonist of these enzyme species does not require an increase in $[Ca^{2+}]_i$ above the basal value.

Some types of cell contain a different type of PtdIns 4,5 P_2-specific phospholipase C. This enzyme is probably not activated by a G protein or phosphorylation but is activated by an increase in $[Ca^{2+}]_i$. Cells which possess this form of the enzyme include the pancreatic β-cell, in which an increase in glucose concentration initiates the hydrolysis of PtdIns 4,5 P_2, and the egg cells of invertebrates.

The entry of a sperm cell to the egg results in the formation of a fertilization envelope which begins at the point of entry of the sperm (Fig. 6.11) and eventually completely surrounds the egg. The envelope is created by the exocytosis of cortical granules which is induced by an increase in $[Ca^{2+}]_i$. The increase in $[Ca^{2+}]_i$ is propagated as a wave which moves through the cytoplasmic space of the egg cell.

There are two mechanisms by which PtdIns 4,5 P_2 hydrolysis is stimulated during the fertilization of an egg cell. Entry of the sperm cell probably activates a G protein which, in turn, stimulates the hydrolysis of PtdIns 4,5 P_2 to form Ins 1,4,5 P_3 and diacylglycerol (Fig. 6.12). Propagation of the wave of increased $[Ca^{2+}]_i$ is thought to be caused by the activation by Ca^{2+} of a Ca^{2+}-activated PtdIns 4,5 P_2-specific phospholipase C. This generates a Ca^{2+}-induced wave of increased Ins 1,4,5 P_3 concentration which propagates the wave of increased $[Ca^{2+}]_i$ (Fig. 6.12).

6.4 The metabolism of inositol trisphosphate

6.4.1 *The dephosphorylation pathway*

Two pathways are responsible for decreasing the intracellular concentration of Ins 1,4,5 P_3. These are the removal of phosphate moieties by hydrolysis and the addition of a phosphate group at position 3 of the inositol ring. Ins 1,4,5 P_3 is rapidly hydrolysed to inositol 1,4-bisphosphate (Ins 1,4 P_2) by Ins 1,4,5 P_3/Ins(1,3,4,5)P_4 5-phosphatase (Fig. 6.13). This enzyme is probably located on the cytoplasmic face of the plasma membrane. Ins 1,4,5 P_3/Ins 1,3,4,5 P_4 5-phosphatase requires Mg^{2+} as a cofactor and has an apparent K_M value for Ins 1,4,5 P_3 of about 30 μM. Inositol polyphosphate-1-phosphatase, which is located in the cytoplasmic space, removes the phosphate moiety at position 1 on the inositol ring of Ins 1,4 P_2 to yield inositol 4-monophosphate (Ins 4 P). This inositol monophosphate is, in turn, further hydrolysed to form inositol in the reaction catalysed by inositol monophosphate phosphatase (Fig. 6.13).

Inositol polyphosphate-1-phosphatase and

PtdIns 4,5 P_2

   ↓ PtdIns 4,5 P_2-specific phospholipase C

Ins 1,4,5 P_3

   ↓ Ins 1,4,5 P_3/Ins 1,3,4,5 P_3-5-phosphatase

Ins 1,4 P_2

Li^+ (I)
F^- (I) ↓ Inositol polyphosphate-1-phosphatase

Ins 4 P

Li^+ (I)
F^- (I) ↓ Inositol monophosphate phosphatase

Inositol

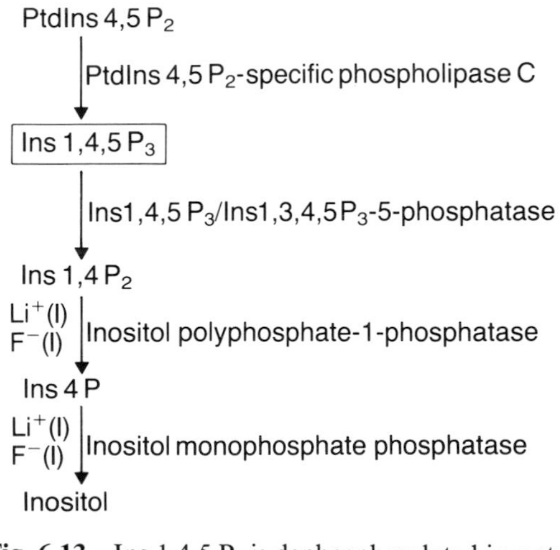

Fig. 6.13 Ins 1,4,5 P_3 is dephosphorylated in a stepwise manner by a series of phosphatases. Inositol polyphosphate-1-phosphatase and inositol monophosphate phosphatase are both inhibited (I) by Li^+ and F^-.

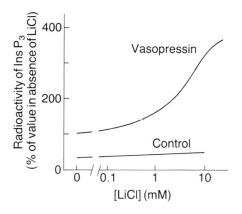

Fig. 6.14 Li$^+$ markedly enhances the increases in [^{3}H]-labelled inositol trisphosphates (Ins P$_3$) induced by the action of vasopressin on hepatocytes labelled with [^{3}H]inositol. From Thomas *et al.* (1984).

inositol monophosphate phosphatase are both inhibited by Li$^+$ and F$^-$ (Fig. 6.13). The effect of Li$^+$ was first observed in studies of inositol metabolism in brain cells (Allison and Stewart 1971; Allison *et al.* 1976; Sherman *et al.* 1981). The inclusion of Li$^+$ during the treatment of cells with an agonist which stimulates PtdIns 4,5 P$_2$ hydrolysis markedly increases the intracellular concentrations of inositol mono-, bis-, and tris-phosphates (Fig. 6.14), and decreases the concentration of inositol. In studies of the effects of agonists on cellular inositol polyphosphate concentrations, Li$^+$ is successfully used to magnify agonist-induced changes in these metabolites.

The enzymatic pathway by which Ins 1,2-(cyclic)4,5 P$_3$ is degraded involves first the successive hydrolysis of the non-cyclic phosphate ester moieties at positions 4 and 5 to form, successively, Ins 1,2-(cyclic)4 P$_2$ and Ins 1,2-(cyclic)P. The phosphate ester bond at position 2 is then hydrolysed with the formation of Ins 1 P, in the reaction catalysed by Ins 1,2(cyclic)P phosphodiesterase. Under the conditions of the cytoplasmic space the cyclic phosphate bond of Ins 1,2(cyclic)P appears to be stable so that hydrolysis of Ins 1,2(cyclic)P is principally due

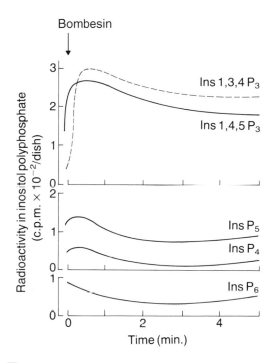

Fig. 6.15 In Swiss 3T3 fibroblasts labelled with [^{3}H]inositol, bombesin induces substantial increases in [^{3}H]Ins 1,4,5 P$_3$ and [^{3}H] Ins 1,3,4 P$_3$ and much smaller increases in [^{3}H]inositol tetraphosphates (Ins P$_4$) and in [^{3}H]inositol pentaphosphate (Ins P$_5$). There is no increase in [^{3}H] inositol hexaphosphate (Ins P$_6$). The increase in [^{3}H]Ins 1,4,5 P$_3$ precedes the increase in [^{3}H]Ins 1,3,4 P$_3$. From Heslop *et al.* (1986).

to this enzymatic reaction rather than the non-enzymatic action of cell water.

6.4.2 *The phosphorylation pathway*

The study of inositol polyphosphate metabolism in animal cells was greatly facilitated by the development of new methods for the chromatographic separation of these molecules. In the early studies, separation of the inositol polyphosphates was achieved by chromatography on columns of anion exchange resin, by high voltage paper electrophoresis, and by the method of descending paper chromatography originally developed by Grado and Ballou (1961). A high-pressure liquid chromatography (HPLC) system, based on anion-exchange column chromatography, was developed by Irvine and his colleagues (Heslop *et al.* 1985) in order to resolve inositol polyphosphates and their isomers more conveniently and more rapidly, and to provide a satisfactory system for the detection of other phosphorylated derivatives of inositol.

Two somewhat surprising observations were made when Irvine and Berridge and their colleagues applied the HPLC separation procedure to extracts of animal cells labelled with [^{3}H]inositol. Firstly, large amounts of the 1,3,4 isomer of inositol trisphosphate, as well as Ins 1,4,5 P_3, were detected (Irvine *et al.* 1984). Secondly, inositol 1,3,4,5-tetrakisphosphate (Ins 1,3,4,5 P_4), inositol pentaphosphate (Ins P_5) and inositol hexaphosphate (Ins P_6) were also found (Heslop *et al.* 1985). It is interesting to note that whilst inositol trisphosphates and higher phosphorylated forms of inositol have only recently been discovered in mammalian cells, the

presence of these compounds in plant cells and in avian red blood cells has been known for many years (Cosgrove 1980).

Agonists which activate PtdIns 4,5 P_2-specific phospholipase C cause substantial increases in Ins 1,3,4 P_3 as well as Ins 1,4,5 P_3 in target cells (Fig. 6.15). The increase in Ins 1,3,4 P_3 is slower in onset and is often greater in magnitude than that in Ins 1,4,5 P_3 (Fig. 6.15). Ins 1,3,4,5 P_4 and Ins P_5 also increase in response to agonists, although the changes are usually much smaller in magnitude than the increases in Ins 1,4,5 P_3 (Fig. 6.15). There is usually little change in the concentration of Ins P_6 (Fig. 6.15).

The observations on agonist-induced changes in higher inositol polyphosphates, together with the elucidation of the properties of the enzymes which metabolize these compounds, led to knowledge of the second pathway for the metabolism of Ins 1,4,5 P_3. This involves the phos-

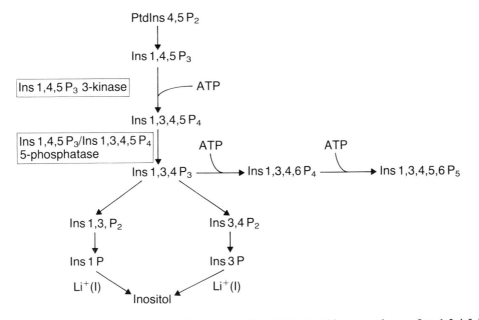

Fig. 6.16 The metabolism of Ins 1,4,5 P_3 through the Ins 1,4,5 P_3 3-kinase pathway. Ins 1,3,4,5 P_4, the product of the phosphorylation of Ins 1,4,5 P_3, is dephosphorylated to form another inositol trisphosphate isomer, Ins 1,3,4 P_3. This, in turn, is sequentially dephosphorylated to inositol in two alternative pathways. In the presence of an agonist which stimulates the hydrolysis of PtdIns 4,5 P_2, some Ins 1,3,4 P_3 is phosphorylated to form Ins 1,3,4,6 P_4 and Ins 1,3,4,5,6 P_5.

phorylation of Ins 1,4,5 P_3 at position 3 of the inositol ring to form Ins 1,3,4,5 P_4, in the reaction catalysed by Ins 1,4,5 P_3 3-kinase (Fig. 6.16). Ins 1,3,4 P_3 is formed by the dephosphorylation of Ins 1,3,4,5 P_4 in the reaction catalysed by Ins 1,4,5 P_3/Ins 1,3,4,5 P_4 5-phosphatase (Fig. 6.16), the same enzyme which removes phosphate from the 5 position of Ins 1,4,5 P_3. There are two alternative pathways for the dephosphorylation of Ins 1,3,4 P_3. The phosphate moiety at either position 1 or position 4 can be removed in reactions catalysed by inositol polyphosphate-1-phosphatase or inositol polyphosphate-4-phosphatase. Both Ins 1,3 P_2 and Ins 3,4 P_2 are further dephosphorylated in successive steps to yield free inositol.

The intracellular concentrations of IP_5 and IP_6 are about 1 mM. This is 100–1000 times the intracellular concentrations of the other inositol polyphosphates. The predominant species of IP_5 present in animal cells is Ins 1,3,4,5,6 P_5. IP_5 and IP_6 are probably formed from inositol by the successive addition of phosphate from ATP, in reactions which are catalysed by a series of

kinases, and separate from the pathways which metabolize Ins 1,4,5 P_3. However, some IP_5 may be formed from Ins 1,3,4 P_3 in reactions catalysed by Ins 1,3,4 P_3 6-kinase and Ins 1,3,4,6 P_4 5-kinase (Fig. 6.16).

6.4.3 *Regulation of inositol trisphosphate concentration*

The intracellular concentration of Ins 1,4,5 P_3 is controlled by the activities of the enzyme which catalyses its formation, PtdIns 4,5 P_2-specific phospholipase C, and the two enzymes which catalyse its removal, Ins 1,4,5 P_3/Ins 1,3,4,5 P_4 5-phosphatase and Ins 1,4,5 P_3 3-kinase (Fig. 6.17). The activities of Ins 1,4,5 P_3/Ins 1,3,4, P_4 5-phosphatase and Ins 1,4,5 P_3 3-kinase are regulated by protein kinase C and Ca^{2+}, respectively. The activity of the phosphatase is increased when the enzyme is phosphorylated (Fig. 6.17). Ins 1,4,5 P_3 3-kinase is activated by combination with the (Ca^{2+} + calmodulin) complex. The regulation of the phosphatase and kinase by protein kinase C and Ca^{2+}, respectively, is thought to constitute a negative-feed-

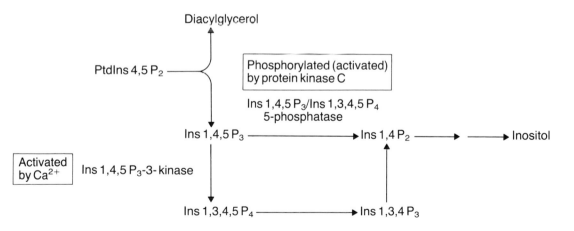

Fig. 6.17 The intracellular concentration of Ins 1,4,5 P_3 is controlled by the reaction which catalyses its formation, PtdIns 4,5 P_2-specific phospholipase C, and by the activities of the enzymes which remove it, Ins 1,4,5 P_3/Ins 1,3,4,5 P_4 5-phosphatase and Ins 1,4,5 P_3 3-kinase. The activity of Ins 1,4,5 P_3/Ins 1,3,4,5 P_4 5-phosphatase is increased by phosphorylation catalysed by protein kinase C. Ins 1,4,5 P_3 kinase is activated by the (Ca^{2+} + calmodulin) complex. These actions of protein kinase C and Ca^{2+} probably constitute a negative-feedback system which limits the duration of the transient increase in Ins 1,4,5 P_3.

back mechanism which limits the increase in the concentration of Ins 1,4,5 P_3 induced by an agonist. The effectiveness of these enzymes in removing Ins 1,4,5 P_3 is demonstrated by the observation that in cells, the half-life of exogenous Ins 1,4,5 P_3 is of the order of seconds, and the transient increase in endogenous Ins 1,4,5 P_3 induced by agonists is very short.

6.5 Regeneration of phosphatidylinositol 4,5-bisphosphate

6.5.1 *The phosphoinositide kinases*

The increase in inositol polyphosphates induced by agonists is maintained for periods of time which are longer than those over which the transient decrease in PtdIns 4,5 P_2 is observed. Moreover, the amount of PtdIns 4,5 P_2 present in the plasma membrane is small in relation to the rate of hydrolysis of this polyphosphoinositide in the presence of an agonist. PtdIns 4,5 P_2 is replenished by two mechanisms. These are utilization of the large reservoir of PtdIns as a precursor of PtdIns 4,5 P_2 and the re-synthesis of PtdIns

and PtdIns 4,5 P_2 from diacylglycerol and inositol.

Two separate kinases are responsible for the successive addition of two phosphate groups to PtdIns to form PtdIns 4 P and PtdIns 4,5 P_2 (Fig. 6.18). The phosphate moieties at positions D-4 and D-5 of the inositol ring of PtdIns 4,5 P_2 can be removed by two phosphomonoesterases (Fig. 6.18). These enzymes, together with the two kinases, catalyse the rapid interconversion of the three polyphosphoinositides. It is these reactions that are responsible for the incorporation of ^{32}P from $[^{32}P]ATP$ into polyphosphoinositides, which is observed when cells are incubated in the presence of $[^{32}P]HPO_4^-$ and an agonist which stimulates PtdIns 4,5 P_2 hydrolysis (Fig. 6.4).

Some cells also possess another phosphoinositide kinase called phosphoinositide 3-kinase. This enzyme phosphorylates the D-3 position of the inositol moiety of PtdIns, PtdIns 4 P and PtdIns 4,5 P_2 to form PtdIns 3 P, PtdIns 3,4 P_2 and PtdIns 3,4,5 P_3, respectively. As described earlier, only very small amounts of

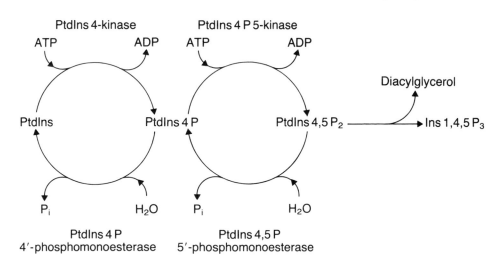

Fig 6.18 The content of PtdIns 4,5 P_2 in the plasma membrane is replenished by the successive phosphorylation of PtdIns and PtdIns 4 P. These reactions are catalysed by PtdIns 4-kinase and PtdIns 4 P 5-kinase, respectively. Cells also contain phosphatases which hydrolyse the phosphomonoester groups at position 5 of PtdIns 4,5 P_2 and position 4 of PtdIns 4 P.

phosphoinositides phosphorylated at the D-3 position are present in animal cells. Moreover, PtdIns 3,4 P_2 and PtdIns 3,4,5 P_3 have only been detected in cells stimulated by growth factors such as PDGF, insulin, CSF-1, or in cells transfected with the *src* oncogene. Phosphoinositide 3-kinase has been found to be very tightly associated with certain protein–tyrosine kinases, including the *src* kinase and the PDGF, insulin, and CSF-1 receptor kinases. The significance of phosphoinositide 3-kinase itself and of its association with the protein–tyrosine kinases is not known. Some investigators have suggested that phosphoinositide 3-kinase could be part of an undiscovered signalling pathway.

6.5.2   *Synthesis of phosphatidylinositol from diacylglycerol and inositol*

The phosphorylation of PtdIns just described contributes to the relatively slow decrease in the concentration of this phosphoinositide which is observed in the presence of an agonist. The supply of PtdIns in the plasma membrane is replenished by its re-synthesis from diacylglycerols and

inositol. The reactions involved in this re-synthesis, together with those for the degradation of Ins 1,4,5 P_3 and the interconversion of PtdIns and PtdIns 4,5 P_2, are shown in Fig. 6.19. These reactions constitute a cycle called the PtdIns cycle which was first detected in pancreatic acinar cells as an agonist-stimulated incorporation of [^{32}P]HPO$_4^-$ into phospholipids by Hokin and Hokin in 1953 (Fig. 6.4).

Diacylglycerol kinase (Fig. 6.19) is predominantly located at the plasma membrane whereas cytidine diphospho-diacylglycerol (CDP-diacylglycerol) synthetase and PtdIns synthetase are located at both the plasma membrane and the endoplasmic reticulum. It is thought that the conversion of a substantial proportion of diacylglycerol to PtdIns takes place near the plasma membrane. The actions of the enzymes at this intracellular location are supplemented by the conversion of phosphatidic acid to PtdIns at the smooth endoplasmic reticulum. The synthesis of PtdIns from phosphatidic acid at the endoplasmic reticulum requires the transport of phosphatidic acid from the plasma membrane to the

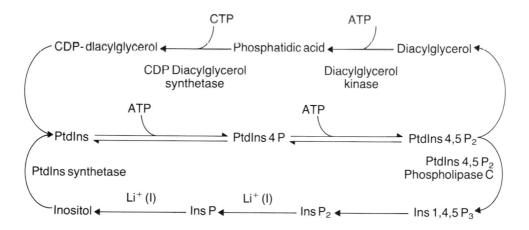

Fig 6.19   The pathway for the regeneration of PtdIns from inositol and diacylglycerol. This pathway is active during the stimulation by an agonist of PtdIns 4,5 P_2 hydrolysis and also during the subsequent phase of recovery after removal of the agonist. The scheme also shows the pathways for the dephosphorylation of Ins 1,4,5 P_3 and phosphorylation of PtdIns and PtdIns 4 P. The sum of all the reactions shown in the scheme constitutes the phosphoinositide cycle. The enzymes which catalyse the dephosphorylation of inositol bis- and monophosphates are inhibited (I) by Li$^+$.

endoplasmic reticulum, and the transport of PtdIns in the opposite direction. The movement of these compounds through the cytoplasmic space is probably mediated by phospholipid-binding proteins.

Not all inositol formed from the hydrolysis of PtdIns 4,5 P_2 and the subsequent degradation of Ins 1,4,5 P_3 is re-converted to PtdIns. In the absence of adequate concentrations of extracellular inositol, significant quantities of intracellular inositol are lost from the cell, and response to the agonist is diminished. This effect was first demonstrated by Fain and Berridge in studies of the effect of 5-hydroxytryptamine on fluid secretion in blowfly salivary glands (Fain and Berridge 1979) (Fig. 6.20). Reference to this work was made earlier in relation to the discovery of Ins 1,4,5 P_3 in animal cells.

The loss of an agonist-induced response in the absence of extracellular inositol is enhanced by the presence of Li^+. This monovalent cation inhibits not only the formation of inositol from Ins 1,4,5 P_3 (Fig. 6.19) but also the conversion of glucose-6-phosphate to inositol, the final step in the *de novo* pathway of inositol synthesis.

6.6 Stimulation by inositol trisphosphate of Ca^{2+} outflow from the endoplasmic reticulum

6.6.1 *Early evidence for the action of inositol trisphosphate*

The work which led to the detection and measurement of Ins 1,4,5 P_3 in animal cells described earlier (Berridge 1983) stemmed from attempts to elucidate the mechanism by which agonists which bind to receptors on the plasma membrane release Ca^{2+} from intracellular stores. However, recognition of the importance of Ins 1,4,5 P_3 as an intracellular messenger also depended on the subsequent discovery of the role of Ins 1,4,5 P_3 in inducing the outflow of Ca^{2+} from intracellular stores.

Ins 1,4,5 P_3 is a water-soluble molecule which does not move through cellular membranes. The experiments conducted to demonstrate that Ins 1,4,5 P_3 releases Ca^{2+} from the endoplasmic reti-

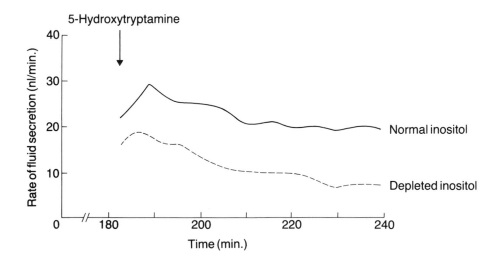

Fig 6.20 The depletion of total cellular inositol substantially diminishes fluid secretion in blowfly salivary glands stimulated by 5-hydroxytryptamine. Cellular inositol was depleted by incubation of the glands for 2 h in the absence of added inositol and in the presence of 5-hydroxytryptamine. From Berridge and Fain (1979).

culum were greatly facilitated by the development of techniques by which the plasma membrane of cells could be made permeable to molecules of low molecular weight. This was successfully achieved by the treatment of cells with saponin or with a high-voltage electric discharge. The plasma membranes of cells treated in this way remain impermeable to molecules of high molecular weight, including the cytoplasmic proteins. This permeabilization technique permits access by exogenous Ins 1,4,5 P_3 to intracellular organelles, with minimal disruption to the cytoplasmic space.

The addition of Ins 1,4,5 P_3 to permeabilized cells causes a net outflow of Ca^{2+} from an intracellular store. As described below, this is probably the endoplasmic reticulum (Fig. 6.21). The concentration of Ins 1,4,5 P_3 which gives half-maximal stimulation of Ca^{2+} outflow is less than 1 µM. This concentration is comparable with the estimated cytoplasmic concentration of Ins 1,4,5 P_3. Ca^{2+} release is not induced by comparable concentrations of Ins 1,3,4 P_3, the other isomer of inositol trisphosphate found in animal cells.

The only other biological compounds which release Ca^{2+} from an intracellular store in this experimental system at concentrations comparable to that which is effective for Ins 1,4,5 P_3 are Ins 1,2-(cyclic)4,5 P_3, Ins 2,4,5 P_3, and GTP. However, the intracellular concentrations of Ins 1,2-(cyclic)4,5 P_3 and Ins 2,4,5 P_3 are too low

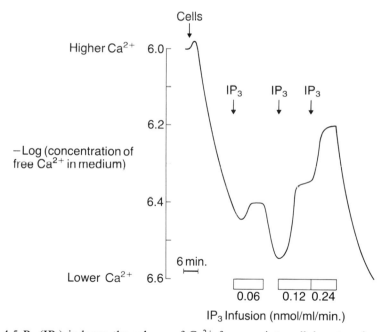

Fig. 6.21   Ins 1,4,5 P_3 (IP$_3$) induces the release of Ca^{2+} from an intracellular store in permeabilized cells. In this experiment Ins 1,4,5 P_3 was added to a suspension of insulinoma cells previously treated with saponin in order to render the plasma membrane freely permeable to inositol polyphosphates and Ca^{2+}. The concentration of Ca^{2+} in the medium surrounding the permeabilized cells was measured using a Ca^{2+}-selective electrode. Addition of cells (in the absence of Ins 1,4,5 P_3) causes a gradual decrease in the concentration of Ca^{2+} in the medium. The infusion of Ins 1,4,5 P_3 at a rate of 0.06 nmol/min per ml for a period of several minutes causes the release of Ca^{2+} from an intracellular store as indicated by an increase in the concentration of Ca^{2+} in the medium. This Ca^{2+} is taken up again by the stores when the infusion of Ins 1,4,5 P_3 is stopped. The amount of Ca^{2+} released into the medium increases as the concentration of Ins 1,4,5 P_3 infused into the cell suspension is increased. From Prentki *et al.* (1985).

to affect Ca^{2+} outflow from the Ins 1,4,5 P_3-sensitive intracellular store and the concentration of GTP does not change during the action of agonists. The possibility that GTP may influence Ca^{2+} release from the Ins 1,4,5 P_3-sensitive intracellular store by influencing the fusion of membranes is described below.

6.6.2 *Intracellular site of action of inositol trisphosphate*

The early experiments on the action of Ins 1,4,5 P_3 in releasing Ca^{2+} from intracellular stores established that Ins 1,4,5 P_3 releases Ca^{2+} from a non-mitochondrial store which was thought to be the endoplasmic reticulum. A variety of techniques have been employed to try to determine more precisely the site from which Ca^{2+} is released in response to Ins 1,4,5 P_3. However, this question has been a difficult one to answer.

The sites of Ins 1,4,5 P_3 action are probably specific regions of the smooth and rough endoplasmic reticulum located near the nucleus and periphery of the cell. Evidence for this conclusion has come from examination of the intracellular distribution of the Ins 1,4,5,P_3 receptor protein, the nature of which is described later, using antibodies to the receptor protein and the techniques of immunohistochemistry. Another approach which also indicates that Ins 1,4,5 P_3 acts at the endoplasmic reticulum has been the analysis of video images of increases in the fluorescence of cells loaded with the intracellular Ca^{2+} chelator fura 2 (Chapter 7, Section 7.6) obtained during the action of Ins 1,4,5, P_3. These increases in $[Ca^{2+}]_i$ correlate with the location of immunological markers for the endoplasmic reticulum.

A different set of experiments has led to speculation that the Ins 1,4,5 P_3-sensitive Ca^{2+} store in non-excitable cells is not part of the endoplasmic reticulum but is a separate organelle which has been called the calciosome. Calciosomes were originally defined as organelles which contain calsequestrin, the Ca^{2+}-binding protein of the sarcoplasmic reticulum of muscle. The location of calciosomes in non-excitable cells was originally determined on the basis of the distribution of calsequestrin detected using immunohistochemical techniques. However, it has now been shown that calciosomes contain calreticulin, a Ca^{2+} binding protein of the endoplasmic reticulum. Thus it is presently unclear whether or not the calciosome is the site of action of Ins 1,4,5 P_3.

6.6.3 *Caged inositol trisphosphate and non-hydrolysable analogues of inositol trisphosphate*

In addition to the stimulation of Ca^{2+} outflow from the endoplasmic reticulum in a wide variety of non-muscle cell types, Ins 1,4,5 P_3 also stimulates Ca^{2+} release from the endoplasmic reticulum of smooth-muscle cells. The release of Ca^{2+} is sufficiently rapid to account for contraction

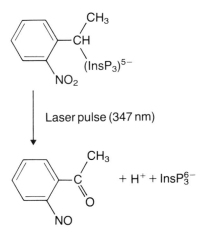

Fig. 6.22 The structure of one form of 'caged' Ins 1,4,5 P_3, inositol 1,4,5-trisphosphate esterified with 1(2-nitrophenyl)diazoethane at the P^5 position. In comparison with non-esterified Ins 1,4,5 P_3, 'caged' Ins 1,4,5 P_3 is hydrolysed very slowly by cellular Ins 1,4,5 P_3/Ins 1,3,4,5 P_4 5-phosphatase. Hence 'caged' Ins 1,4,5 P_3 is considerably more stable in the cytoplasmic space than is Ins 1,4,5 P_3. The ester bond can be very rapidly hydrolysed by photolysis, induced for example by a laser pulse. This releases Ins 1,4,5 P_3.

of the muscle induced by the action of an agonist at receptors on the plasma membrane.

The action of Ins 1,4,5 P_3 in smooth-muscle cells has been most elegantly demonstrated by the use of a derivative of Ins 1,4,5 P_3 in which the phosphate moiety at either position 4 or 5 is esterified with 1(2-nitropheny)diazoethane. The resulting ester (Fig. 6.22) has been termed 'caged' Ins 1,4,5 P_3. The esterified phosphate group is protected from hydrolysis by cellular Ins 1,4,5 P_3/Ins 1,3,4,5 P_4 5-phosphatase. Caged Ins 1,4,5 P_3 cannot release Ca^{2+} from the endoplasmic reticulum.

When introduced into a cell, the esterified form of Ins 1,4,5 P_3 can be very rapidly converted to Ins 1,4,5 P_3 by photolysis using a laser beam (Fig. 6.22). In smooth-muscle cells this results in the rapid release of Ca^{2+} from the

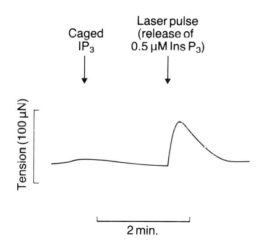

Fig. 6.23 The transient increase in tension of a strip of smooth muscle from the main pulmonary artery of the rabbit, which follows a very rapid increase in the concentration of Ins 1,4,5 P_3 within the cytoplasmic space. The plasma membrane of the muscle cells was made permeable to small molecules by treatment with saponin. At the time indicated, 'caged' Ins 1,4,5 P_3 (IP3), the structure of which is shown in Fig. 6.22, was added. After a further period of time, the 1(2-nitrophenyl)ethyl ester group on the P^5 position of 'caged' Ins 1,4,5 P_3 was removed by irradiation at 347 nm using a laser pulse, leading to the rapid generation of Ins 1,4,5 P_3. From Walker *et al.* (1987).

endoplasmic reticulum and contraction of the muscle (Fig. 6.23).

Whilst these experiments indicate that Ins 1,4,5 P_3 acts as an intracellular messenger in smooth-muscle cells, experiments which have employed 'caged' Ins 1,4,5 P_3 and the use of other techniques indicate that it is unlikely that Ins 1,4,5 P_3 induces the release of Ca^{2+} from the sarcoplasmic reticulum of skeletal and heart muscle.

Another approach to the study of the role of Ins 1,4,5 P_3 in inducing the outflow of Ca^{2+} from the endoplasmic reticulum in a variety of cell types has been to use non-metabolizable analogues of Ins 1,4,5 P_3 which can both bind to the endoplasmic reticulum with high affinity and induce the release of Ca^{2+}. The use of these compounds overcomes the problem of the rapid metabolism of Ins 1,4,5 P_3 in the cell under test. Two such analogues which have been synthesized are inositol 1,4,5-triphosphorothioate and inositol 1,4-bisphosphate-5-phosphorothioate. In each of these compounds one or more phosphate groups (PO_4^{2-}) is replaced by the phosphorothioate moiety (PO_3S^{2-}). The non-metabolizable analogues of Ins 1,4,5 P_3 are useful in generating a prolonged signal for Ca^{2+} outflow and in avoiding the formation of other inositol polyphosphates which could potentially act as intracellular messengers.

6.6.4 *Mechanism of action of inositol trisphosphate*

Ins 1,4,5 P_3 binds to a receptor protein in the membrane of the endoplasmic reticulum and opens a Ca^{2+} channel which is part of the receptor protein. This allows Ca^{2+} to flow into the cytoplasmic space (Fig. 6.24). The receptor protein, to which Ins 1,4,5 P_3 binds with a high affinity, is a glycoprotein with a molecular weight of 260 kDa (Chapter 7, Section 7.4.3). The binding of Ins 1,4,5 P_3 to its receptor and the opening of the Ca^{2+} channel are inhibited in a competitive manner by the glycosaminogly-can, heparin. The action of Ins 1,4,5 P_3 in releasing Ca^{2+} from the endoplasmic reticulum does not involve an Ins 1,4,5 P_3-sensitive protein kinase or inhibition of the $(Ca^{2+} + Mg^{2+})$-ATPase Ca^{2+} pump.

In permeabilized cells and in isolated microsomes composed of vesicles of endoplasmic reticulum, the ability of Ins 1,4,5 P_3 to induce Ca^{2+} outflow from the endoplasmic reticulum is enhanced by GTP. This effect, as well as the ability of GTP to induce Ca^{2+} release from the endoplasmic reticulum in the absence of Ins 1,4,5 P_3 described earlier, is most likely due to the action of GTP in inducing the fusion of membranes of components of the endoplasmic reticulum. This may result in the transfer of Ca^{2+} from regions of the endoplasmic reticulum which are not responsive to Ins 1,4,5 P_3 to regions which are responsive to the actions of this molecule. This action of GTP is probably related to the monomeric GTP-binding proteins which are involved in the fusion of transport vesicles with target membranes (Chapter 2, Section 2.6.6).

6.7 Possible functions of other inositol polyphosphates as intracellular messengers

As described earlier, cells stimulated with an appropriate agonist contain many inositol polyphosphates in addition to Ins 1,4,5 P_3, which has a clearly defined function as an intracellular messenger. In response to an agonist which increases the concentration of Ins 1,4,5 P_3, the concentrations of Ins 1,3,4 P_3, Ins 1,3,4,5 P_4, Ins 1,3,4,5,6 P_5, and of inositol bis- and mono-phosphates also increase although often with time-courses which differ from the time-course for the changes in Ins 1,4,5 P_3. Do any of these other inositol polyphosphates act as intracellular messengers? The answer so far is that, with the possible exception of Ins 1,3,4,5 P_4, there is no compelling evidence for an intracellular messenger function for any of these molecules. On the basis of the results of experiments in which Ins 1,3,4,5 P_4 has been introduced to cells by microinjection and Ca^{2+} movement across the plasma membrane measured by the patch-clamp technique (described in Chapter 7, Section

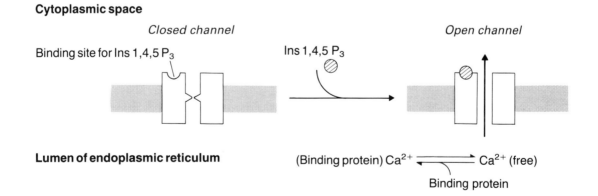

Fig. 6.24 The proposed mechanism for the action of Ins 1,4,5 P_3 in releasing Ca^{2+} from the endoplasmic reticulum. Ins 1,4,5 P_3 formed at the plasma membrane diffuses through the cytoplasmic space and binds to a specific site on the cytoplasmic face of the Ins 1,4,5 P_3-sensitive Ca^{2+} channel in the endoplasmic reticulum. This, in turn, opens the channel and allows Ca^{2+} to move from the lumen of the endoplasmic reticulum to the cytoplasmic space. Within the lumen, Ca^{2+} is probably stored as a complex with a Ca^{2+}-binding protein.

7.3.3), some investigators have suggested that Ins 1,3,4,5 P_4 activates Ca^{2+} inflow across the plasma membrane in some types of cell. Other experiments have suggested that Ins 1,3,4,5 P_4 mediates the transfer of Ca^{2+} from a region of the endoplasmic reticulum which is insensitive to Ins 1,4,5 P_3 to one which is sensitive to this molecule. However, further experiments are required in order to show whether these ideas are correct.

Whilst there is no evidence to indicate that Ins P_5 and Ins P_6 function as intracellular messengers, some experiments suggest that they may act in an extracellular manner as possible neurotransmitters or local hormones in the central nervous system. Evaluation of this idea will also require further experiments.

6.8   The formation of diacylglycerols with intracellular messenger function

The increases in cellular diacylglycerols caused by the action of agonists on cells have been measured in lipid extracts of cells using either gas chromatography or HPLC to estimate the chemical mass of the diacylglycerols, or as radioactively labelled diacylglycerols in cells labelled with [^{3}H]- or [^{14}C]arachidonic acid or [^{3}H]glycerol. Gas chromatography, which permits the nature and amount of the fatty acids in diacylglycerols to be measured, has been used to determine the fatty-acid composition of cellular diacylglycerols. In many cells, of which the platelet is one example, the increase in *sn*-1,2-diacylglycerols observed upon combination of an agonist with its receptor is rapid in onset and transient (Fig. 6.25). Prolonged increases in *sn*-1,2-diacylglycerols which occur more slowly are observed in some other cells, of which smooth muscle and liver are examples (Fig. 6.25).

A complex network of pathways, the details of which are not yet fully resolved, seems to be involved in the formation of diacylglycerols which activate protein kinase C. The initial increase in diacylglycerols in response to an agonist is probably chiefly due to the hydrolysis of

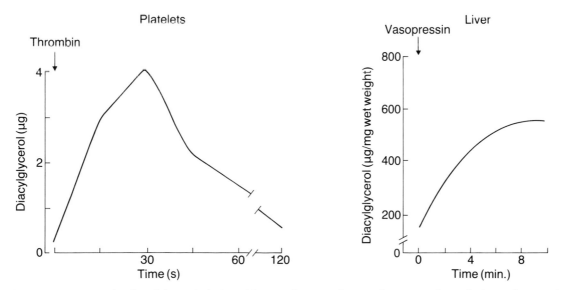

Fig. 6.25   Increases in diacylglycerols induced by agonists may be transient or prolonged, depending on the nature of the target cell. In platelets, thrombin induces a transient increase in diacylglycerols (Rittenhouse-Simmons 1979), whereas the action of vasopressin on hepatocytes induces a sustained increase in diacylglycerols (Bocckino *et al.* 1985).

PtdIns 4,5 P_2 in the reaction catalysed by PtdIns 4,5 P_2-specific phospholipase C. Later, several additional pathways contribute to the formation of diacylglycerols. These are the hydrolysis of PtdIns 4 P and PtdIns, and the hydrolysis of phosphatidylcholine and some other non-inositol phospholipids. The relative contribution of each of these pathways to the formation of diacylglycerol varies from one cell type to another. Within a given cell type it may also depend on the nature of the agonist.

The hydrolysis of PtdIns and PtdIns 4 P is catalysed by one or more phosphoinositide-specific phospholipases C. These reactions were described earlier in the context of agonist-induced decreases in PtdIns and PtdIns 4 P (Section 6.3.2). The hydrolysis of phosphatidylcholine is catalysed by a phospholipase C enzyme specific for this phospholipid species (Fig. 6.26). Another route of phosphatidylcholine hydrolysis is the sequential actions of phospholipase D and phosphatidate phosphohydrolase (Fig. 6.26). Phosphatidic acid is an intermediate in this alternative pathway. The reaction catalysed by phospholipase D is probably the regulated step.

The stimulation, by an agonist, of diacylglycerol formation requires activation of the phospholipase C or phospholipase D. As described earlier, PtdIns 4,5 P_2-specific phospholipase C is activated by a G protein or by phosphorylation in the case of receptors which are protein–tyrosine kinases. The activation by agonists of other phospholipases C and phospholipases D is not understood so well. The PtdIns-, PtdIns 4 P- and phosphatidylcholine-specific phospholipases C are probably activated by a G protein and by protein kinase C. Phospholipase D is thought to be activated by an increase in $[Ca^{2+}]_i$, by protein kinase C, and by a G protein.

Evidence which indicates that diacylglycerols formed in response to an agonist are derived

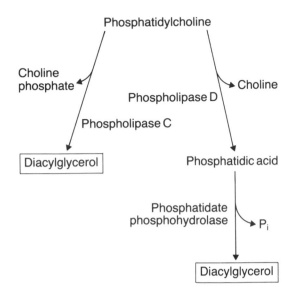

Fig. 6.26   In some cells, the hydrolysis of phosphatidylcholine and other non-inositol phospholipids is responsible for a prolonged agonist-induced increase in diacylglycerols with intracellular messenger function. There are two alternative pathways for the hydrolysis of phosphatidylcholine. One involves phosphatidylcholine-specific phospholipase C whilst the other employs phospholipase D. Phosphatidic acid formed by the action of phospholipase D can be converted to diacylglycerol in the reaction catalysed by phosphatidate phosphohydrolase. Phosphatidylcholine-specific phospholipase C is probably activated by the action of a G protein and protein kinase C whilst phospholipase D may be activated by protein kinase C, a G protein and Ca^{2+}.

from both phosphoinositides and non-inositol phospholipids has come from analyses of the fatty-acid composition of the newly formed diacylglycerols. Those formed from the hydrolysis of phosphoinositides are enriched in stearic and arachidonic acids at positions 1 and 2, respectively, while diacylglycerols formed from the hydrolysis of non-inositol phospholipids contain a smaller proportion of arachidonic and stearic acids and a larger proportion of other fatty acids such as palmitate.

6.9   The metabolism of diacylglycerols

The *sn*-1,2-diacylglycerols formed from phospholipids in the plasma membrane are removed by the actions of diacylglycerol kinase and diacylglycerol lipase (Fig. 6.27). Monoacylglycerol formed by the action of diacylglycerol

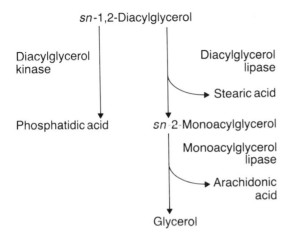

Fig. 6.27 Diacylglycerol formed as a result of the combination of an appropriate agonist with its receptor is rapidly metabolized to either phosphatidic acid or monoacylglycerol. Some cells possess both pathways whilst in other cells one pathway predominates. Monoacylglycerol can be further de-acylated to yield arachidonic acid and glycerol.

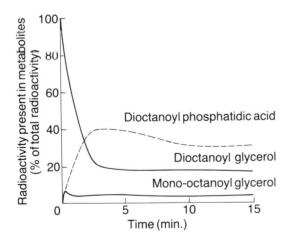

Fig. 6.28 In platelets, the synthetic diacylglycerol, dioctanoylglycerol, is rapidly metabolized to dioctanoylphosphatidic acid and a small amount of mono-octanoylglycerol. The formation of these metabolites was followed using [^{3}H]dioctanoylglycerol. From Bishop and Bell (1986).

lipase is further hydrolysed to yield a fatty acid, predominantly arachidonic acid, and glycerol. This is one of two pathways for the release of arachidonic acid which, as described in Chapter 9, gives rise to a series of arachidonic acid metabolites with extracellular and possibly intracellular messenger function.

The transient nature of the increase in diacylglycerols observed when an agonist binds to cells is due, in part, to the rapid metabolism of *sn*-1,2-diacylglycerols by diacylglycerol kinase and diacylglycerol lipase. An illustration of the ability of these two enzymes to metabolize diacylglycerol is the rapid decrease in the concentration of the synthetic diacylglycerol, dioctanoylglycerol, and increases in dioctanoyl phosphatidic acid and mono-octanoylglycerol observed when dioctanoylglycerol is added to platelets (Fig. 6.28). Presumably in cells in which agonists induce an increase in diacylglycerol by the activation of phospholipase D and the formation of phosphatidic acid as an intermediate, the flux through diacylglycerol kinase is considerably less than that through phosphatidate phosphohydrolase during the period in which diacylglycerol is increased.

Increases in the cellular concentration of diacylglycerols are often associated with increases in phosphatidic acid. This is formed either through the hydrolysis of phospholipids by phospholipase D or by the action of diacylglycerol kinase on diacylglycerol in the reactions described earlier. Some investigators have suggested that phosphatidic acid may function as an intracellular and an extracellular messenger. However, there is presently no compelling evidence to support these suggestions.

6.10   The activation of protein kinase C by diacylglycerol

A central piece of evidence which indicates that *sn*-1,2-diacylglycerols formed in a cell can acti-

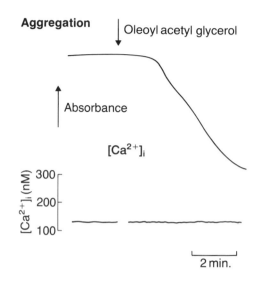

Fig. 6.29 Addition of the synthetic diacylglycerol, *sn*-1-oleoyl-2-acetylglycerol, to platelets induces aggregation of the platelets as revealed by a decrease in absorbance. In this experiment, no increase in $[Ca^{2+}]_i$, measured using the fluorescent intracellular Ca^{2+} indicator quin 2, was detected upon the addition of oleoylacetylglycerol. From Rink *et al.* (1983).

vate protein kinase C was the observation that the addition of synthetic *sn*-1,2-diacylglycerols to cells induces cellular responses which can be attributed to the activation of protein kinase C. This was first shown by Rink and his colleagues (Rink *et al.* 1983) who induced the aggregation of platelets by *sn*-1,2-oleoyl-acetylglycerol in the absence of an apparent increase in $[Ca^{2+}]_i$ (Fig. 6.29).

Synthetic diacylglycerols which activate protein kinase C in intact cells must be able to both permeate the plasma membrane and bind to the diacylglycerol-binding site on protein kinase C. A comparison of the effects of three synthetic *sn*-1,2-diacylglycerols on the activation of protein kinase C in platelets, as assessed by the phosphorylation of a 40 kDa target protein for protein kinase C, is shown in Fig. 6.30. Medium-chain diacylglycerols, such as dihexanoyl-glycerol, dioctanoylglycerol and didecanoyl-glycerol, but not short-chain diacylglycerols

such as dibutyrylglycerol, can both readily pass through the plasma membrane and activate protein kinase C. Medium-chain diacylglycerols are the most effective activators of protein kinase C in intact cells. As described earlier, oleoylace-tylglycerol is also a very effective activator of protein kinase C in intact cells. The effective synthetic activators of protein kinase C are more hydrophilic than *sn*-1-stearoyl-2-arachidonyl glycerol, the most common natural species of diacylglycerol which activates the enzyme.

In the absence of agonists and hence at a basal concentration of diacylglycerol in the plasma membrane, most protein kinase C is located in the cytoplasmic space and is not bound to the plasma membrane. The amount of *sn*-1,2-diacylglycerols formed in the plasma membrane as a result of agonist-induced phospholipid hydrolysis is a very small percentage of the total

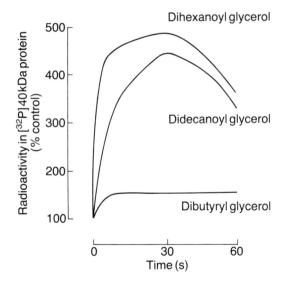

Fig. 6.30 Comparison of the abilities of three synthetic diacylglycerols to activate protein kinase C in intact platelets. The activity of protein kinase C was assayed indirectly by measurement of the degree of phosphorylation of a 40 kDa protein which is known to be phosphorylated by protein kinase C. The diacylglycerols are *sn*-1,2-dibutyrylglycerol, *sn*-1,2-dihexanoylglycerol, and *sn*-1,2-didecanoylglycerol. From Lapetina *et al.* (1985).

membrane phospholipids. How does this small increase in diacylglycerols in the plasma membrane lead to activation of protein kinase C present in the cytoplasmic space? Only a partial answer to this question has so far been obtained.

The activation of protein kinase C by diacylglycerol takes place on the cytoplasmic face of the plasma membrane. Agonist-induced activation of the protein kinase is associated with an increase in the amount of the kinase which is combined with the plasma membrane (Fig. 6.31). In the presence of Ca^{2+}, an increase in the concentration of *sn*-1,2-diacylglycerols in the plasma membrane probably increases the affinity of the membrane for protein kinase C and consequently increases the amount of enzyme bound to the plasma membrane (Fig. 6.32).

The mechanism by which Ca^{2+}, diacylglycerol, and membrane lipids activate protein kinase C is not completely understood. In the presence of both diacylglycerols and Ca^{2+}, diacylglycerol binds to an allosteric site (Chapter 4, Section 4.6.3) on the membrane-bound pro-

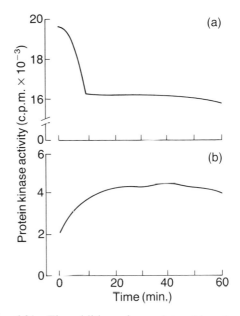

Fig. 6.31   The addition of gonadotrophin-releasing hormone to pituitary gonadotroph cells decreases the activity of protein kinase C subsequently measured in the cytosolic fraction (a) and increases the activity of the enzyme in the membrane fraction (b). The fractions were prepared after homogenization of the cells. From Hirota *et al.* (1985).

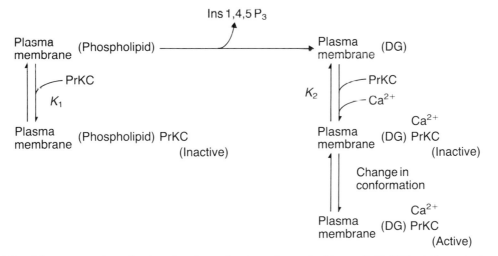

Fig. 6.32   The proposed mechanism for the activation of protein kinase C (PrKC) at the cytoplasmic face of the plasma membrane. In the absence of an agonist-induced increase in diacylglycerol (DG) the affinity (K_1) of the membrane for the kinase is low. In the presence of an increase in the concentration of plasma-membrane diacylglycerol induced by an agonist and at resting $[Ca^{2+}]_i$, the affinity (K_2) of the membrane for protein kinase C is increased so that more enzyme binds to the membrane. The binding of diacylglycerol to an allosteric site on membrane-bound protein kinase C alters the conformation of the enzyme so that the active site can interact with substrates.

tein kinase C. This causes the enzyme to undergo a conformational change from an inactive to an active form (Fig. 6.32). Although the activation of protein kinase C can occur at resting concentrations of $[Ca^{2+}]_i$, in some cells the activation of protein kinase C by diacylglycerol seems to depend on the increase in $[Ca^{2+}]_i$ induced by the action of the agonist.

On the basis of studies with artificial membrane systems, Bell and his colleagues (Ganong *et al.* 1986) have proposed that the conformational change which leads to activation of protein kinase C requires the combination of at least four molecules of phosphatidylserine, and one molecule each of diacylglycerol and Ca^{2+} to each molecule of the protein kinase (Fig. 6.33). It is thought that Ca^{2+} forms bonds with phosphatidylserine, diacylglycerol, and the protein kinase C.

In intact cells, protein kinase C can be activated by a group of non-physiological compounds, the tumour-promoting phorbol esters.

These probably bind to the allosteric site for diacylglycerol (Chapter 4, Section 4.6.3). Like diacylglycerol they induce association of the enzyme with the plasma membrane and subsequent activation of the enzyme. The incubation of cells with phorbol esters, such as tetradecanoyl phorbol acetate or phorbol dibutyrate, for periods of time ranging from about 1 to 30 minutes has been used as an experimental procedure to artificially activate protein kinase C. Longer exposure of cells to one of these tumour-promoting phorbol esters, for example for 24 h, leads to a dramatic decrease in the total amount of protein kinase C in the cells. In some cases all the enzyme is depleted. The loss of enzyme activity is due to proteolytic degradation of the protein kinase C (Chapter 4, Section 4.6.4). The prolonged treatment of cells with tumour-promoting phorbol esters has been used as an experimental manipulation to deplete cells of protein kinase C.

Diacylglycerols may not be the only physiolo-

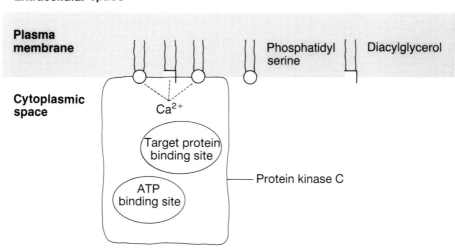

Fig 6.33 Formation of the active conformation of protein kinase C bound to the cytoplasmic face of the plasma membrane probably requires the combination of Ca^{2+}, diacylglycerol, and phosphatidylserine, or other phospholipids of the plasma membrane, to specific sites on the protein kinase C polypeptide chain. Adapted from Ganong *et al.* (1986).

gical regulators of protein kinase C. Other possible regulators are the activator arachidonic acid and the inhibitor sphingosine.

Protein kinase C phosphorylates a wide range of target enzymes. The nature of these and the mechanisms by which it is thought that protein kinase C located at the plasma membrane phosphorylates target enzymes within the interior of the cell are described in Chapter 4 (Section 4.6.5).

6.11 Dual action of inositol trisphosphate and diacylglycerols in inducing cellular responses

6.11.1 *The bifurcating signalling pathway*
The responses induced by the actions of agonists on many types of cells seem to require parallel increases in Ins 1,4,5 P_3 and diacylglycerols (Fig. 6.34). This observation has led to the idea that the activation of (Ca^{2+} + calmodulin)-dependent protein kinases by Ca^{2+} (increased as a result of the action of Ins 1,4,5 P_3) and the activation by diacylglycerol of protein kinase C represents a bifurcating signalling system in which the bifurcation occurs at the site of hydrolysis

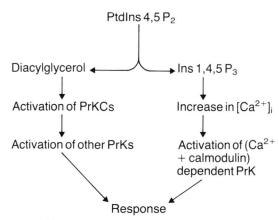

Fig. 6.34 Increases in the intracellular concentrations of both Ins 1,4,5 P_3 and diacylglycerol are required for the actions of a number of agonists on target cells. The formation and action of these two intracellular messengers has been called a bifurcating signalling pathway.

of PtdIns 4,5 P_2, a molecule of which yields two intracellular messengers.

The concept of the bifurcating signalling system involving Ins 1,4,5 P_3 and diacylglycerol has been emphasized by Berridge (1987) and Nishizuka (1984). Although this is a useful concept it may be an over-simplification of the true picture in some cases. Two examples which illustrate the concept of the bifurcating signalling system well are the action of agonists in inducing the aggregation of platelets and the actions of mitogens in stimulating cell division.

6.11.2 *Aggregation of platelets*
Agonists which use the Ins 1,4,5 P_3 and diacylglycerol bifurcating signalling system in platelets include thrombin, collagen, ADP, vasopressin, and thromboxane A_2. Each binds to a specific receptor on the platelet plasma membrane, induces the hydrolysis of PtdIns 4,5 P_2, and induces increases in Ins 1,4,5 P_3, $[Ca^{2+}]_i$, and diacylglycerol (Fig. 6.35). The magnitude of the maximal change in any of these intracellular messengers, and the onset and duration of the change, depends on the given agonist. The targets for protein kinase C include several enzymes which catalyse cell aggregation and the release of secretory granules. One of the consequences of the increase in $[Ca^{2+}]_i$ induced by Ins 1,4,5 P_3 is a change in the structure of the cytoskeleton.

6.11.3 *Mitogenic stimulation of cell division*
Another example of the roles of Ins 1,4,5 P_3 and diacylglycerol as dual intracellular messengers is the action of mitogens in stimulating cell division. A mitogen is defined as an agonist which is capable of stimulating DNA synthesis and cell division. A major class of mitogens are the growth factors. A given growth factor may be able to act as a mitogen alone or in combination with other growth factors. Many studies of the actions of mitogens have been conducted using

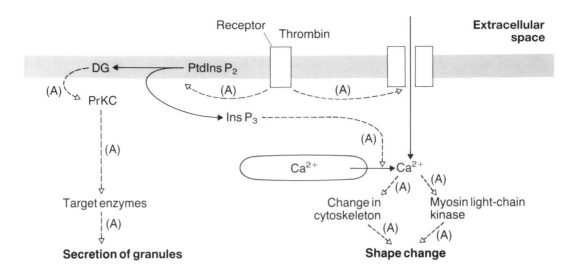

Fig. 6.35 Activation of the Ins 1,4,5 P_3 and diacylglycerol bifurcating signalling pathway in platelets by thrombin. The combination of thrombin with its receptor stimulates the hydrolysis of PtdIns 4,5 P_2. This results in the formation of diacylglycerol (DG) and Ins 1,4,5 P_3 (InsP$_3$), an increase in [Ca^{2+}]$_i$, the activation of protein kinase C (PrKC) and (Ca^{2+} + calmodulin)-dependent protein kinases, and the combination of Ca^{2+} with Ca^{2+}-binding proteins. Protein kinase C phosphorylates enzymes required for the stimulation of granule secretion. Actions of activated (Ca^{2+} + calmodulin)-dependent protein kinases and the Ca^{2+}-binding proteins include changes in the activities of enzymes which alter the structure of the cytoskeleton and lead to changes in platelet shape. The symbol (A) represents the activation of a pathway. There are, most likely, other target proteins for protein kinase C, (Ca^{2+} + calmodulin)-dependent protein kinases, and Ca^{2+}. However, the functions of many of these have not yet been elucidated.

established lines of cultured fibroblasts. Swiss 3T3 fibroblasts have often been used although other fibroblasts, for example Chinese hamster lung fibroblasts, have also been employed. As described in Chapter 11 (Section 11.1.2), these cells have undergone at least one mutation in a critical gene, probably the normal counterpart of an oncogene, which enables them to grow indefinitely *in vitro* under appropriate conditions.

In the presence of adequate amounts of serum, which supplies growth factors, Swiss 3T3 cells continue to undergo cycles of DNA synthesis and division. If the supply of serum is depleted, cell division stops and the cells become quiescent. DNA synthesis and cell division can be re-initiated by the re-addition of serum or the addition to the medium of one or more defined growth factors.

Bombesin and PDGF are the only known growth factors which, when added alone to the cell culture, can induce DNA re-synthesis and cell division in Swiss 3T3 fibroblasts. Insulin and one of several other growth factors can act synergistically to induce DNA re-synthesis and cell division. Growth factors which synergize with insulin include prostaglandin E1 (PGE$_1$), PDGF, EGF, and vasopressin. Insulin also greatly enhances the mitogenic action of bombesin. The known pathways of intracellular communication activated by these growth factors are those which involve receptor protein–tyrosine kinases (insulin, PDGF, and EGF), Ins 1,4,5 P_3 and Ca^{2+} (bombesin and PDGF), diacylglycerol (bombesin, PDGF, and vasopressin), and cyclic AMP (PGE$_1$).

As a result of his studies with Swiss 3T3 cells, Rozengurt (1986) has concluded that each single

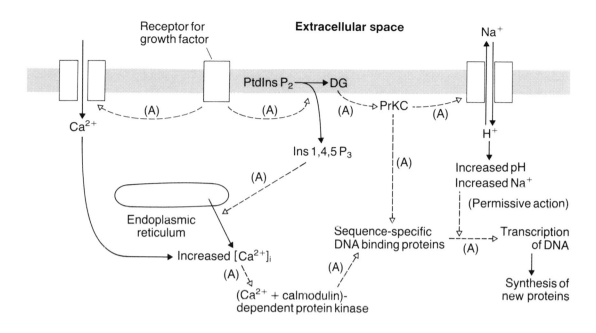

Fig. 6.36   The interaction of some mitogenic growth factors, including bombesin, thrombin, and vasopressin, with their receptors causes parallel increases in Ins 1,4,5 P_3 (and hence in $[Ca^{2+}]_i$) and diacylglycerols (DG) in target cells such as quiescent fibroblasts. Target proteins for protein kinase C (PrKC) include the Na^+–H^+ exchange system of the plasma membrane and sequence-specific DNA-binding proteins. Activation of the Na^+–H^+ exchanger, possibly by phosphorylation of the exchange protein itself, leads to increases in intracellular pH_i and $[Na^+]_i$. These changes in pH_i and $[Na^+]_i$ probably act in a permissive manner to stimulate DNA synthesis and cell division. The increase in $[Ca^{2+}]_i$ probably acts, through $(Ca^{2+}$ + calmodulin)-dependent protein kinases and Ca^{2+}-binding proteins, to stimulate reactions of the cell cycle. The symbol (A) represents the activation of an enzyme or pathway.

mitogenic growth factor, or a mitogenic combination of two or more growth factors, activates more than one pathway of intracellular communication. Co-operation between at least two of these pathways is required to induce DNA re-synthesis and cell division. These actions of mitogens in stimulating cell proliferation are discussed from a different perspective in Chapter 12.

Some mitogenic growth factors, such as bombesin in the case of Swiss 3T3 cells, or thrombin, bombesin, vasopressin, or bradykinin in the case of lung fibroblasts, have as a major or sole component of their action the stimulation of the formation of diacylglycerol and Ins 1,4,5 P_3. As shown in Fig. 6.36, these intracellular mess-

engers act together through $(Ca^{2+}$ + calmodulin)-dependent protein kinases, Ca^{2+}-binding proteins, and protein kinase C to stimulate the re-initiation of DNA synthesis and cell division.

Two important targets of protein kinase C are sequence-specific DNA-binding proteins in the nucleus and the Na^+–H^+ exchange protein in the plasma membrane. The phosphorylation of sequence-specific DNA-binding proteins and their mechanism of action are described in Chapter 10 (Section 10.4.3). Activation of Na^+–H^+ exchange by protein kinase C probably involves either direct phosphorylation of the Na^+–H^+ exchanger or the phosphorylation of another protein with which the exchange protein interacts. As described in Chapter 8 (Section

8.6.2), the resulting increase in cytoplasmic pH is thought to have a permissive effect on DNA synthesis.

6.12 Summary

Inositol 1,4,5-trisphosphate (Ins 1,4,5 P_3) and diacylglycerol act as intracellular messengers in a wide variety of cell types. Ins 1,4,5 P_3 is formed at the plasma membrane by the hydrolysis of phosphatidylinositol 4,5-bisphosphate (PtdIns 4,5 P_2) in the reaction catalysed by PtdIns 4,5 P_2-specific phospholipase C. This phospholipase is activated by a GTP-binding regulatory protein which can couple to an appropriate agonist–receptor complex. Two pathways are responsible for the metabolism of Ins 1,4,5 P_3. In the first, Ins 1,4,5 P_3 is dephosphorylated in successive steps to form Ins 1,4 P_2, Ins 4 P and inositol. In the second, Ins 1,4,5 P_3 is phosphorylated to form Ins 1,3,4,5 P_4 which is then successively dephosphorylated to form Ins 1,3,4 P_3 (another isomer of inositol trisphosphate), inositol bisphosphates, inositol monophosphates, and inositol. The metabolism of Ins 1,4,5 P_3 is regulated by protein kinase C and (Ca^{2+} + calmodulin)-dependent protein kinase. Li^+ is a pharmacological inhibitor of the dephosphorylation of inositol monophosphates and Ins 1,4 P_2.

During the action of an agonist which stimulates the hydrolysis of PtdIns 4,5 P_2, and in the subsequent recovery phase after removal of the agonist, the supply of PtdIns 4,5 P_2 in the plasma membrane is replenished from the much larger reservoir of PtdIns. This involves the addition of successive phosphate groups at positions D-4 and D-5 of the inositol moiety in reactions catalysed by PtdIns 4-kinase and PtdIns 4 P 5-kinase. The supply of PtdIns at the plasma membrane is maintained by its re-synthesis from CDP–diacylglycerol and inositol. The reactions involved in the hydrolysis of PtdIns 4,5 P_2, degradation of Ins 1,4,5 P_3, re-synthesis of PtdIns and phosphorylation of PtdIns constitute a cycle called the phosphatidylinositol cycle.

The function of Ins 1,4,5 P_3 is to release Ca^{2+} from a specific region of the endoplasmic reticulum. The combination of Ins 1,4,5 P_3 with a receptor protein on the endoplasmic reticulum membrane opens a Ca^{2+} channel which facilitates the movement of Ca^{2+} from the lumen of the endoplasmic reticulum to the cytoplasmic space. The pathways for the interconversion of inositol polyphosphates in animal cells are complex. Future investigations will probably define these pathways further and may reveal that some inositol polyphosphates other than Ins 1,4,5 P_3 function as intracellular messengers.

The role of diacylglycerol as an intracellular messenger is confined to the hydrophobic environment of the plasma membrane and possibly some intracellular membranes rather than the cytoplasmic space. In response to the action of certain agonists, diacylglycerols with intracellular messenger function are formed at the plasma membrane by several pathways. These are the hydrolysis of PtdIns 4,5 P_2 (the reaction which forms Ins 1,4,5 P_3), the hydrolysis of PtdIns and PtdIns 4 P, and the hydrolysis of phosphatidylcholine and other non-inositol phospholipids. The hydrolysis of phosphatidylcholine is catalysed by a phosphatidylcholine-specific phospholipase C or, under some circumstances, by the combination of phospholipase D, which yields phosphatidic acid, and phosphatidate phosphohydrolase, which converts phosphatidic acid to diacylglycerol. The pathways which hydrolyse non-inositol phospholipids are not yet fully understood. Once formed, diacylglycerols may be rapidly converted to phosphatidic acid, in the reaction catalysed by diacylglycerol kinase, or to monoacylglycerols and free fatty acids, in the reaction catalysed by diacylglycerol lipase.

The intracellular messenger function of diacylglycerol is to activate protein kinase C on the cytoplasmic face of the plasma membrane. In the absence of an agonist which stimulates the formation of diacylglycerol, the majority of protein kinase C is located in the cytoplasmic space and has a low affinity for the plasma membrane. An increase in the concentration of diacylglycerol in the plasma membrane enhances the affinity of the plasma membrane for protein kinase C and leads to an increase in the binding of this enzyme to the membrane. The interaction of protein kinase C with diacylglycerol, Ca^{2+}, and phosphatidylserine, a component of the phospholipid bilayer, causes a conformational change which leads to activation of the enzyme. Activated protein kinase C phosphorylates a number of target proteins in the plasma membrane, cytoplasmic space, and nucleus. There are many aspects of the mechanism of activation of protein kinase C and of the processes by which this enzyme phosphorylates target proteins that are not yet defined.

In many types of cell, there are parallel increases in the intracellular concentrations of Ins 1,4,5 P_3 and diacylglycerols in response to an agonist. This is thought to constitute a bifurcating intracellular signalling pathway. Examples of processes in which the bifurcating pathway probably operates are induction of the aggregation of platelets by agonists such as thrombin, and the stimulation by mitogens of protein and DNA synthesis and cell division.

References

Abdel-Latif, A. A., Akhtar, R. A., and Hawthorne, J. N. (1977). Acetylcholine increases the breakdown of triphosphoinositide of rabbit iris muscle pre-labelled with [^{32}P]phosphate. *Biochem. J.*, **162**, 61–73.

Allison, J. H. and Stewart, M. A. (1971). Reduced brain inositol in lithium-treated rats. *Nature*, **233**, 267–8.

Allison, J. H., Blisner, M. E., Holland, W. H., Hipps, P. P., and Sherman, W. R. (1976). Increased brain *myo*-inositol 1-phosphate in lithium-treated rats. *Biochem. Biophys. Res. Commun.*, **71**, 664–70.

Berridge, M. J. (1983). Rapid accumulation of inositol-trisphosphate reveals that agonists hydrolyse polyphosphoinositides instead of phosphatidylinositol. *Biochem. J.*, **212**, 849–58.

Berridge, M. J. (1987). Inositol trisphosphate and diacylglycerol: two interacting second messengers. *Ann. Rev. Biochem.*, **56**, 159–93.

Berridge, M. J. and Fain, J. N. (1979). Inhibition of phosphatidylinositol synthesis and the inactivation of calcium entry after prolonged exposure of the blowfly salivary gland to 5-hydroxytryptamine. *Biochem. J.*, **178**, 59–69.

Bishop, W. R. and Bell, R. M. (1986). Attenuation of *sn*-1,2-diacylglycerol second messengers. Metabolism of exogenous diacylglycerols by human platelets. *J. Biol. Chem.*, **261**, 12513–19.

Bocckino, S. B., Blackmore, P. F., and Exton, J. H. (1985). Stimulation of 1,2-diacylglycerol accumulation in hepatocytes by vasopressin, epinephrine and angiotensin II. *J. Biol. Chem.*, **260**, 14201–7.

Cosgrove, D. J. (1980). *Inositol phosphates: their chemistry, biochemistry and physiology*. Elsevier, Amsterdam.

De Robertis, E. (1971). Molecular biology of synaptic receptors. *Science*, **171**, 963–71.

Durell, J., Garland, J. T., and Friedel, R. O. (1969). Acetylcholine action: biochemical aspects. *Science*, **165**, 862–6.

Fain, J. N. and Berridge, M. J. (1979). Relationship between phosphatidylinositol synthesis and recovery of 5-hydroxytryptamine-responsive Ca^{2+} flux in blowfly salivary glands. *Biochem. J.*, **180**, 655–61.

Ganong, B. R., Loomis, C. R., Hannun, Y. A., and Bell, R. M. (1986). Specificity and mechanism of protein kinase C activation by *sn*-1,2-diacylglycerols. *Proc. Natl Acad. Sci. USA*, **83**, 1184–8.

Gilkey, J. C., Jaffe, L. F., Ridgway, E. B., and Reynolds, G. T. (1978). A free calcium wave traverses the activating egg of the medaka, *Oryzias latipes*. *J. Cell Biol.*, **76**, 448–66.

Grado, C. and Ballou, C. E. (1961). Myo-inositol

phosphates obtained by alkaline hydrolysis of beef brain phosphoinositide. *J. Biol. Chem.*, **236**, 54–60.

Heslop, J. P., Irvine, R. F., Tashjian Jr, A. H., and Berridge, M. J. (1985). Inositol tetrakis and pentakis phosphates in GH$_4$ cells. *J. Exp. Biol.*, **119**, 395–401.

Heslop, J. P., Blakeley, D. M., Brown, K. D., Irvine, R. F., and Berridge, M. J. (1986). Effects of bombesin and insulin on inositol (1,4,5)trisphosphate and inositol (1,3,4)trisphosphate formation in Swiss 3T3 cells. *Cell*, **47**, 703–9.

Hirota, K., Hirota, T., Aguilera, G., and Catt, K. J. (1985). Hormone-induced redistribution of calcium-activated phospholipid-dependent protein kinase in pituitary gonadotrophs. *J. Biol. Chem.*, **260**, 3243–6.

Hokin, M. R. and Hokin, L. E. (1953). Enzyme secretion and the incorporation of ^{32}P into phospholipids of pancreas slices. *J. Biol. Chem.*, **203**, 967–77.

Inoue, M., Kishimoto, A., Takai, Y., and Nishizuka, Y. (1977). Studies on a cyclic nucleotide-independent protein kinase and its proenzyme in mammalian tissues. *J. Biol. Chem.*, **252**, 7610–16.

Irvine, R. F., Letcher, A. J., Lander, D. J., and Downes, C. P. (1984). Inositol trisphosphates in carbachol-stimulated rat parotid glands. *Biochem. J.*, **223**, 237–43.

Kikkawa, U., Takai, Y., Tanaka, Y., Miyake, R., and Nishizuka, Y. (1983). Protein kinase C as a possible receptor protein of tumour-promoting phorbol esters. *J. Biol. Chem.*, **258**, 11442–5.

Kishimoto, A., Takai, Y., Mori, T., Kikkawa, U., and Nishizuka, Y. (1980). Activation of calcium and phospholipid-dependent protein kinase by diacylglycerol, its possible relation to phosphatidylinositol turnover. *J. Biol. Chem.*, **255**, 2273–6.

Lapetina, E. G. and Michell, R. H. (1973). Phosphatidylinositol metabolism in cells receiving extracellular stimulation. *FEBS Lett.*, **31**, 1–10.

Lapetina, E. G., Reep, B., Ganong, B. R., and Bell, R. M. (1985). Exogenous *sn*-1,2-diacylglycerols containing saturated fatty acids function as bioregulators of protein kinase C in human platelets. *J. Biol. Chem.*, **260**, 1358–61.

Michell, R. H. (1975). Inositol phospholipids and cell surface receptor function. *Biochim. Biophys. Acta*,

415, 81–147.

Michell, R. H., Kirk, C. J., Jones, L. M., Downes, C. P., and Creba, J. A. (1981). The stimulation of inositol lipid metabolism that accompanies calcium mobilization in stimulated cells: defined characteristics and unanswered questions. *Phil. Trans. Roy. Soc. London*, B **296**, 123–37.

Morgan, R. O., Chang, J. P., and Catt, K. J. (1987). Novel aspects of gonadotropin-releasing hormone action on inositol polyphosphate metabolism in cultured pituitary gonadotrophs. *J. Biol. Chem.*, **262**, 1166–71.

Nishizuka, Y. (1984). The role of protein kinase C in cell surface signal transduction and tumour promotion. *Nature*, **308**, 693–8.

Prentki, M., Corkey, B. E., and Matschinsky, F. M. (1985). Inositol 1,4,5-trisphosphate and the endoplasmic reticulum Ca^{2+} cycle of a rat insulinoma cell line. *J. Biol. Chem.*, **260**, 9185–90.

Rebecchi, M. J. and Gershengorn, M. C. (1983). Thyroliberin stimulates rapid hydrolysis of phosphatidylinositol 4,5-bisphosphate by a phosphodiesterase in rat mammotropic pituitary cells. Evidence for an early Ca^{2+}-independent action. *Biochem. J.*, **216**, 287–94.

Rink, T. J., Sanchez, A., and Hallam, T. J. (1983). Diacylglycerol and phorbol ester stimulate secretion without raising cytoplasmic free calcium in human platelets. *Nature*, **305**, 317–19.

Rittenhouse-Simmons, S. (1979). Production of diglyceride from phosphatidylinositol in activated human platelets. *J. Clin. Invest.*, **63**, 580–7.

Rozengurt, E. (1986). Early signals in the mitogenic response. *Science*, **234**, 161–6.

Sherman, W. R., Leavitt, A. L., Honchar, M. P., Hallcher, L. M., and Phillips, B. E. (1981). Evidence that lithium alters phosphoinositide metabolism: chronic administration elevates primarily D-*myo*-inositol-1-phosphate in cerebral cortex of the rat. *J. Neurochem.*, **36**, 1947–51.

Streb, H., Irvine, R. F., Berridge, M. J., and Schulz, I. (1983). Release of Ca^{2+} from a non-mitochondrial intracellular store in pancreatic acinar cells by inositol-1,4,5-trisphosphate. *Nature*, **306**, 67–9.

Thomas, A. P., Alexander, J., and Williamson, J. R. (1984). Relationship between inositol polyphosphate production and the increase of cytosolic free Ca^{2+} induced by vasopressin in isolated hepatocytes. *J. Biol. Chem.*, **259**, 5574–84.

Walker, J. W., Somlyo, A. V., Goldman, Y. E., Somlyo, A. P., and Trentham, D. R. (1987). Kinetics of smooth and skeletal muscle activation by laser pulse photolysis of caged inositol 1,4,5-trisphosphate. *Nature*, **327**, 249–52.

Further reading

Bansal, V. S. and Majerus, P. W. (1990). Phosphatidylinositol-derived precursors and signals. *Ann. Rev. Cell Biol.,* **6**, 41–67.

Berridge, M. J. (1985). The molecular basis of communication within the cell. *Sci. Am.*, **253**, 124–34.

Berridge, M. J. and Irvine, R. F. (1989). Inositol phosphates and cell signalling. *Nature*, **341**, 197–205.

Hokin, L. E. (1985). Receptors and phosphoinositide-generated second messengers. *Ann. Rev. Biochem.*, **54**, 205–35.

Kikkawa, U., Kishimoto, A., and Nishizuka, Y. (1989). The protein kinase C family: heterogeneity and its implications. *Ann. Rev. Biochem.*, **58**, 31–44.

Putney Jr, J. W. (1986). *Phosphoinositides and receptor mechanisms.* Alan R. Liss Inc., New York.

7 Calcium

7.1 Ca²⁺ as an intracellular messenger in both electrically excitable and non-excitable cells

7.1.1 General features of the role of Ca²⁺ as an intracellular messenger

Changes in the concentration of free Ca^{2+} in the cytoplasmic space ($[Ca^{2+}]_i$) act as an intracellular messenger in most animal cells. These include both electrically excitable cells, for example muscle, nerve, and a number of secretory cells, and non-electrically-excitable cells, for example parenchymal cells of the liver, and white blood cells (Table 7.1).

The principles which govern the action of Ca^{2+} as an intracellular messenger are shown in Fig. 7.1. The combination of the agonist with its receptor causes an increase in $[Ca^{2+}]_i$. This, in turn, alters the activities of Ca^{2+}-dependent protein kinases and other target proteins by binding to Ca^{2+}-binding sites on these enzymes or proteins. There are two sources of agonist-induced increases in $[Ca^{2+}]_i$. These are the endoplasmic reticulum (or the sarcoplasmic reticulum) and the extracellular fluid. In addition to the regulation of processes in the cytoplasmic space, changes in the concentration of free Ca^{2+} in the mitochondrial matrix contribute to the regulation of the activity of Ca^{2+}-sensitive enzymes in this compartment. These changes in free Ca^{2+} are induced by corresponding changes in $[Ca^{2+}]_i$.

Ca^{2+} appears to have evolved as an intracellular messenger because it can form quite specific complexes with certain proteins, the Ca^{2+}-binding proteins. This question has been considered in some detail by Williams and his colleagues

Table 7.1 *Examples of some cellular responses mediated by changes in the concentration of Ca^{2+} in the cytoplasmic space*

Cellular response	Cell type	Agonist
Contraction	Skeletal muscle	Various neurotransmitters
	Smooth muscle	Norepinephrine
Glycogenolysis	Liver parenchymal	Adrenalin
Secretion of proteins and ions	Pancreatic acinar cell	Acetylcholine
	Pituitary cell	Thyroid-releasing hormone
Shape change	Platelets	Thrombin
Growth (proliferation)	Fibroblasts	Platelet-derived growth factor
Ion transport	Blowfly salivary gland	5-Hydroxytryptamine
	Photoreceptor cells	Photons
Fertilization	Sea-urchin eggs	Spermatozoa

(Williams 1976). As explained later in Section 7.8.2, this involves the formation of a co-ordination complex between Ca^{2+} and eight oxygen atoms, seven of which are provided by amino-acid residues. Mg^{2+}, Na^+, and K^+, which are far more plentiful than Ca^{2+} within cells, cannot form such a specific complex.

7.1.2 Discovery of the role of Ca^{2+} as an intracellular messenger

Elucidation of the role of Ca^{2+} as an intracellular messenger began over one hundred years ago with the observation by Ringer (1883) that the contraction of cardiac muscle requires the presence of extracellular Ca^{2+}. In the period 1940 to 1950 Heilbrunn (1940) and Heilbrunn and Wiercinski (1947) showed that Ca^{2+} induces the contraction of myofibrils. Subsequent experiments by many investigators established that the role of Ca^{2+} in heart and skeletal muscle is to couple the depolarization of the sarcolemma to the contraction of myofibrils. A central contribution to knowledge of the mechanism of

this coupling was the discovery in 1965 of troponin, the protein which binds Ca^{2+} and interacts with myosin (Ebashi and Kodama 1965). Investigation of the mechanism by which neurotransmitters induce the contraction of smooth-muscle cells revealed that an increase in $[Ca^{2+}]_i$ is also responsible for contraction in these cells (Szent-Györgyi et al. 1973; Dabrowska et al. 1978).

During the decade beginning in 1970, evidence was obtained which suggested that changes in $[Ca^{2+}]_i$ are required for coupling between extracellular stimuli and cellular responses in non-muscle cells. These experiments showed that the response to an agonist was substantially reduced in the absence of extracellular Ca^{2+} and was abolished in cells pre-treated with EGTA, a Ca^{2+} chelator. Furthermore, the action of an agonist could often be mimicked by the Ca^{2+}-selective ionophore A23187, which facilitates the movements of Ca^{2+} across biological membranes. In many cases, the actions of the agonists being tested were not associated with changes in the concentrations of the other known intracellular

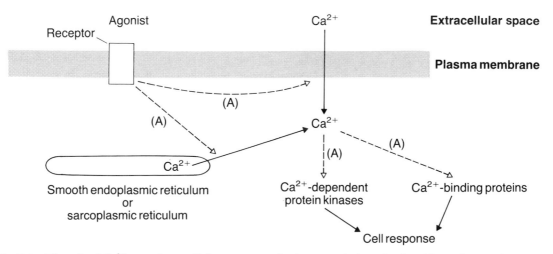

Fig. 7.1 The role of Ca^{2+} as an intracellular messenger in the transmission of a signal from the agonist–receptor complex on the plasma membrane through the cytoplasmic space to intracellular target proteins. Combination of the agonist with its receptor leads to an increase in net Ca^{2+} movement to the cytoplasmic space from both the extracellular space and the endoplasmic reticulum. This results in an increase in $[Ca^{2+}]_i$. Ca^{2+} activates Ca^{2+}-dependent protein kinases and other target proteins by binding to allosteric sites on these molecules. The symbol (A) represents the activation of a pathway.

messengers, cyclic AMP, and cyclic GMP. With the advent of a widely applicable technique for the measurement of $[Ca^{2+}]_i$ in the cytoplasmic space (Tsien 1981), it became possible to directly measure changes in $[Ca^{2+}]_i$ induced by agonists in many cell types.

In parallel with experiments which indicated that certain agonists require increases in $[Ca^{2+}]_i$ for their action was the discovery by Cheung (1970) of the intracellular Ca^{2+}-binding protein, calmodulin. This protein is present in almost all cells, and plays an important role in transmitting the effects of increased $[Ca^{2+}]_i$ to intracellular enzymes. Many other Ca^{2+}-binding proteins, in addition to troponin C and calmodulin, have now been discovered.

In this chapter, the mechanisms by which agonists increase $[Ca^{2+}]_i$, the nature of Ca^{2+}-binding proteins, and the interaction of Ca^{2+} with these proteins will be described. In order to appreciate fully the actions of agonists on $[Ca^{2+}]_i$ it is useful to consider the processes which control the amount of Ca^{2+} present in a cell, and the distribution of this Ca^{2+} between the intracellular Ca^{2+} stores and the cytoplasmic space. These processes will be considered first.

7.2 Components of the systems which control the free cytoplasmic Ca^{2+} concentration

7.2.1 *The gradient of Ca^{2+} across the plasma membrane*

One of the most striking features of Ca^{2+} homeostasis in animal cells is the large gradient of Ca^{2+} between the extracellular fluid and the cytoplasmic space. The value of $[Ca^{2+}]_i$ is about 0.1 μM whereas the concentration of free Ca^{2+} in the interstital fluid is greater than 1mM. Thus the gradient of free Ca^{2+} concentrations across the plasma membrane is 10 000:1. The low value of $[Ca^{2+}]_i$ is a reflection of the specificity and high affinity of regulatory Ca^{2+}-binding proteins and Ca^{2+} transporters for Ca^{2+}.

There are at least two possible reasons for the maintenance of $[Ca^{2+}]_i$ at such a low value. Firstly, this prevents the precipitation of calcium phosphate in the cytoplasmic space. Secondly, considerably less energy is required to reversibly increase $[Ca^{2+}]_i$ by 5–10-fold than would be expended if the resting value of free $[Ca^{2+}]_i$ was substantially higher than 0.1 μM.

7.2.2 *The intracellular stores of Ca^{2+}*

All animal cells contain two main intracellular stores of Ca^{2+}. These are the endoplasmic or sarcoplasmic reticulum and the mitochondria. In addition, a considerable amount of Ca^{2+} is bound to components of the cytoplasmic space (Fig. 7.2). In many cells substantial amounts of Ca^{2+} are bound to the glycocalyx on the outside of the plasma membrane. Langer and his colleagues have shown that for myocardial muscle, this pool of extracellular Ca^{2+} is probably necessary for normal cell function (Langer 1978). However, in most cells it probably does not play a role in the regulation of intracellular Ca^{2+} concentrations.

It has been difficult to obtain reliable estimates for the amounts of Ca^{2+} present in the intracellular stores and cytoplasmic space. In many early experiments the calcium content of subcellular fractions isolated from broken cell preparations was determined. However, recent examination of this approach has indicated that, with some exceptions, the results cannot be extrapolated to intact cells because considerable redistribution of Ca^{2+} may occur during isolation of the subcellular fractions. Recently, other techniques, which do not involve disruption of the cell, have been used. These techniques include electron probe microanalysis and the analysis of steady-state $^{45}Ca^{2+}$ exchange curves. Although non-disruptive, these approaches also have disadvantages. The use of $^{45}Ca^{2+}$ is indirect and the estimation of calcium by electron probe microanalysis is a relatively insensitive measure of intracellular Ca^{2+}.

Values for the concentration of total calcium in different parts of smooth-muscle cells, obtained using the electron probe, are shown in Table 7.2. The concentration of total calcium in the endoplasmic reticulum and mitochondria is substantially greater than that present in the cytoplasmic space.

Table 7.2   *The distribution of total Ca^{2+}, measured by electron probe X-ray microanalysis, within the relaxed smooth-muscle cell. Taken from Kowarski et al. (1985)*

Intracellular location	Amount of Ca^{2+} present $(mmol\,kg^{-1}\,dry\,wt\,tissue)$
Endoplasmic reticulum	1.6
Mitochondria	2.6
Cytoplasmic space	0.25
Nucleus	0.4
Whole cell	3.6

7.2.3   *The network of channels and transporters which interconnect Ca^{2+} in the extracellular space, cytoplasmic space, and intracellular stores*

$[Ca^{2+}]_i$ and the concentration of Ca^{2+} in the intracellular stores are controlled by the network of Ca^{2+} channels shown in Fig. 7.2. The network permits the movement of Ca^{2+} between the cytoplasmic space and the extracellular fluid and between the cytoplasmic space and intracellular Ca^{2+} stores. The plasma membrane, the membranes of the endoplasmic reticulum or the sarcoplasmic reticulum, and the mitochondrial inner membrane each possess at least one type of Ca^{2+} transporter and one type of Ca^{2+} channel. These permit the movement of Ca^{2+} in opposite directions across the same membrane, as shown in Fig. 7.2. As a result of this arrangement there is a considerable Ca^{2+} flux due to the cycling of Ca^{2+} across cellular membranes. This system of transporters and channels pro-

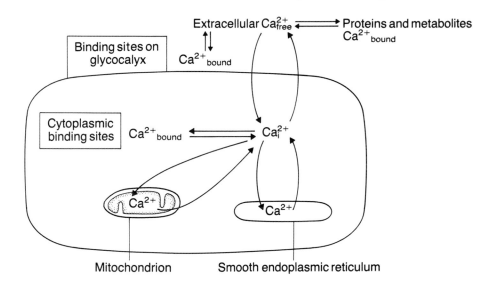

Fig. 7.2   The networks of Ca^{2+} channels and transporters and Ca^{2+} stores which control $[Ca^{2+}]_i$. The movement of Ca^{2+} across the plasma membrane, the membrane of the endoplasmic reticulum or sarcoplasmic reticulum, and the mitochondrial inner membrane is facilitated by one or more channels which permit Ca^{2+} to move down the concentration gradient, and by one or more Ca^{2+} transporters which facilitate the transport of Ca^{2+} against the concentration gradient. The magnitude of changes in $[Ca^{2+}]_i$ is influenced by the buffering capacity of anionic binding sites for Ca^{2+} in the cytoplasmic space. These sites are present on inorganic anions, metabolites, proteins, and phospholipids. On the external side of the plasma membrane of most cells there are substantial quantities of Ca^{2+} bound to the glycocalyx.

vides a fine control of $[Ca^{2+}]_i$. This control is achieved at the expense of the utilization of energy required to maintain the Ca^{2+} gradients and the cycling of the cation across membranes.

Ca^{2+} channels and transporters in the plasma membrane have two major roles. Firstly, they maintain the gradient of Ca^{2+} between the extracellular fluid and the cytoplasmic space, and secondly, they provide long-term control of the total amount of Ca^{2+} in the cell. Ca^{2+} stored in the endoplasmic or sarcoplasmic reticulum is used for the initial rapid increases in $[Ca^{2+}]_i$ induced by agonists. These stores contribute to the removal of this Ca^{2+} from the cytoplasmic space when the agonist is no longer present. While the activity of the intracellular Ca^{2+} stores is limited by the capacities of the stores to take up Ca^{2+}, the extracellular space provides an unlimited source of Ca^{2+} and an unlimited sink for the removal of Ca^{2+}.

The apparent K_M value for Ca^{2+} of the $(Ca^{2+}+Mg^{2+})$ATPase of the sarcoplasmic or endoplasmic reticulum, about 0.2 µM, is similar to the value of the apparent K_M for Ca^{2+} of the plasma-membrane $(Ca^{2+} + Mg^{2+})$ATPase. This means that the $(Ca^{2+} + Mg^{2+})$ATPases in the plasma membrane and endoplasmic or sarcoplasmic reticulum are chiefly responsible for maintenance of the value of $[Ca^{2+}]_i$ at the basal value of about 0.1 µM.

The total amount of Ca^{2+} and the concentration of free Ca^{2+} in the mitochondrial matrix are closely controlled by $[Ca^{2+}]_i$ and the mitochondrial Ca^{2+} transporters and channels. In contrast to the endoplasmic or sarcoplasmic reticulum, mitochondria are not a source of the increase in $[Ca^{2+}]_i$ induced by agonists. However, Ca^{2+} does move into the mitochondrial matrix when $[Ca^{2+}]_i$ rises, and out of the matrix when $[Ca^{2+}]_i$ falls. Although the affinity of the mitochondrial Ca^{2+} transporter for Ca^{2+} is lower than that of the endoplasmic or sarcoplasmic reticulum, mitochondria have a much higher

capacity to store Ca^{2+}. This capacity is utilized in physiological conditions in which $[Ca^{2+}]_i$ is increased for prolonged periods of time, and in pathological states, in which the movement of Ca^{2+} into the cytoplasmic space from the extracellular fluid is increased as a result of damage to the plasma membrane.

7.2.4 Binding sites for Ca^{2+} in the cytoplasmic space

Components of the cytoplasmic space which bind Ca^{2+} include the Ca^{2+}-binding proteins, other proteins present in the cytoplasmic space or in membranes, membrane phospholipids, metabolites (for example ATP and citrate), and inorganic ions (for example HPO_4^{3-}). Ca^{2+} which is unbound is described as free Ca^{2+} while Ca^{2+} which has formed an ionic complex with an anionic binding site is described as bound Ca^{2+} (Fig. 7.3).

The majority of Ca^{2+} present in the cytoplasmic space and in the lumen of organelles such as the endoplasmic reticulum, the sarcoplasmic reticulum, and mitochondria, is in the bound form. In the cytoplasmic space, the concentration of free Ca^{2+} is estimated to be between 0.1 and 1 per cent of the total Ca^{2+} present in this space. Likewise, the amount of free Ca^{2+} present in the matrix of the mitochondria and lumen of the endoplasmic reticulum is a small

$$Ca^{2+} \; + \; \text{(Anionic binding site)}^{n-} \rightleftharpoons Ca^{2+}\text{(Anionic binding site)}^{n-}$$

Free ionized form of Ca^{2+}	Protein Phospholipid Metabolite or Inorganic ion	Bound form of Ca^{2+}

Fig. 7.3 The combination of free ionized Ca^{2+} with anionic binding sites within the cytoplasmic space or the lumen of an organelle forms an ionic complex which is defined as 'bound Ca^{2+}'. Anionic binding sites are provided by metabolites, inorganic anions such as phosphate, proteins, and phospholipids.

fraction of the total Ca^{2+} present in these organelles. During transient increases in $[Ca^{2+}]_i$, such as those induced by many agonists, the maximum value of $[Ca^{2+}]_i$ achieved depends on the buffering capacity of Ca^{2+}-binding sites in the cytoplasmic space.

It is the concentration of the free Ca^{2+} in the cytoplasmic space and in the lumen of organelles which determines the fractional saturation of the Ca^{2+}-binding sites on Ca^{2+}-binding proteins. This means that knowledge of the various processes which determine the concentration of free Ca^{2+} in these spaces is important in understanding the role of Ca^{2+} as an intracellular messenger. These will now be considered in turn.

7.3 The Ca^{2+} channels and transporters of the plasma membrane

7.3.1 *An overview of Ca^{2+} movement across the plasma membrane*

The plasma membranes of most animal cells possess at least one type of system which facilitates the inflow of Ca^{2+} to the cytoplasmic space, and one or two types of transporter which move Ca^{2+} from the cytoplasmic space to the extracellular medium (Fig. 7.4). For the majority of animal cells, Ca^{2+} inflow into the cell can be subdivided into two general processes. These are basal Ca^{2+} inflow, which is independent of external stimuli such as depolarization of the membrane or the binding of an agonist to its receptor, and agonist-stimulated inflow which is initiated by an external signal (Fig. 7.4). The relative contribution of basal and agonist-stimulated Ca^{2+} inflow in a particular cell differs according to the type of cell. For example, in nerve and muscle cells Ca^{2+} inflow takes place predominantly in response to agonists, in red blood cells by only the basal process of Ca^{2+} inflow, and in liver cells by both the basal mechanism and in response to agonists.

Ca^{2+} inflow across the plasma membrane in response to extracellular stimuli is facilitated by voltage-operated Ca^{2+} channels and receptor-activated Ca^{2+} inflow systems. Most types of

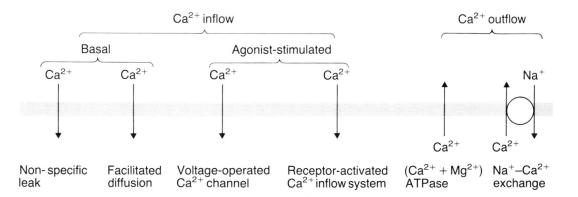

Fig. 7.4 The Ca^{2+} channels and transporters which facilitate the movement of Ca^{2+} across the plasma membrane, or the sarcolemma of muscle cells. In most cells significant quantities of Ca^{2+} move into the cell in the absence of an agonist or depolarization of the plasma membrane. This basal Ca^{2+} inflow may be facilitated by a specific Ca^{2+} channel, or may represent permeation of the membrane by Ca^{2+} in a non-specific manner. Agonist-stimulated Ca^{2+} inflow may be mediated by either a voltage-operated Ca^{2+} channel or a receptor-activated Ca^{2+} inflow system. The energy for the transport of Ca^{2+} out of the cell is derived from the hydrolysis of ATP either directly, as in the case of the $(Ca^{2+} + Mg^{2+})$ATPase, or indirectly through the gradient of Na^+ across the plasma membrane, as in the case of the Na^+–Ca^{2+} exchange system. Not all the channels or transporters shown are present in every cell type.

electrically excitable cells possess voltage-operated Ca^{2+} channels. Receptor-activated Ca^{2+} inflow systems are present in the plasma membranes of many non-excitable cells as well as many electrically excitable cells.

There are two types of plasma-membrane Ca^{2+} outflow transporter. These are the Na^+–Ca^{2+} exchange system and the $(Ca^{2+} + Mg^{2+})$-ATPase Ca^{2+} transporter (Fig. 7.4). The latter is present in all cells so far investigated while the former mode of outflow has so far been detected only in electrically excitable cells. A number of experiments indicate that the role of the Na^+–Ca^{2+} exchange system is to facilitate the rapid outflow of large amounts of Ca^{2+}

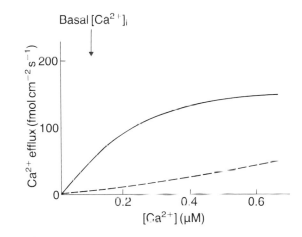

Fig. 7.5 Evidence which indicates that the $(Ca^{2+} + Mg^{2+})$ATPase Ca^{2+} transporter is responsible for the movement of the majority of Ca^{2+} from the cytoplasmic space of the squid axon to the extracellular fluid at basal values of $[Ca^{2+}]_i$. In the experiment shown, the ionic composition of the cytoplasmic space of the giant axon of the squid *Loligo pealei* was controlled by internal dialysis. At values of $[Ca^{2+}]_i$ near the basal value (0.1 µM), there is little Ca^{2+} movement out of the axon when ATP is absent from the cytoplasmic space and Na^+ is present in the extracellular medium (broken line) (conditions which favour Na^+–Ca^{2+} exchange). However, in the presence of ATP and in the absence of external Na^+ (solid line) (conditions which favour the $(Ca^{2+} + Mg^{2+})$ATPase) there is a substantial movement of Ca^{2+} out of the axon at basal $[Ca^{2+}]_i$. From DiPolo and Beauge (1979).

which have entered a cell and have induced an elevation of $[Ca^{2+}]_i$ following the opening of voltage-operated Ca^{2+} channels. The role of the $(Ca^{2+} + Mg^{2+})$ATPase is to maintain $[Ca^{2+}]_i$ near the basal value over more prolonged periods of time. An example of the evidence which indicates that the two Ca^{2+} outflow transporters have different roles in excitable cells is an experiment conducted by DiPolo and Beauge (1979) with dialysed giant-nerve axons from squid. They showed that at basal $[Ca^{2+}]_i$, the amount of Ca^{2+} which flows from the axoplasm to the extracellular medium through the $(Ca^{2+} + Mg^{2+})$ATPase is much greater than that which flows through the Na^+–Ca^{2+} exchange system (Fig. 7.5).

7.3.2   *Mechanisms of Ca^{2+} inflow in the absence of agonists*

There seem to be at least two components of the basal process of Ca^{2+} inflow. These are facilitated diffusion, thought to occur via a specific protein channel, and a non-specific leak of Ca^{2+} (Fig. 7.4). In terms of moles of Ca^{2+} transported per unit area of plasma membrane, the flux of Ca^{2+} into cells by facilitated diffusion through a specific protein channel is very low in some cells, such as nerve, muscle, and red blood cells, and apparently high in others, such as liver cells. The process of Na^+–Ca^{2+} exchange (the inward movement of Ca^{2+} in exchange for the outward movement of Na^+) may also contribute to Ca^{2+} inflow in some types of cell although further experiments are required to verify the existence of this mode of Ca^{2+} inflow.

Basal Ca^{2+} inflow to the cytoplasmic space by non-specific leakage probably includes the diffusion of Ca^{2+} through the phospholipid bilayer itself, through gap junctions, as well as Ca^{2+} inflow mediated in a non-specific manner by proteins involved in the movement of other ions. Ca^{2+} inflow mediated by the non-specific pathway is increased in some pathological states.

7.3.3 *The physiological properties of voltage-operated Ca^{2+} channels*

Studies of Ca^{2+} movement through voltage-operated Ca^{2+} channels have been greatly assisted by the use of the patch-clamp technique modified so that the movement of Ca^{2+} ions through a single channel can be studied. This technique, which was developed by Neher and Sakmann and their colleagues (Hammill *et al.*, 1991), involves the isolation of a patch of membrane by pressing a small heat-polished glass pipette, which contains Ba^{2+}, against the membrane. A successful patch requires the formation of a very tight seal between the membrane and the pipette. The patch of membrane can remain attached to the cell or can be detached from the cell. A depolarizing potential is applied and maintained (clamped) for a period of milliseconds in order to depolarize the membrane. The resulting movement of Ba^{2+} through open Ca^{2+} channels is detected as a brief increase in current. If the diameter of the pipette is sufficiently small, a single Ca^{2+} channel can be isolated in the patch. Success of the technique depends on the tightness of the seal formed between the membrane and pipette.

Experiments using the patch-clamp technique have shown that there are at least four types of voltage-operated Ca^{2+} channel, designated the L, T, N, and P-type channels. These are distinguished by the change in membrane potential required to induce opening of the channel, the rate of inactivation of the channel, and the sensitivity of the channel to inhibiton by members of the dihydropyridine family of drugs and ω-conotoxin.

L-type channels are opened by a strong depolarization, allow Ca^{2+} currents of long duration, and are sensitive to inhibition by some dihydropyridines or activation by other dihydropyridines. These channels are the predominant voltage-operated Ca^{2+} channels present in cardiac and skeletal muscle cells. T-type channels are activated by a weak depolarization, are rapidly inactivated in a voltage-dependent manner, and are relatively insensitive to dihydropyridines which inhibit L-type channels.

A relatively strong depolarization is required to activate N-type channels. Inactivation of these channels is moderately rapid. They are inhibited by ω-conotoxin and are insensitive to dihydropyridines. N-type channels are present in neurones. P-type channels are distinguished by their susceptibility to inhibition by funnel web spider toxin, lack of susceptibility to inhibition by dihydropyridines and ω-conotoxin, and activation by a medium depolarization of the plasma membrane.

It is envisaged that a given voltage-operated Ca^{2+} channel exists in at least three states. These are the closed, open, and inactivated states (Fig. 7.6). The inactivated state represents the form of the channel which has closed after being opened. The likelihood of a particular channel being in the open state at any given time is described by a probability term, p_{open}. The value of p_{open} is zero when the membrane is fully polarized and approaches 1 when the membrane is completely depolarized. Depolarization of the

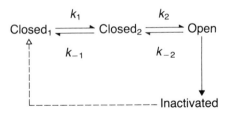

Fig. 7.6 At any given instant an individual voltage-operated Ca^{2+} channel probably exists in one of two closed states, an open state or an inactivated state. The inactivated state is reached when the open channel is inactivated. A probability term, p_{open}, is used to describe the probability that an individual channel is in the open state. When the membrane is fully polarized, p_{open} is zero. Depolarization from a resting membrane potential of about $-70\,mV$ to values between 0 and $+30\,mV$ increases p_{open} to its maximum value (approaching 1) by increasing the rate constants for opening, k_1 and k_2, and by decreasing those for closing, k_{-1} and k_{-2}.

plasma membrane leads to the opening of an individual Ca^{2+} channel for a very brief period. The channels are thought to be inactivated by re-polarization of the membrane and by the movement of the Ca^{2+} ions through the channel.

The flux of Ca^{2+} through open voltage-operated channels depends on the membrane potential and the Ca^{2+} concentration gradient across the membrane. Each Ca^{2+} ion is thought to bind momentarily to the channel protein as it passes through the channel. On the basis of the theory proposed by Hodgkin and Katz (1949), the flux of Ca^{2+} through open voltage-operated Ca^{2+} channels is described by the equation.

Inward Ca^{2+} flux =
$$P\exp(-2FE/RT)[Ca^{2+}]_o{}^F - P[Ca^{2+}]_i{}^F$$

where the inward Ca^{2+} flux is expressed in mol $cm^{-2}s^{-1}$, $[Ca^{2+}]_o{}^F$ and $[Ca^{2+}]_i{}^F$ represent the con-

centrations (M) of free Ca^{2+} in the extracellular medium and cytoplasmic space, respectively, P (cm s^{-1}) is a permeability constant, F ($=9.652 \times 10^4$ C mol^{-1}) is the Faraday constant, E (V) is the membrane potential, R ($=8.31$ J mol^{-1} K^{-1}) is the gas constant, and T(K) is the absolute temperature.

The movement of Ca^{2+} through voltage-operated Ca^{2+} channels is inhibited by La^{3+} and divalent metal ions as well as Ca^{2+} channel blockers. These inhibitors and their proposed modes of action are listed in Table 7.3. Some dihydropyridines, for example the compounds Bay K 8644 and CGP 28392, increase the probability of channel opening and hence stimulate Ca^{2+} inflow.

On the basis of the results of electrophysiological experiments, the voltage-operated Ca^{2+} channel is viewed as a water-filled pore through

Table 7.3   *Inhibitors of voltage-operated Ca^{2+} channels*

Inhibitor group	Examples	Nature of inhibition
Dihydropyridines	Nifedipine, nitrendipine	Bind to α_1 subunit Modify probability of channel opening, preferentially bind to inactivated state Preferentially inhibit L-type channels
Phenylalkylamines	Verapamil	Bind to α_1 subunit Require open channel, preferentially bind to inactivated state Preferentially inhibit L-type channels
Benzothiazepines	Diltiazem	Bind to α_1 subunit Act from the cytoplasmic face of channel, preferentially bind to inactivated state, interfere with gating mechanism Preferentially inhibit L-type channels
Metal ions	La^{3+}, Mn^{2+} Co^{2+}, Ni^{2+}	May occupy putatiave Ca^{2+} binding site within channel

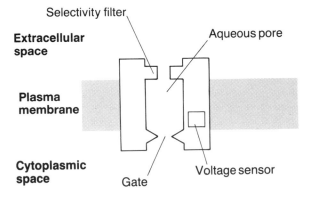

Fig. 7.7 Structural features of the voltage-operated Ca^{2+} channel which have been proposed on the basis of electrophysiological data. One subunit of the channel protein is thought to form an aqueous pore through which Ca^{2+} ions can move. Postulated components of the channel include a selectivity filter, which determines the nature of the ions admitted, and a gate which determines whether the channel is opened or closed. The gate is probably linked to a component of the channel which acts as a sensor to detect changes in the membrane potential. In L-type Ca^{2+} channels, the subunit which forms the Ca^{2+} pore also contains the binding site for dihydropyridine Ca^{2+} antagonists. From Stanfield (1986).

which Ca^{2+} can move (Fig. 7.7). The movement of Ca^{2+} is regulated by a gating mechanism which determines whether the channel is open or closed, and by a selectivity filter which determines the nature of the ions which are admitted. The gating mechanism is linked to a voltage sensor. These are shown only in schematic form in Fig. 7.7 because their molecular nature and mode of action are not yet known. The Ca^{2+} channel excludes most ions except Ca^{2+}, Ba^{2+}, Sr^{2+}, and some other divalent cations. In experimental systems, Ba^{2+} and Sr^{2+} are transported more rapidly than Ca^{2+}. By contrast, Mg^{2+} is transported very poorly.

7.3.4 *The molecular structure of voltage-operated Ca^{2+} channels*

The voltage-operated Ca^{2+}-channel protein complexes present in a number of types of cells have been isolated. Successful channel-protein

isolation has been dependent upon the development of a suitable method for the assay of the channels. Fortunately this problem was solved by making use of compounds such as [³H]nitrendipine, [³H]nimodipine, the photoaffinity label [³H]azidopin, and other radioactively labelled Ca^{2+} antagonists which bind tightly and specifically to voltage-operated Ca^{2+} channels (Glossmann and Ferry 1983).

The L-type voltage-operated Ca^{2+} channel is an oligomeric glycoprotein with a molecular weight of about 390 kDa. The oligomer is composed of one each of five subunits named a_1 (175 kDa), α_2 (105 kDa), β (54 kDa), γ (30kDa), and a much smaller subunit, δ. The probable arrangement of these subunits in the plasma membrane is shown in Fig. 7.8. The α_1 subunit is a membrane-spanning protein which creates the water-filled pore through which, on the basis of the electrophysiological data described earlier, it is proposed that Ca^{2+} moves. The a_1 subunit also contains the binding site for 1,4-dihydropyridines and is thought to contain a voltage sensor. The α_2 and γ subunits also contain membrane-spanning domains and are glycosylated. The hydrophilic β subunit is probably attached to the cytoplasmic side of the oligomer and the hydrophilic and glycosylated δ subunit to the extracellular side. The α_1 and β subunits each contain sites which can be phosphorylated by cyclic AMP-dependent protein kinase (Fig. 7.8).

The amino-acid sequence of the α_1 subunit of the rabbit skeletal muscle L-type voltage-operated Ca^{2+} channel has been deduced from the base sequence of the cDNA which encodes this polypeptide chain (Tanabe *et al.* 1987). The polypeptide chain is folded into four motifs each of which consists of six membrane-spanning sequences. One charged membrane-spanning sequence from each motif may line the water-filled pore of the channel while a second membrane-spanning sequence from each motif may

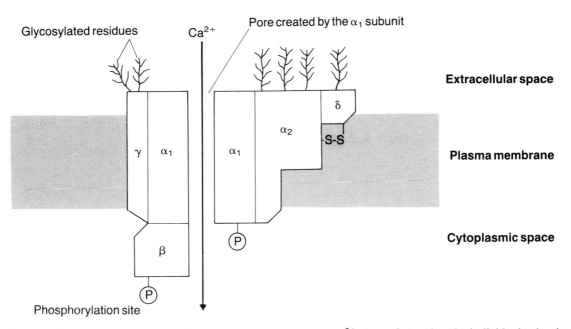

Fig. 7.8 The subunit structure of the L-type voltage-operated Ca^{2+} channel showing the individual subunits and their proposed relationships to the plasma membrane. The phosphorylation sites represent serine or threonine residues phosphorylated by cyclic AMP-dependent protein kinase. From Campbell *et al.* (1988).

constitute the voltage detector. Elucidation of the structure of the voltage-operated Ca^{2+} channel was aided by knowledge of the structure of the voltage-operated channels for Na^+ and K^+ which had been determined previously.

7.3.5 *The receptor-activated Ca^{2+} inflow systems*

The opening of receptor-activated Ca^{2+} inflow systems requires the binding of an agonist to its receptor, and is not dependent on depolarization of the plasma membrane. This type of Ca^{2+} inflow system is sometimes called a receptor-operated Ca^{2+} channel. Some receptor-activated Ca^{2+} inflow systems are inhibited by the Ca^{2+} antagonists listed in Table 7.3. However, the concentrations of a given antagonist which inhibit receptor-activated Ca^{2+} inflow systems are generally considerably higher than those which inhibit voltage-operated Ca^{2+} channels.

A number of experiments have suggested that there may be at least two types of receptor-activated Ca^{2+} inflow system. These are channels which are opened by an intracellular messenger, such as an inositol polyphosphate or Ca^{2+} itself, and channels which are opened by interaction of the channel protein with a GTP-binding regulatory protein. Another possibility is that for some receptor-activated Ca^{2+} inflow systems the Ca^{2+} channel is part of the receptor protein itself and is opened by a conformational change in the receptor protein induced by the binding of an agonist. Such a putative 'ligand-induced' Ca^{2+} channel would be similar in its general structure to the nicotinic acetylcholine Na^+ channel described in Chapter 3.

7.3.6 *The $(Ca^{2+} + Mg^{2+})ATPases$*

The $(Ca^{2+} + Mg^{2+})ATPase$ Ca^{2+} transporter which facilitates the outflow of Ca^{2+} across the plasma membrane of non-muscle cells or the sarcolemma of muscle cells was first characterized

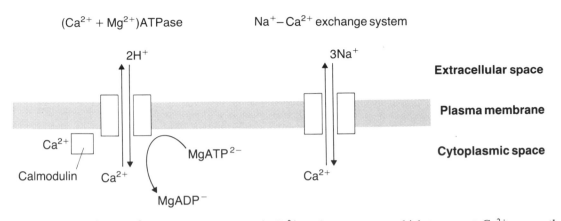

Fig. 7.9 The $(Ca^{2+} + Mg^{2+})$ATPase and the $Na^+–Ca^{2+}$ exchange system which transport Ca^{2+} across the plasma membrane against the Ca^{2+} concentration gradient. All cells possess a $(Ca^{2+} + Mg^{2+})$ATPase Ca^{2+} transporter, and many electrically excitable cells and some other cells also possess an $Na^+–Ca^{2+}$ exchange system. In some but not all cells, the $(Ca^{2+} + Mg^{2+})$ATPase Ca^{2+} transporter is activated by the binding of calmodulin to the enzyme in the presence of Ca^{2+}.

by Schatzmann and Vincenzi (1969). They studied the properties of the enzyme present in red blood cells. Subsequently Caroni and Carafoli (1981) purified the $(Ca^{2+} + Mg^{2+})$ATPases present in red blood cells and myocardial muscle cells and conducted extensive investigations of the properties of these enzymes.

The plasma-membrane $(Ca^{2+} + Mg^{2+})$ATPase protein has a molecular weight of about 140 kDa. The enzyme catalyses the electroneutral transport of one Ca^{2+} ion for two H^+ ions (Fig. 7.9). Therefore the movement of Ca^{2+} by this transporter is independent of membrane potential. The energy required to move Ca^{2+} ions against the Ca^{2+} concentration gradient is provided by the hydrolysis of ATP. Mg^{2+} is required as a cofactor. In many cell types this reaction is sensitive to inhibition by orthovanadate (VO_4^{3-}) and some other species of vanadate ions.

The plasma-membrane $(Ca^{2+} + Mg^{2+})$ATPase Ca^{2+} transporters present in a number of cells, including red blood cells and myocardial muscle cells, bind calmodulin. This is shown schematically in Fig. 7.9. The binding of the $(Ca^{2+} + calmodulin)$ complex leads to a marked

decrease in the apparent K_M of the $(Ca^{2+} + Mg^{2+})$ATPase for Ca^{2+} and to an increase in the maximum activity of the enzyme (Fig. 7.10). In the presence of calmodulin, the apparent K_M for Ca^{2+} for the enzyme from red blood cells is about 1 μM and the plot of the rate of Ca^{2+}-stimulated ATP hydrolysis as a function of free Ca^{2+} concentration is sigmoidal (Fig. 7.10). Calmodulin does not bind to the $(Ca^{2+} + Mg^{2+})$ATPase Ca^{2+} transporters present in the plasma membranes of liver cells and a number of other types of cell. The affinity for Ca^{2+} of these $(Ca^{2+} + Mg^{2+})$ATPases is comparable with that of the $(Ca^{2+} + Mg^{2+})$ATPases which do bind calmodulin when the affinity for Ca^{2+} is measured in the presence of calmodulin.

In addition to the action of calmodulin, plasma-membrane $(Ca^{2+} + Mg^{2+})$ATPases are also activated by proteolytic cleavage, by interaction with the acidic molecule phosphatidylinositol 4,5-bisphosphate, and by phosphorylation by protein kinases. Whilst the physiological role of the first two processes is unclear, protein phosphorylation, like the action of calmodulin, has an important physiological role in the regulation of Ca^{2+} outflow across the

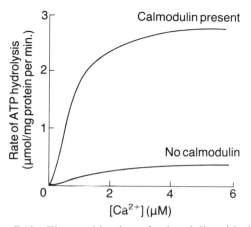

Fig. 7.10 The combination of calmodulin with the plasma-membrane $(Ca^{2+} + Mg^{2+})$ATPase Ca^{2+} transporter isolated from red blood cells increases the maximum reaction velocity and decreases the apparent K_M for Ca^{2+}. In this example, the purified enzyme was reconstituted with phospholipids by insertion in phosphatidylcholine liposomes. From Niggli *et al.* (1981).

plasma membrane. This is discussed further in Section 7.7.2.

7.3.7 *The Na^+–Ca^{2+} exchange system*

In the Na^+–Ca^{2+} exchange system, each Ca^{2+} ion moves out of the cell in exchange for three Na^+ ions (Fig. 7.9). Since the movement of the charge is not balanced, this transport system is electrogenic. Energy for the outward movement of Ca^{2+} is derived from both the Na^+ concentration gradient across the plasma membrane and the membrane potential. The Na^+–Ca^{2+} exchange system has a high capacity to transport Ca^{2+} (in terms of ion equivalents of Ca^{2+} transported per unit area of cell surface). It has been estimated that in a single heart cell, Na^+–Ca^{2+} exchange systems transport 3×10^9 Ca^{2+} ions per second.

7.4 The Ca^{2+} channels and transporters of the endoplasmic and sarcoplasmic reticulum

7.4.1 *The reticular network as a Ca^{2+} store*

The smooth and rough endoplasmic reticulum and the sarcoplasmic reticulum are extensive tubular networks which ramify through the cell. Sections of the reticular network in the liver cell are shown in Fig. 7.11. Glycogen granules are surrounded by smooth endoplasmic reticulum. The reticular membranes enclose a space which is separate from the cytoplasmic space. The uptake, storage, and release of Ca^{2+} is one of a number of functions of the endoplasmic reticulum. It appears to be the sole function of the sarcoplasmic reticulum in skeletal and heart muscle cells.

The reticular network provides a system by which $[Ca^{2+}]_i$ can be altered near the intracellular sites at which changes in $[Ca^{2+}]_i$ are required for the regulation of target enzymes. The dis-

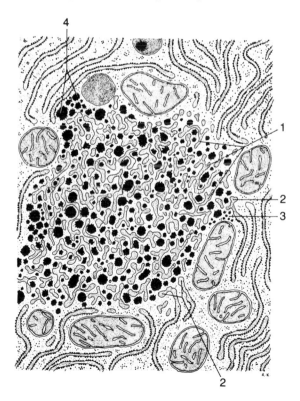

Fig. 7.11 An example of the ramifying network of the endoplasmic reticulum. In the liver cell, tubules of the smooth endoplasmic reticulum (1) originate from the rough endoplasmic reticulum (2) and lie between glycogen granules (3,4). From Krstic (1979).

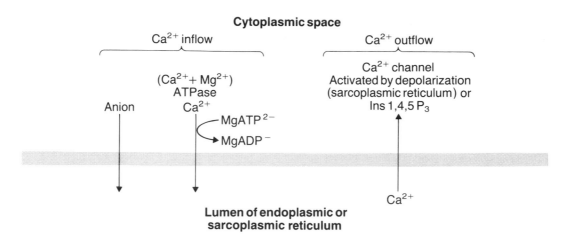

Fig. 7.12 The Ca^{2+} channels and transporters which facilitate the movement of Ca^{2+} across the membranes of the smooth endoplasmic reticulum and the sarcoplasmic reticulum. Ca^{2+} is transported from the cytoplasmic space to the lumen by a $(Ca^{2+} + Mg^{2+})ATPase$. It is thought that the increase in positive charge caused by the electrogenic movement of Ca^{2+} into the lumen is balanced by the movement of anions in the same direction. The movement of Ca^{2+} from the lumen to the cytoplasmic space is facilitated by at least two types of channel. These may be opened by Ins 1,4,5 P_3 (endoplasmic reticulum) or by depolarization of the sarcolemma (sarcoplasmic reticulum).

tance within a cell over which Ca^{2+} must diffuse from the site of its release to its site of action is thus greatly reduced by the presence of the endoplasmic and sarcoplasmic reticulum. Some experiments with smooth-muscle cells have led to the suggestion that the smooth endoplasmic reticulum may also provide an avenue through which external Ca^{2+} can move to internal sites in the cell without entering the cytoplasmic space. In skeletal muscle cells, the T tubules, an extension of the plasma membrane, perform this function. A further advantage to the cell of a Ca^{2+} store in the endoplasmic or sarcoplasmic reticulum is that less energy is expended in transporting Ca^{2+} from the cytoplasmic space to this Ca^{2+} store than would be expended in the transport of Ca^{2+} to the extracellular fluid against the large Ca^{2+} gradient at the plasma membrane.

7.4.2   *The $(Ca^{2+} + Mg^{2+})ATPases$ of the endoplasmic and sarcoplasmic reticulum*

Ca^{2+} is transported from the cytoplasmic space

to the lumen of the endoplasmic reticulum by a $(Ca^{2+} + Mg^{2+})ATPase$ (Fig. 7.12). This Ca^{2+} is stored in the lumen as a complex with specific Ca^{2+}-binding proteins. In the sarcoplasmic reticulum of skeletal muscle, the major Ca^{2+}-binding protein is calsequestrin. The structure and properties of this protein were elucidated by MacLennan and his colleagues (MacLennan and Wong 1971).

There are two isoforms of the sarcoplasmic and endoplasmic $(Ca^{2+} + Mg^{2+})ATPase$. One form is predominant in cardiac and slow-twitch muscle while the second form is present in smooth muscle and in most other types of cell. Some types of cell, including brain neurones, possess both isoforms. The two forms are generated from the same gene by alternative splicing of the transcribed RNA.

Studies of the molecular properties of the $(Ca^{2+} + Mg^{2+})ATPase$ Ca^{2+} transporter in the sarcoplasmic reticulum have been facilitated by the fact that 70 per cent of the total protein in the sarcoplasmic reticulum is the $(Ca^{2+} +$

Mg^{2+})ATPase enzyme. The molecular weight of this enzyme is about 100 kDa. In contrast to the $(Ca^{2+} + Mg^{2+})$ATPase from the sarcolemma, the transport of Ca^{2+} by the reticulum enzyme is electrogenic. In most types of cell the enzyme from the reticular network is much more sensitive to the inhibitory effects of vanadate than is the plasma-membrane $(Ca^{2+} + Mg^{2+})$ATPase.

The mechanism of the reaction catalysed by the sarcoplasmic reticulum $(Ca^{2+} + Mg^{2+})$ATPase has been studied in detail and is shown in Fig. 7.13. The cycles of Ca^{2+} movement and ATP hydrolysis begin with the sequential combination of Ca^{2+} and $MgATP^{2-}$ with the enzyme at the cytoplasmic face of the membrane. Subsequent hydrolysis of ATP and concomitant phosphorylation of the enzyme induces a conformation change in the enzyme, the movement of Ca^{2+} across the membrane, and the release of Ca^{2+} into the lumen of the reticulum. The enzyme-phosphate bond is then hydrolysed and the enzyme returns to the original conformation.

Electron micrographs show that the sarcoplasmic reticulum $(Ca^{2+} + Mg^{2+})$ATPase Ca^{2+} transporter is spherical and attached to the membrane by a narrow stalk. The transmembrane domain of the molecule is composed of ten membrane-spanning helices (Fig. 7.14). Five of the α-helices extend into the cytoplasmic space to create the stalk region. The hydrophilic sphere in the cytoplasmic domain contains the binding site for ATP and the ATPase catalytic site. Glutamate and aspartate residues in a number of the transmembrane domains may create binding sites for Ca^{2+} in the pathway through which Ca^{2+} traverses the membrane.

Whilst $[Ca^{2+}]_i$ is the main parameter which determines the activity of the $(Ca^{2+} + Mg^{2+})$ATPase of the endoplasmic and sarcoplasmic reticulum, an additional regulatory mechanism is present in the sarcoplasmic reticulum. This involves the interaction of a small integral membrane protein called phospholamban with the

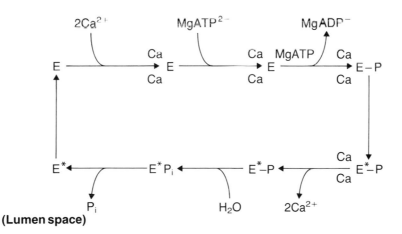

(Cytoplasmic space)

(Lumen space)

Fig. 7.13 Reaction sequences for the transport of Ca^{2+} from the cytoplasmic space to the lumen of the sarcoplasmic reticulum by the $(Ca^{2+} + Mg^{2+})$ATPase which is present in skeletal and heart muscle. Ca^{2+} and $MgATP^{2-}$ bind at the cytoplasmic side of the membrane. Phosphorylation of the enzyme (E) leads to a conformational change (to the form E*–P) which is associated with the movement of Ca^{2+} from the cytoplasmic space to the luminal side of the membrane where the Ca^{2+} is subsequently released. Hydrolysis of E*–P occurs on the cytoplasmic side of the membrane. Adapted from de Meis (1981).

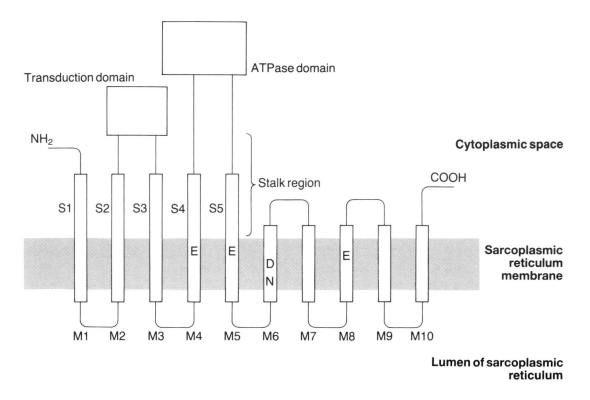

Fig. 7.14 A schematic view of the secondary structure of the $(Ca^{2+} + Mg^{2+})$ATPase of skeletal muscle sarcoplasmic reticulum. The structure is represented as a planar diagram and does not reflect the true three-dimensional structure of the molecule. The membrane-spanning domain is composed of 10 helices (named M1 to M10). This region is connected to the ATPase domain and another cytoplasmic domain, which is called the transduction domain, by a region of five α-helices (S1 to S5) called the stalk region. The cytoplasmic domain is globular in shape. A number of charged residues, including aspartate (D), glutamate (E), and asparagine (N) in the transmembrane helices probably contribute to the formation of high-affinity binding sites for Ca^{2+}. Adapted from Clarke *et al.* (1989).

$(Ca^{2+} + Mg^{2+})$ATPase. Phospholamban is an amphipathic peptide with a molecular weight of 6 kDa. In the isolated form of the protein, five of these phospholamban monomers form a complex. In the sarcoplasmic reticulum membrane one molecule of phospholamban is present for every molecule of $(Ca^{2+} + Mg^{2+})$ATPase. The phosphorylation of phospholamban by either cyclic AMP-dependent protein kinase or by a specific $(Ca^{2+} + calmodulin)$-dependent protein kinase leads to an activation of the $(Ca^{2+} + Mg^{2+})$ATPase and hence to an increase in the rate of Ca^{2+} transport at a given value of $[Ca^{2+}]_i$.

7.4.3 *The Ca^{2+} channels of the endoplasmic and sarcoplasmic reticulum*

For most types of cell there is a small flow of Ca^{2+} from the lumen of the endoplasmic reticulum or sarcoplasmic reticulum to the cytoplasmic space in the absence of an extracellular agonist. This Ca^{2+} flow is greatly enhanced by the action of an appropriate agonist. The outflow of Ca^{2+} from the sarcoplasmic reticulum in skeletal and heart muscle cells and from the endoplasmic reticulum in other cells in response to the action of an agonist at the plasma membrane is a rapid process. This indicates that the channels which facilitate the movement of Ca^{2+} out of these organelles have a large capacity for the movement of Ca^{2+}. There are at least two types of Ca^{2+} channel. These are the inositol 1,4,5-trisphosphate-sensitive Ca^{2+} channel of the endoplasmic reticulum and the Ca^{2+} channel of the sarcoplasmic reticulum of skeletal and heart muscle. The sarcoplasmic reticulum Ca^{2+} channel is also known as the junctional 'foot protein' and the ryanodine receptor.

The Ins 1,4,5 P_3-sensitive Ca^{2+} channel of the endoplasmic reticulum is a tetrameric glycoprotein which binds heparin and concanavalin A as well as Ins 1,4,5 P_3 (Chapter 6, Section 6.6.4). Each monomer has a molecular weight of 250 kDa and probably contains seven membrane-spanning sequences. The carboxy terminus is located in the lumen of the endoplasmic reticulum while the amino terminus and a large amino-terminal hydrophilic domain are located in the cytoplasmic space.

There is considerable homology between regions of the sarcoplasmic reticulum Ca^{2+} channel and the Ins 1,4,5 P_3-sensitive Ca^{2+} channel. The sarcoplasmic reticulum Ca^{2+} channel is located in the terminal cisternae of the sarcoplasmic reticulum. Under the electron microscope these channels can be seen as 'foot' structures associated with the junctional face of the membrane. Like the Ins 1,4,5 P_3-sensitive Ca^{2+} channel, the sarcoplasmic reticulum Ca^{2+} channel is also a tetramer. The monomers have a molecular weight of 360–450 kDa and probably possess four membrane-spanning sequences. In contrast to the Ins 1,4,5 P_3-sensitive Ca^{2+} channel, the carboxy terminus, the amino terminus, and an associated large amino-terminal hydrophilic domain are located in the cytoplasmic space. The sarcoplasmic reticulum Ca^{2+} channel is inhibited by the toxic alkaloid ryanodine which binds to the channel with high affinity and in a specific manner. This property has been used as an assay for the channel during its purification.

7.5 The Ca^{2+} channels and transporters of the mitochondria

The inner mitochondrial membrane is selectively permeable to Ca^{2+} and other cations and anions whereas the outer membrane appears to be freely permeable to ions and metabolites. In 1962, Vasington and Murphy observed that isolated mitochondria avidly accumulate Ca^{2+}. Subsequently, the mechanism by which Ca^{2+} is transported from the cytoplasmic space to the mitochondrial matrix across the inner membrane was characterized by Lehninger and his colleagues (Lehninger *et al.* 1967) and by many others. However, some time elapsed before it was realized that the mitochondrial inner membrane also possesses Ca^{2+} outflow systems which are separate in structure and mechanism of action from the Ca^{2+} inflow transporter.

The term Ca^{2+} uniporter is used to describe the pathway by which Ca^{2+} is transported from the cytoplasmic space to the mitochondrial matrix. The transfer of charge carried by Ca^{2+} is not directly compensated by the co-transport of an anion or exchange of Ca^{2+} with another cation so that the movement of Ca^{2+} through the uniporter is electrogenic (Fig. 7.15). The energy required to move Ca^{2+} against the concentration gradient is derived from the membrane potential and the pH gradient across the mitochondrial inner membrane. Thus, in contrast to the movement of Ca^{2+} to the lumen of the endoplasmic and sarcoplasmic reticulum, a $(Ca^{2+} + Mg^{2+})$ATPase is not involved in the uptake of Ca^{2+} to the mitochondrial matrix.

Under experimental conditions in which isolated mitochondria take up large amounts of Ca^{2+}, the inflow of Ca^{2+} is accompanied by the movement of an anion, usually HPO_4^-, from the extra-mitochondrial medium to the matrix. Movement of HPO_4^- is catalysed by the phosphate–OH^- exchanger (Fig. 7.15). The large inflow of Ca^{2+} is due to the formation of insolu-

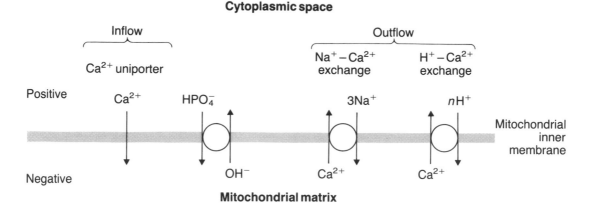

Fig. 7.15 The channels and transporters which move Ca^{2+} across the mitochondrial inner membrane. Ca^{2+} is transported from the cytoplasmic space to the mitochondrial matrix against the Ca^{2+} concentration gradient by the Ca^{2+} uniporter. The required energy is derived from the electrochemical gradient across the mitochondrial inner membrane. The electrogenic movement of Ca^{2+} into the matrix may be accompanied by the movement of HPO_4^- through the HPO_4^-–OH^- exchange transporter. A Ca^{2+}–Na^+ or Ca^{2+}–H^+ exchange system facilitates the movement of Ca^{2+} from the mitochondrial matrix to the cytoplasmic space. These exchange proteins are separate from the Ca^{2+} uniporter.

ble calcium phosphate in the mitochondrial matrix and to compensation of the charge carried by Ca^{2+} by the movement of HPO_4^-.

The movement of Ca^{2+} from the mitochondrial matrix to the cytoplasmic space is facilitated by an Na^+–Ca^{2+} or H^+–Ca^{2+} exchange system (Fig. 7.15). In the mitochondria of myocardial muscle cells and of cells of the central nervous system, Na^+–Ca^{2+} exchange predominates. In liver-cell mitochondria, the major process of Ca^{2+} outflow appears to be H^+–Ca^{2+} exchange. The movement of three Na^+ or several H^+ in exchange for Ca^{2+} more than compensates for the transfer of the charge carried by Ca^{2+}. This means that Ca^{2+} cannot flow into the mitochondrial matrix through the Na^+–Ca^{2+} or H^+–Ca^{2+} exchange systems. (If the movement of Ca^{2+} were not fully compensated by the movement of Na^+ or H^+ in the opposite direction, the Na^+–Ca^{2+} or H^+–Ca^{2+} exchange systems would permit the movement of Ca^{2+} into the mitochondrial matrix down the gradient of charge across the membrane.)

7.6 The increase in the cytoplasmic free Ca^{2+} concentration induced by agonists

7.6.1 *Measurement of agonist-induced increases in the cytoplasmic free Ca^{2+} concentration*

Although it was realized for many years that the intracellular concentration of free rather than total Ca^{2+} is the key parameter in the regulation of enzyme activity by this cation, measurement of the changes in free Ca^{2+} and direct verification of the hypothesis that agonists increase $[Ca^{2+}]_i$ proved difficult. This was due chiefly to the small volume of the cytoplasmic space, difficulties encountered in the introduction of detectors of free Ca^{2+} into the cytoplasmic space, the presence of a large proportion of intracellular Ca^{2+} in a bound form, and the heterogeneous distribution of both free and bound Ca^{2+} within the cell. Early estimates of $[Ca^{2+}]_i$ were made using Ca^{2+}-selective microelectrodes or photoproteins such as aequorin. The last-mentioned protein, which is extracted

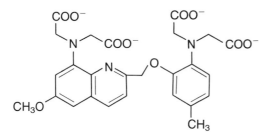

Quin 2

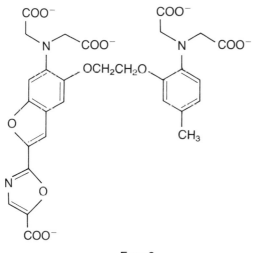

Fura 2

Fig. 7.16 Structures of quin 2 and fura 2, two fluorescent Ca²⁺ chelators developed by Tsien and his colleagues (Tsien 1980; Grynkiewicz *et al.* 1985) for the measurement of $[Ca^{2+}]_i$.

from the jellyfish *Aequorea forskalea*, emits luminescence when it binds Ca^{2+}. However, the application of these techniques to a wide variety of cell types was limited.

The development in 1980 of a family of intracellular fluorescent Ca^{2+} chelators by Tsien provided a technique which could be applied to the measurement of $[Ca^{2+}]_i$ in many different types of cell (Tsien 1980; 1981). The two members of this family which have been used most extensively are quin 2 and fura 2 (Fig. 7.16). These compounds have structural features which are similar to the structure of EGTA, and bind Ca^{2+}

with high affinity and specificity. Tsien modified the basic structure of EGTA by introducing cyclic groups so that the binding of Ca^{2+} would be accompanied by an increase in fluorescence of the molecule.

Quin 2 was the first of the intracellular fluorescent Ca^{2+} chelators to be developed. However, intracellular concentrations of about 1 mM quin 2 are necessary for adequate measurement of $[Ca^{2+}]_i$. In some experiments, the presence of high concentrations of quin 2 interfered with the measurement of changes in $[Ca^{2+}]_i$ by acting as an intracellular Ca^{2+} buffer. Subsequent modification of the structure of quin 2, and the synthesis of fura 2, indo 1, and other molecules of this family has enabled $[Ca^{2+}]_i$ to be measured using lower intracellular concentrations of the Ca^{2+} chelator. The success of the technique invented by Tsien was also due to the development of a procedure in which small cells could be loaded with a fluorescent Ca^{2+} chelator by incubation with the lipid-soluble acetoxymethylester of the chelator.

Although there are some limitations to the use of the fluorescent intracellular Ca^{2+} chelators developed by Tsien, the technique has been invaluable in studies of the role of Ca^{2+} as an intracellular messenger. Changes in $[Ca^{2+}]_i$ have been measured either in stirred cell suspensions in the cuvette of a spectrofluorimeter or in individual cells using a fluorescence microscope and the techniques of image analysis.

7.6.2 *The biphasic increase in cytoplasmic free Ca²⁺ concentration induced by agonists*

In most types of cell, the increase in $[Ca^{2+}]_i$ induced by agonists occurs in two phases when changes in $[Ca^{2+}]_i$ are measured in cell suspensions (Fig. 7.17). After a large initial increase, which is rapid in onset and often transient, $[Ca^{2+}]_i$ is maintained for a more prolonged period at a value greater than the basal value. The second phase of $[Ca^{2+}]_i$ increase is substantially

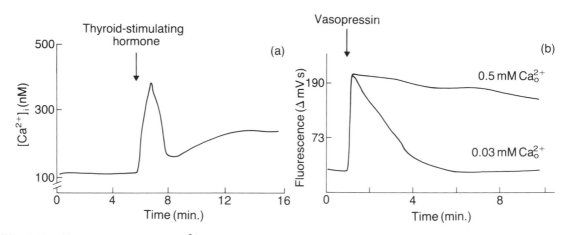

Fig. 7.17 Changes observed in $[Ca^{2+}]_i$ in suspensions of cultured GH_3 pituitary cells following the addition of thyrotropin-releasing hormone (a), and in suspensions of isolated hepatocytes following addition of vasopressin (b). $[Ca^{2+}]_i$ was measured using fura 2 (a) and quin 2 (b). The experiment with hepatocytes shows that maintenance of increased $[Ca^{2+}]_i$ at longer times after the addition of vasopressin depends on the presence of physiological concentrations of Ca^{2+} (Ca_o^{2+}) in the extracellular medium. From Kolesnick and Gershengorn (1985) (GH_3 cells) and Charest *et al.* (1985) (isolated hepatocytes).

reduced by the removal of extracellular Ca^{2+}, as shown in Fig. 7.17 for the action of vasopressin on hepatocytes.

In heart muscle, some nerve cells, and in some other types of cell, agonist-induced depolarization of the plasma membrane induces transient increases in $[Ca^{2+}]_i$ with a duration as short as one second. In contrast to these transient increases of short duration, $[Ca^{2+}]_i$ is increased above the basal value for much longer periods during the action of mitogens on quiescent cells.

7.7 The mechanisms by which agonists increase the cytoplasmic free Ca^{2+} concentration

7.7.1 *Enhanced Ca^{2+} inflow across the plasma membrane and release of Ca^{2+} from the endoplasmic or sarcoplasmic reticulum*

The increase in $[Ca^{2+}]_i$ which results from the binding of agonists to receptors on the plasma membrane, or from depolarization of the plasma membrane, is caused by increases in the rates of net Ca^{2+} movement to the cytoplasmic space across two membranes. These are the plasma membrane and the membrane of the endoplas-

mic (or sarcoplasmic) reticulum (Fig. 7.18). Although both processes contribute to the initial increase in $[Ca^{2+}]_i$, only the former is responsible for the prolonged maintenance of $[Ca^{2+}]_i$ above

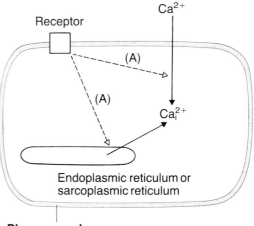

Fig. 7.18 In many types of cell the combination of an agonist with its receptor on the plasma membrane causes an increase in $[Ca^{2+}]_i$ by increasing the rate of movement of Ca^{2+} to the cytoplasmic space across two membranes. These are the plasma membrane and the membrane of the endoplasmic reticulum or sarcoplasmic reticulum.

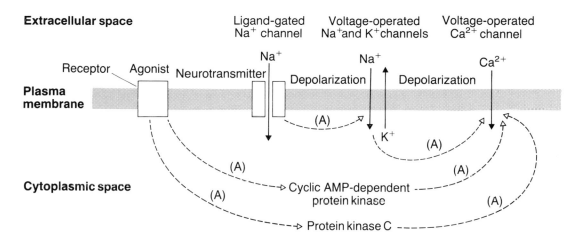

Fig. 7.19   In excitable cells there are two pathways by which agonists can influence the inward movement of Ca^{2+} through voltage-operated Ca^{2+} channels. Neurotransmitters open voltage-operated Ca^{2+} channels by inducing the movement of ions across the plasma membrane, such as the inward movement of Na^+ through a ligand-gated Na^+ channel. This causes a depolarization of the plasma membrane which is propagated by the opening of voltage-operated Na^+ and K^+ channels. In the second pathway, agonists can enhance the response of voltage-operated Ca^{2+} channels to depolarization by inducing phosphorylation of the channel protein through the activation of a protein kinase such as cyclic AMP-dependent protein kinase or protein kinase C. The symbol (A) represents activation.

the basal value. While the increase in $[Ca^{2+}]_i$ induced by agonists is caused by increases in both Ca^{2+} inflow across the plasma membrane and Ca^{2+} release from intracellular stores, the relative contribution of these two pathways varies from one cell type to another. For example, in skeletal muscle, most of the increase in $[Ca^{2+}]_i$ is derived from the sarcoplasmic reticulum.

The increase in net Ca^{2+} inflow across the plasma membrane is mediated by receptor-activated Ca^{2+} inflow systems and by voltage-operated Ca^{2+} channels. The possible mechanisms by which agonist–receptor complexes open plasma-membrane receptor-activated Ca^{2+} inflow systems were described earlier in Section 7.3.5, whilst the properties of voltage-operated Ca^{2+} channels have also been described (Sections 7.3.3 and 7.3.4). Agonists such as neurotransmitters open voltage-operated Ca^{2+} channels by inducing a depolarization of the plasma membrane (Fig. 7.19). Examples of this type of activation of voltage-operated Ca^{2+}

channels include the actions of thyroid-stimulating hormone on pituitary cells and of acetylcholine on smooth-muscle cells.

Another mechanism by which agonists can stimulate net Ca^{2+} inflow through voltage-operated Ca^{2+} channels is through phosphorylation of the channel protein (Fig. 7.19). This increases the probability that a particular Ca^{2+} channel is in the open state at a given membrane potential (Fig. 7.20). In heart muscle cells, adrenalin and other β-adrenergic agonists induce phosphorylation of the voltage-operated Ca^{2+} channel protein through activation of cyclic AMP-dependent protein kinases. In other cell types, the phosphorylation of voltage-operated Ca^{2+} channels by protein kinase C increases the frequency of opening of the channels.

The increase in net Ca^{2+} outflow across the membrane of the endoplasmic reticulum is mediated by Ins 1,4,5 P_3-sensitive channels. The nature of these channels was described earlier in Section 7.4.3 and the reactions by which Ins

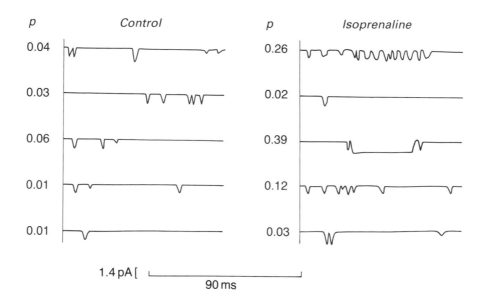

Fig. 7.20 A demonstration of the ability of the β-adrenergic agonist, isoprenaline, to increase the probability of opening of a single voltage-operated Ca^{2+} channel in a cultured rat heart cell. Current carried through a single Ca^{2+} channel was measured in a patch-clamp experiment in which a depolarizing clamp of 60 mV was applied for 90 ms. The downward defection indicates an increase in current caused by the open state of the channel. The value of p_{open} is given alongside each trace. For most of the traces obtained in the presence of isoprenaline the value of p_{open} is greater than the value for traces obtained in the absence of agonist. From Reuter (1983).

1,4,5 P_3 is synthesized and metabolized are described in Chapter 6 (Sections 6.3 and 6.4).

In skeletal and heart muscle cells, net Ca^{2+} outflow from the sarcoplasmic reticulum is initiated by depolarization of the sarcolemma. This probably involves some form of interaction between the voltage-operated Ca^{2+} channel (dihydropyridine receptor) in the sarcolemma and the sarcoplasmic reticulum Ca^{2+} channel (ryanodine receptor) which is located, as described earlier in Section 7.4.3, on the junctional face of the terminal cisternae. In this model it is proposed that depolarization of the sarcolemma leads to a conformational change in the voltage-operated Ca^{2+} channel which subsequently induces a conformation change in the neighbouring sarcoplasmic reticulum Ca^{2+} channel. This results in opening of the sarcoplasmic reticulum Ca^{2+} channel.

Another model which has been proposed to explain the process of Ca^{2+} release from the sarcoplasmic reticulum hypothesizes that a small increase in $[Ca^{2+}]_i$, caused by the opening of voltage-operated Ca^{2+} channels in the sarcolemma, results in the binding of Ca^{2+} to the sarcoplasmic reticulum Ca^{2+} channel and the opening of this channel. This idea is called the Ca^{2+}-induced Ca^{2+} release hypothesis. While this is an attractive proposal there are some observations which suggest that it is unlikely to be correct.

7.7.2 *Modulation of the agonist-induced increase in cytoplasmic free Ca^{2+} concentration*
The maintenance of increased $[Ca^{2+}]_i$ for periods longer than about a minute probably requires inhibition of some of the processes which normally remove Ca^{2+} from the cytoplasmic space. These processes include the transport of Ca^{2+}

from the cytoplasmic space to the extracellular space, the endoplasmic reticulum, mitochondria, and to an Ins 1,4,5 P_3-insensitive store (Fig. 7.21). This store may be a region of the endoplasmic reticulum, or another organelle such as the calciosome.

Ins 1,4,5 P_3 inhibits the net inflow of Ca^{2+} to the endoplasmic reticulum as a consequence of the stimulation by this molecule of the outflow of Ca^{2+} from this organelle (Fig. 7.21). There is some evidence to indicate that in some types of cell the plasma-membrane (Ca^{2+} + Mg^{2+}) ATPase Ca^{2+} transporter is also inhibited during the action of agonists (Fig. 7.21).

Whilst some mechanisms seem to have evolved to prolong agonist-induced increases in

[Ca^{2+}]$_i$ under appropriate conditions, there are others that reduce the maximum value and duration of the increase. In cardiac muscle cells, the activation of (Ca^{2+} + calmodulin)-dependent protein kinase, which results from the increase in [Ca^{2+}]$_i$, leads to phosphorylation and activation of the (Ca^{2+} + Mg^{2+})ATPase Ca^{2+} transporters of the sarcolemma and sarcoplasmic reticulum and hence to the removal of Ca^{2+} from the myoplasm. Similar mechanisms, involving the (Ca^{2+} + Mg^{2+})ATPase Ca^{2+} transporters of the plasma membrane and endoplasmic reticulum, act to reduce the increase in [Ca^{2+}]$_i$ in smooth-muscle cells. These (Ca^{2+} + Mg^{2+})ATPase Ca^{2+} transporters can also be activated by cyclic AMP-dependent protein kinase.

7.7.3 *Spatial distribution and oscillatory behaviour of agonist-induced changes in cytoplasmic free Ca^{2+} concentration*

Most of the information on the effect of agonists on [Ca^{2+}]$_i$ has come from studies of cell suspensions. In these experiments, the observed value of [Ca^{2+}]$_i$ represents the average value of [Ca^{2+}]$_i$ in all cells in the sample being investigated. Measurement of the changes in [Ca^{2+}]$_i$ in individual cells has revealed further complexities in the processes which control [Ca^{2+}]$_i$ during the action of agonists. In many types of cell differences between individual cells of the same type are observed in the time-courses for the agonist-induced increase in [Ca^{2+}]$_i$ and in the maximum values of the increase. In some types of cell, regional variations in the increase in [Ca^{2+}]$_i$ in response to agonists have been observed within a given cell (Fig. 7.22).

Another type of behaviour observed in individual cells in response to the action of an agonist is oscillatory changes in [Ca^{2+}]$_i$. For example, in individual hepatocytes a series of rapid transient increases in [Ca^{2+}]$_i$ is observed in the presence of low concentrations of certain agonists

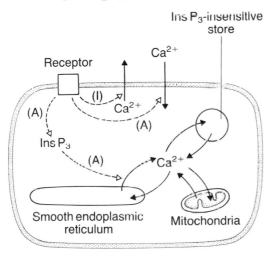

Fig. 7.21 The maintenance of increased [Ca^{2+}]$_i$ over a period of time exceeding one or two minutes probably requires inhibition of the removal of Ca^{2+} from the cytoplasmic space as well as a maintained increase in the rate of Ca^{2+} inflow across the plasma membrane. During periods in which [Ca^{2+}]$_i$ is increased above the basal value, Ca^{2+} is transported from the cytoplasmic space to the extracellular medium, endoplasmic reticulum or sarcoplasmic reticulum, mitochondria, and probably to other Ins 1,4,5 P_3-insensitive stores. Ca^{2+} inflow to the smooth endoplasmic reticulum is inhibited by the action of Ins 1,4,5 P_3. Ca^{2+} outflow across the plasma membrane may also be inhibited. The symbols (A) and (I) represent activation and inhibition, respectively.

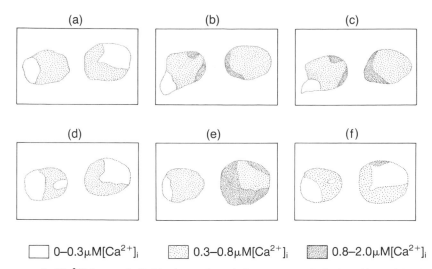

$\square$ 0–0.3μM[Ca²⁺]ᵢ $\boxed{}$ 0.3–0.8μM[Ca²⁺]ᵢ $\blacksquare$ 0.8–2.0μM[Ca²⁺]ᵢ

Fig. 7.22 Increases in $[Ca^{2+}]_i$ in two individual rat adrenal glomeruosa cells induced by K^+ (a–c) or angiotensin II (d–f). The distribution of $[Ca^{2+}]_i$ throughout the cytoplasmic space is represented by the degree of shading, as shown in the boxes below the panels. Panels (a), (b), and (c) represent $[Ca^{2+}]_i$ at 0, 1.5, and 2 min. after depolarization of the plasma membrane with extracellular K^+. Panels (d), (e), and (f) represent $[Ca^{2+}]_i$ at 0, 0.5, and 1.0 min. after the addition of angiotensin II. Adapted from Connor *et al.* (1987).

(Fig. 7.23). Agonist-induced oscillations in $[Ca^{2+}]_i$ in individual cells are observed in many excitable cells and in many non-excitable cells. It is not known exactly how oscillations in $[Ca^{2+}]_i$ are generated. Three possible mechanisms are the successive activation and inactivation of voltage-operated Ca^{2+} channels in excitable cells, the generation of transient increases in Ins 1,4,5 P_3, and the successive uptake and release of Ca^{2+} by an Ins 1,4,5 P_3-insensitive store in non-excitable cells.

The observation that agonist-induced increases in $[Ca^{2+}]_i$ are heterogeneous within the cytoplasmic space, and the detection of agonist-induced oscillations in $[Ca^{2+}]_i$, indicate that the mechanisms by which $[Ca^{2+}]_i$ is controlled are more complex than those described earlier. Resolution of this complexity will require knowledge of the spatial distribution of the intracellular Ca^{2+} stores, Ca^{2+} channels, and Ca^{2+} transporters which control $[Ca^{2+}]_i$, a description of the interactions between the various intracellular processes which regulate $[Ca^{2+}]_i$, and knowledge of the rates of diffusion of Ca^{2+}

within the cytoplasmic space.

The rate of Ca^{2+} diffusion determines the region of the cytoplasmic space though which

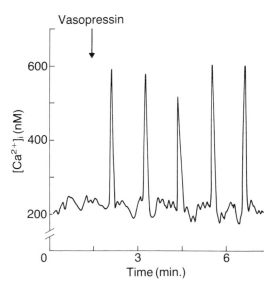

Fig. 7.23 Agonist-induced oscillations in $[Ca^{2+}]_i$. A low concentration of vasopressin induces transient pulses of increased $[Ca^{2+}]_i$ in a single hepatocyte loaded with aequorin. From Woods *et al.* (1987).

Ca^{2+} released from a given site moves. The rate of diffusion of Ca^{2+} is slow relative to the rates for the monovalent cations. The apparent diffusion coefficient for Ca^{2+} in the myoplasm of skeletal muscle and in the axoplasm of nerve is about 10^{-5} mm^{2}s^{-1}. This is only 2 per cent of the value for the apparent diffusion coefficient for Ca^{2+} in a pure aqueous solution. The main factors which impede the movement of Ca^{2+} through the interior of a cell are the binding of Ca^{2+} to components of the cytoplasmic space and the ability of intracellular organelles to remove Ca^{2+} from the cytoplasmic space when [Ca^{2+}]$_i$ is above the basal value.

The rate of diffusion of Ca^{2+} through the interior of a cell will determine the time required for a front of increased [Ca^{2+}]$_i$, generated at a given intracellular surface, to reach a target protein which is some distance away from that surface.

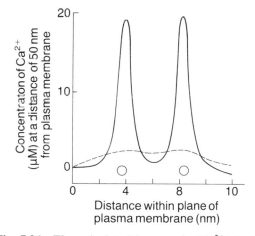

Fig. 7.24 The calculated increase in [Ca^{2+}]$_i$ in the cytoplasmic space in the vicinity of two individual voltage-operated Ca^{2+} channels (indicated by the circles) following the opening of the channels for a period of 2 ms induced by depolarization of the plasma membrane. The value of [Ca^{2+}]$_i$ in a plane parallel to that of the membrane at a distance of 50 nm from the plasma membrane has been plotted as a function of distance in the plane of the membrane. The curves represent [Ca^{2+}]$_i$ at 1 ms (full curve) and 3.4 ms (broken curve) after opening of the channels. From Zucker and Fogelson (1986).

For example, simulation studies suggest that when an individual voltage-operated Ca^{2+} channel is opened, the resulting increase in [Ca^{2+}]$_i$ in the adjacent cytoplasmic space is confined to a region close to the channel (Fig. 7.24).

On a larger scale, regions of elevated [Ca^{2+}]$_i$ called 'Ca^{2+} hotspots' have been observed following the opening of L-type voltage-operated Ca^{2+} channels in the growth cones of nerve cells (Fig. 7.25). The localization of these increases in [Ca^{2+}]$_i$ is probably due to the presence of clusters of L-type voltage-operated Ca^{2+} channels and to restrictions on the diffusion of Ca^{2+} from regions of the cytoplasmic space adjacent to these clusters. These localized regions of high [Ca^{2+}]$_i$, which result from electrical activity at the plasma membrane, may induce a change in the spatial direction of growth of the neuronal growth cone.

7.8 The Ca^{2+}-modulated proteins

7.8.1 *Classification of the Ca^{2+}-modulated proteins*

The increase in [Ca^{2+}]$_i$ induced by agonists alters the activity of intracellular enzymes and other proteins by binding to Ca^{2+}-binding sites on Ca^{2+}-modulated proteins. The term Ca^{2+}-modulated protein refers to any protein which is a target for increased [Ca^{2+}]$_i$ and is used in order to distinguish this group of proteins from other intracellular Ca^{2+}-binding proteins, such as parvalbumins and calbindins, which have different functions. The calbindins are vitamin D-dependent intestinal Ca^{2+}-binding proteins which are designated by the names 9 K (mammals) and 28 K or D (birds). The functions of the parvalbumins and calbindins may include the buffering of [Ca^{2+}]$_i$ and the trans-cellular movement of Ca^{2+}.

The Ca^{2+}-modulated proteins can be divided into two groups (Table 7.4) on the basis of whether or not the Ca^{2+}-binding site has a struc-

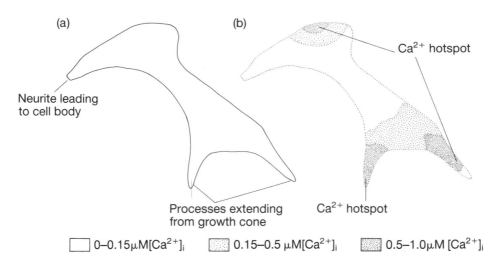

Fig. 7.25 Localized increases in $[Ca^{2+}]_i$ in the growth cone of a cultured NIE-115 neuroblastoma cell. Values of $[Ca^{2+}]_i$, represented by the degree of shading as shown by the boxes below the panels, are shown for a growth cone under control conditions (panel (a)) and at 0.5 s after the opening of L-type voltage-operated Ca^{2+} channels (panel (b)). The localized increases in $[Ca^{2+}]_i$ have been called 'Ca^{2+} hotspots'. $[Ca^{2+}]_i$ was measured using fura 2 and an excitation wavelength of 380 nm. Adapted from Silver *et al.* (1990).

Table 7.4 *Classification of Ca^{2+}-modulated proteins on the basis of the structure of the Ca^{2+}-binding site*

Class of Ca^{2+}-modulated protein	Members of the class
Helix–loop–helix structure, component of many different oligomeric proteins	Calmodulin
Helix–loop–helix structure, component of only one oligomeric protein	Troponin C S100 proteins Calpains α-Actinins
Non-helix–loop–helix structures	Protein kinase C Annexins ((Ca^{2+} + phospholipid) Ca^{2+}-binding proteins) Ca^{2+}-activated ion channels Phospholipase A_2 and D Mitochondrial Ca^{2+}-responsive enzymes (pyruvate dehydrogenase phosphatase, α-ketoglutarate dehydrogenase and isocitrate dehydrogenase)

ture called the helix–loop–helix motif. This motif, which is also called the E–F hand structure, is described in Section 7.8.2.

Each Ca^{2+}-modulated protein that possesses a helix–loop–helix Ca^{2+}-binding site is a subunit of an oligomeric protein. The other subunit or subunits of the oligomeric protein possess enzymatic or other functions. Calmodulin is a regulatory subunit of a large number of different oligomeric proteins and is responsible for conferring on each of these proteins the ability to respond to $[Ca^{2+}]_i$. Each of the other Ca^{2+}-modulated proteins that possess a helix–loop–helix Ca^{2+}-binding site is a subunit of only one type of oligomeric protein. Some other proteins such as myosin regulatory light chain and the B subunit of phosphoprotein phosphatase 2B (calcineurin), possess sequences of amino acids that are very similar to the helix–loop–helix sequence. However, these proteins either do not bind Ca^{2+} (myosin regulatory light chain) or bind Ca^{2+} without a known physiological effect (phosphoprotein phosphatase 2B).

7.8.2 *Structure of the helix–loop–helix Ca^{2+}-binding motif*

The helix–loop–helix (HLH) Ca^{2+}-binding motif consists of a loop of 12 contiguous amino-acid residues flanked by two α-helices. The arrangement of the four HLH motifs in calmodulin is shown in Fig. 7.26. The Ca^{2+} ion is bound as a co-ordination complex with eight oxygen atoms (Fig. 7.27), each of which donates a pair of electrons to the Ca^{2+} ion. Seven of these oxygen atoms are provided by amino-acid residues and one by water (Fig. 7.27). Hydrogen bonding between a number of amino-acid residues of the Ca^{2+}-binding loop helps to stabilize the structure of the loop.

The HLH motif is also called the E–F hand structure because it resembles the index finger (E helix), a curled second finger (loop), and thumb (F helix) of the right hand. The HLH

Ca^{2+}-binding motifs occur in closely linked pairs. Most Ca^{2+}-modulated proteins, for example calmodulin (Fig. 7.26), have four motifs whilst some, for example the S100 proteins, have two motifs. The HLH motif is also present in Ca^{2+}-binding proteins which do not modulate protein function, including parvalbumin, the calbindins, and aequorin.

When compared with other ions, the greater specificity and higher affinity of the metal-binding site of the HLH motif and other types of Ca^{2+}-binding sites for Ca^{2+} are thought to be chiefly due to the presence of the two positive charges on Ca^{2+} and the small ionic radius of this cation. These features allow Ca^{2+} to bind much more tightly to the Ca^{2+}-binding proteins than do monovalent cations or mono- or divalent anions.

Mg^{2+}, which is the most abundant divalent cation present in cells, might also be expected to bind to Ca^{2+}-modulated proteins. However, the ionic radius of Mg^{2+} is much smaller than that of Ca^{2+}. In order to adapt to the Mg^{2+} ion,

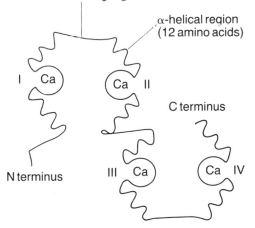

Fig. 7.26 The four helix–loop–helix motifs which bind Ca^{2+} in the calmodulin polypeptide chain. The co-ordination complex between Ca^{2+} and oxygen atoms derived from the amino-acid residues of the Ca^{2+}-binding loop is shown in Fig. 7.27. From England (1986).

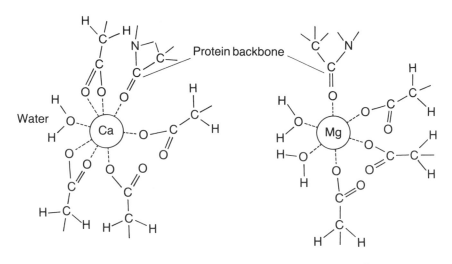

Fig. 7.27 The structures of the co-ordination complexes formed between the Ca^{2+}-binding loop of the helix–loop–helix motif of a Ca^{2+}-binding protein and Ca^{2+} (left) and Mg^{2+} (right). The complete Ca^{2+}-binding site is composed of a loop of 12 amino-acid residues. Only those residues which provide oxygen atoms that interact directly with the divalent metal ion are shown. The Ca^{2+} co-ordination complex involves a total of eight oxygen atoms. Six of these are from amino-acid residues which constitute the Ca^{2+}-binding loop, one is from an amino-acid residue in one of the α-helices (the protein backbone), and one is from water. The bond between the metal-binding site and Mg^{2+} is much weaker than that for Ca^{2+}. In the case of Mg^{2+}, a total of only six co-ordinate bonds are formed. Two of these are with water molecules. From Carafoli and Penniston (1985).

the orientation of atoms at the metal-binding site of a Ca^{2+}-modulated protein must change. However, the oxygen atoms lack the flexibility to do this, so that some of the co-ordination bonds potentially available to Mg^{2+} are formed with water instead of the protein (Fig. 7.27). This results in a much weaker bond between the cation-binding sites on the protein and Mg^{2+} than the bond formed between the cationic binding site and Ca^{2+}. Consequently, under the conditions of the cytoplasmic space, little Mg^{2+} is bound to Ca^{2+}-binding proteins.

7.8.3 *Calmodulin*

The discovery of calmodulin by Cheung (1970) arose from an investigation of unexpected changes in the activity of cyclic nucleotide phosphodiesterase observed during the purification of this enzyme. Investigation of this phenomenon led to the identification of calmodulin as

an activator of cyclic AMP phosphodiesterase. At the same time, Kakiuchi and Yamazaki (1970) identified calmodulin as an activator of an enzyme which they called Ca^{2+}-regulated cyclic nucleotide phosphodiesterase. Subsequently, Teo and Wang (1973) showed that calmodulin binds Ca^{2+} with a high affinity. Further investigation showed that the (Ca^{2+} + calmodulin) complex activates a large number of enzymes and other proteins.

Calmodulin is a single polypeptide chain with a molecular weight of 16.7 kDa. The polypeptide is acidic, has a pI of 4.2, and is relatively stable to heat. As described earlier, there are four helix–loop–helix Ca^{2+}-binding motifs in each molecule of calmodulin (Fig. 7.26). The amino-acid sequence around the Ca^{2+}-binding site is highly conserved in calmodulins isolated from different animal species, and also in calmodulins from plants and protozoa. Calmodulin may have evolved by successive duplication of an ancestral gene which coded for a protein with a single Ca^{2+}-binding site.

Experiments using fluorescently labelled antibodies to calmodulin have shown that in many types of cell, calmodulin is located near the plasma membrane, in the nucleus, and in association with specialized structures in the cytoplasmic space such as glycogen granules, muscle filaments, and components of the cytoskeleton. The total intracellular concentration of calmodulin has been estimated to be about 10–50 μM. In some cells, the total amount of calmodulin and the intracellular distribution of the protein change during different phases of cell growth.

7.8.4 *The calmodulin-binding proteins*

A large number of different enzymes and other proteins are activated by the $(Ca^{2+}$ + calmodulin) complex (Table 7.5). The multifunctional $(Ca^{2+}$ + calmodulin)-dependent protein kinase permits Ca^{2+} to affect a large number of target enzymes within a cell. This role of the $(Ca^{2+}$ + calmodulin)-dependent protein kinase in transmitting the effects of Ca^{2+} is analogous to that of the cyclic AMP-dependent protein kinases in mediating the effects of cyclic AMP.

The interaction of the $(Ca^{2+}$ + calmodulin) complex with adenylate cyclase and cyclic nucleotide phosphodiesterase provides a mechanism by which Ca^{2+} can regulate the concentration of cyclic nucleotides in cells in which calmodulin-sensitive forms of these enzymes are present. As described earlier in Section 7.7.2, activation by $(Ca^{2+}$ + calmodulin) of $(Ca^{2+}$ + $Mg^{2+})$ATPase Ca^{2+} transporters is one of the mechanisms by which the removal of Ca^{2+} from the cytoplasmic space is enhanced when $[Ca^{2+}]_i$ is increased. The actions of $(Ca^{2+}$ + calmodulin) on enzymes or proteins associated with the cytoskeleton are

Table 7.5 *Enzymes and other proteins regulated by direct interaction with the (Ca^{2+} + calmodulin) complex*

Enzyme or other protein	Function

$(Ca^{2+}$ + calmodulin)-dependent protein kinases
    Multifunctional kinase (kinase II)
    Kinases I and III
    Myosin light-chain kinase
    Glycogen phosphorylase kinase
	Regulation of enzyme activity through phosphorylation of target enzymes

Phosphoprotein phosphatase 2B (calcineurin)	Regulation of enzyme activity through dephosphorylation of target phosphoenzymes
Cyclic nucleotide phosphodiesterases	Degradation of cyclic AMP and cyclic GMP
Adenylate cyclase (a form found only in some cell types)	Formation of cyclic AMP
$(Ca^{2+}$ + $Mg^{2+})$ATPase Ca^{2+} transporters	Regulation of intracellular free Ca^{2+} concentration

Proteins of the microtubular network
    Tubulin
    Tau factor
    MAP-2
	Regulation of microtubular network

Actin-binding proteins
    Fodrin
    Spectrin
    Caldesmon
	Regulation of cytoskeleton structure

thought to mediate a number of the effects of Ca^{2+} on the exocytotic secretion of proteins and ions, and on cell growth and differentiation.

The enzymes and other proteins listed in Table 7.5 were originally identified as calmodulin-binding proteins by demonstrating the direct interaction of (Ca^{2+} + calmodulin) with the enzyme or protein. This interaction was detected as a change in activity of the enzyme or protein with which calmodulin interacts. Since these observations were made, a number of other techniques for the detection of calmodulin-binding proteins in cells have been developed. One of these involves the separation of proteins present in a cell extract by polyacrylamide gel electrophoresis and the identification of the calmodulin-binding proteins by overlaying [^{125}I]-labelled calmodulin. The use of this technique has led to the identification of a number of additional enzymes and other proteins which bind calmodulin.

7.8.5 *Interaction of calmodulin with calmodulin-binding proteins*

The interaction of calmodulin with most target proteins is initiated by an increase in $[Ca^{2+}]_i$. At basal values of $[Ca^{2+}]_i$ most calmodulin present in the cell is probably in the free state. Since the intracellular concentrations of total calmodulin and total calmodulin-binding sites are approximately equal, the majority of calmodulin is probably bound to calmodulin-binding proteins immediately following an agonist-induced increase in $[Ca^{2+}]_i$. For some calmodulin-binding proteins, for example glycogen phosphorylase kinase, calmodulin is tightly bound at basal values of $[Ca^{2+}]_i$. As described in Chapter 4 (Section 4.5.2), calmodulin is one of the four different types of subunit which compose glycogen phosphorylase kinase. In addition to these tightly bound calmodulin subunits, further molecules of calmodulin, or molecules of troponin C, bind to glycogen phosphorylase kinase

in the presence of increased $[Ca^{2+}]_i$.

The binding of Ca^{2+} to calmodulin and the binding of the (Ca^{2+} + calmodulin) complex to a calmodulin-binding protein (Enz) takes place in the following sequence:

$$\text{Calmodulin} + 4Ca^{2+} \rightleftharpoons \text{Calmodulin} (Ca^{2+})_4$$

$$\text{Calmodulin} (Ca^{2+})_4 + \text{Enz}_{\text{inactive}} \rightleftharpoons [\text{Calmodulin} (Ca^{2+})_4]\text{Enz}_{\text{active}}.$$

Interaction of the (Ca^{2+} + calmodulin) complex with the protein causes changes in the conformation and activity of the protein. For example in the case of cyclic nucleotide phosphodiesterase, the binding of (Ca^{2+} + calmodulin) induces an increase of 6–10 fold in the maximum velocity of the reaction without a change in the apparent K_M for cyclic nucleotides. The activation of some calmodulin-binding proteins requires more than one molecule of (Ca^{2+} + calmodulin) complex per molecule of protein.

The conformational change induced in calmodulin by the binding of Ca^{2+} involves an increase in the content of the α-helical component of the polypeptide chain and alterations in the environment of specific amino-acid residues. The conformational changes occur in a stepwise manner following the successive

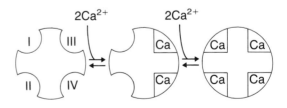

Fig. 7.28 The successive binding of two pairs of Ca^{2+} ions to calmodulin causes a series of conformational changes in the polypeptide. The four binding sites for Ca^{2+} are designated I to IV. The sequence shown was deduced on the basis of results obtained for the effects of Ca^{2+} and other divalent cations on the structure of the calmodulin polypeptide monitored by absorption and fluorescence spectroscopy, ^{113}Cd$^+$ nuclear magnetic resonance spectroscopy, and Tb^{3+} binding. From Klee *et al.* (1983).

addition of two and four molecules of Ca^{2+} (Fig. 7.28). The dissociation constant of free calmodulin for Ca^{2+} is about $4\,\mu M$. However, when complexed with a calmodulin-binding protein, Ca^{2+} is bound with a 50-fold higher affinity.

The dissociation constant for the combination of calmodulin with calmodulin-binding proteins varies from about 10^{-10} to $10^{-6}\,M^{-1}$, depending on the nature of the calmodulin-binding protein. The region on the calmodulin polypeptide chain which interacts with the binding protein is small in area, hydrophobic in character, and susceptible to proteolysis. Different calmodulin-binding proteins probably interact with the protein-binding region of calmodulin in slightly different ways.

7.8.6   *Pharmacological inhibitors of calmodulin action*

There are a number of drugs which bind to calmodulin and inhibit the activation of calmodulin-binding proteins by the $(Ca^{2+} + calmodulin)$ complex. These drugs include phenothiazines and other anti-psychotic drugs with a related structure, smooth-muscle relaxants, α-adrenergic antagonists, a number of antidepressant drugs and anaesthetics, calmidazolium, and a drug called compound 48/80 which is also an inhibitor of the movement of Ca^{2+} through intracellular membranes. The inhibition of calmodulin by phenothiazines was reported by Levin and Weiss in 1976. The structures of two drugs in this group, chlorpromazine and penfluridol, are shown in Fig. 7.29. A common structural feature of many drugs which inhibit the action of calmodulin is the presence of a large hydrophobic ring and a side-chain which contains an amino group.

The action of the drugs which inhibit calmodulin is dependent on the presence of Ca^{2+}. The drugs interact only with the $(Ca^{2+} + calmodulin)$ complex and not with free calmodulin. In the case of the phenothiazines, there are two binding sites for the drug on each molecule of calmodulin. The combination of two molecules of phenothiazine per molecule of calmodulin completely inhibits the binding of $(Ca^{2+} + cal$-

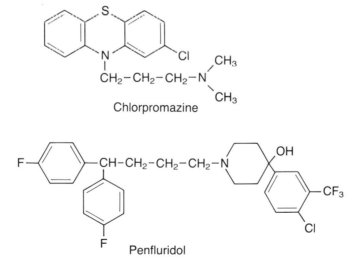

Chlorpromazine

Penfluridol

Fig. 7.29   The structures of chlorpromazine, a phenothiazine, and penfluridol, a diphenylbutylpiperidine, which inhibit the interaction of $(Ca^{2+} + calmodulin)$ with calmodulin-binding proteins. The concentrations of the drugs which give 50 per cent inhibition of the Ca^{2+}-induced response are about $40\,\mu M$ for chlorpromazine and $2.5\,\mu M$ for penfluridol.

modulin) to all calmodulin-binding proteins whereas the combination of one molecule of drug per molecule of calmodulin inhibits the binding of (Ca^{2+} + calmodulin) to some but not to other calmodulin-binding proteins.

Trifluoperazine and related phenothiazines, calmidazolium, and other drugs which interact with calmodulin have been employed to elucidate the role of calmodulin in intact cells and tissues. However, most of these drugs are not specific for calmodulin and interact with other proteins, including Ca^{2+}-binding proteins other than calmodulin, and certain plasma-membrane receptors. This has complicated the interpretation of the results obtained from this type of experiment.

7.8.7   *Other helix–loop–helix Ca^{2+}-modulated proteins*

In addition to calmodulin, the other known helix–loop–helix Ca^{2+}-modulated proteins are troponin C, the S100 group of proteins, the calpains, and the α-actinins (Table 7.4). Troponin C is present only in heart and skeletal muscle. Together with troponins I and T, troponin C constitutes the oligomeric protein called troponin. The troponin–tropomyosin complex is responsible for the contraction of striated-muscle fibres. The troponin oligomer provides a mechanism by which Ca^{2+} can control the activity of tropomyosin. Troponin C is an acidic polypeptide which has a molecular weight of 18 kDa and possesses four HLH Ca^{2+}-binding motifs. The binding of Ca^{2+} to troponin C induces a conformational change in this polypeptide which, in turn, affects its interaction with troponin I.

The S100 family of Ca^{2+}-binding proteins contains a large number of members. These include proteins designated S100α, S100β, and p11 as well as a number of other Ca^{2+}-modulated proteins associated with regulation of the cell cycle and cell differentiation. Each of the S100 pro-

teins probably functions by interacting with another enzyme or protein and conferring on this second protein the ability of Ca^{2+} to regulate its activity. Thus the S100 proteins may act in a manner similar to calmodulin. Each S100 protein contains two HLH Ca^{2+}-binding motifs and two hydrophobic domains. S100 proteins are probably required for the regulation by Ca^{2+} of a number of processes including reactions involved in microtubule polymerization and depolymerization, reactions which control the cell cycle and cell differentiation, and regulation of the activities of some other enzymes.

The calpains are a group of Ca^{2+}-dependent proteases which cleave substrates at a cysteine residue. Each calpain protease is composed of a catalytic and a regulatory subunit. These subunits have molecular weights of 80 and 30 kDa, respectively. Each calpain protease is found as two isoforms which differ in the molecular weight of the catalytic subunit.

Each regulatory and catalytic subunit of the calpain dimer contains two HLH Ca^{2+}-binding motifs. Activation of the calpain protease is probably initiated by an increase in $[Ca^{2+}]_i$. This leads to association of the calpain with the plasma membrane. The interaction of calpain with Ca^{2+}, membrane phospholipids, and possibly another protein called an activator protein, is required for full activation of the proteolytic activity of calpain. The process of activation of calpain by its interaction with Ca^{2+} and the plasma membrane has some similarities with the mechanism of activation of protein kinase C at the plasma membrane (Chapter 6, Section 6.10).

Activated calpains may exert their intracellular effects by the proteolytic cleavage of protein kinase C to yield a constitutively active form, protein kinase M (Chapter 4, Section 4.6.4), and by degradation of components of the cytoskeleton, for example, fodrin. Further experiments are required to establish the intracellular physiological actions of calpain.

7.8.8 *Ca^{2+}-modulated proteins which do not possess the helix–loop–helix Ca^{2+}-binding motif*

The Ca^{2+}-modulated proteins which do not possess the helix–loop–helix Ca^{2+}-binding motif (Table 7.4) have a variety of different structures and functions. For most of the proteins in this group, the polypeptide chain on which the Ca^{2+}-binding site is located also possesses the catalytic site of the enzyme or the ion channel (Fig. 7.30). Ca^{2+}-activated ion channels are located at the plasma membrane and include a K$^+$ channel, a non-specific monovalent cation channel, and a Cl$^-$ channel. All of the proteins which do not possess the helix–loop–helix Ca^{2+}-binding motif are activated by concentrations of free Ca^{2+} in the range of 1 μM. The combination of Ca^{2+} with

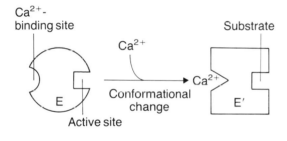

Fig. 7.30 A schematic description of the structure of Ca^{2+}-modulated proteins which do not possess a helix–loop–helix Ca^{2+}-binding motif. Proteins in this group are listed in Table 7.4. For most of these proteins the polypeptide chain on which the Ca^{2+}-binding sites are located has at least one other function in addition to the binding of Ca^{2+}. These other functions include the catalysis of chemical reactions and facilitation of the movement of ions. Upon the binding of Ca^{2+}, the protein undergoes a conformational change which, in the case of an enzyme, allows the substrate to interact with the active site.

the allosteric Ca^{2+}-binding site induces a conformational change in the protein which leads to an increase in catalytic activity (Fig. 7.30) or to a change in the function of the protein.

The mitochondrial Ca^{2+}-responsive enzymes are located in the mitochondrial matrix. They include pyruvate dehydrogenase phosphatase, α-ketoglutarate dehydrogenase, and isocitrate dehydrogenase. These enzymes are activated by an increase in the free Ca^{2+} concentration in the mitochondrial matrix which probably occurs as a result of an increase in [Ca^{2+}]$_i$ (Section 7.2.2).

The annexins include proteins called synexins I and II, calelectrin, endonexins I and II, calpactin I (lipocortin II) and calpactin II (lipocortin I), the calcimedins, and the protein p70 (also called protein III). Since the activation of these proteins also involves interaction of the protein with phospholipids, the anexins have also been called the (Ca^{2+} + phospholipid)-dependent membrane-binding proteins. Members of the annexin family are involved in mediating Ca^{2+}-induced changes in the structure of the cytoskeleton and in the exocytosis of secretory granules. The calpactins (lipocortins) are inhibitors of phospholipase A$_2$. In addition to regulation by [Ca^{2+}]$_i$, the activity of a number of the annexins is probably also regulated by phosphorylation catalysed by protein–serine and protein–tyrosine kinases.

Investigation of the interaction of Ca^{2+} with some Ca^{2+}-modulated proteins in cells has been facilitated by the use of photosensitive Ca^{2+} chelators which exhibit a marked decrease in affinity for Ca^{2+} upon photolysis. An example of this group of compounds, which have been named photosensitive 'caged-Ca^{2+}' molecules, is nitr-5. The introduction of nitr-5 to the cytoplasmic space provides a reservoir of bound Ca^{2+}. Upon photolysis this Ca^{2+} is released causing a transient increase in [Ca^{2+}]$_i$ which is very rapid in onset. The photosensitive Ca^{2+} chelators have been particularly useful in studying the consequences of a rapid increase in [Ca^{2+}]$_i$. For example, experiments conducted with *Aplysia californica* bursting-pacemaker neurons loaded with nitr-5 have enabled a study of the effect of increased in [Ca^{2+}]$_i$ on opening of the Ca^{2+}-activated K$^+$ channel.

7.9 Summary

An increase in the concentration of free Ca^{2+} in the cytoplasmic space ($[Ca^{2+}]_i$) acts as an intracellular messenger for the action of many agonists. This Ca^{2+} binds to sites on target proteins leading to alterations in enzyme activity and protein function.

$[Ca^{2+}]_i$ is controlled by the rates of movement of Ca^{2+} between the cytoplasmic space and both the extracellular space and intracellular stores. The main intracellular stores are the endoplasmic reticulum (or sarcoplasmic reticulum) and mitochondria. A large proportion of Ca^{2+} present in the cytoplasmic space and in the lumen of the endoplasmic reticulum, sarcoplasmic reticulum, and in the mitochondrial matrix is bound to proteins, metabolites, and membrane phospholipids. The remaining unbound Ca^{2+} is described as free or ionized Ca^{2+}.

Ca^{2+} can move in both directions across the plasma membrane and across each of the membranes of the intracellular Ca^{2+} stores by two different processes. One is responsible for Ca^{2+} movement against the Ca^{2+} concentration gradient and the other for Ca^{2+} movement in the direction of the gradient. Ca^{2+} flows into the cytoplasmic space across the plasma membrane through basal and agonist-stimulated Ca^{2+} inflow systems. Agonist-stimulated Ca^{2+} inflow is facilitated by voltage-operated Ca^{2+} channels or receptor-activated Ca^{2+} inflow systems. Ca^{2+} outflow from the cytoplasmic space to the extracellular fluid is facilitated by a (Ca^{2+} + Mg^{2+})ATPase Ca^{2+} transporter and an Na^+–Ca^{2+} exchange system.

The main function of the endoplasmic or sarcoplasmic reticular Ca^{2+} stores is to release Ca^{2+} to the cytoplasmic space in response to the binding of an agonist to a plasma-membrane receptor. The reticular networks ramify through the cell and probably provide a source of Ca^{2+} near intracellular sites of Ca^{2+} action. Ca^{2+} is transported from the cytoplasmic space to the lumen of the endoplasmic or sarcoplasmic reticulum by a (Ca^{2+} + Mg^{2+})ATPase. Ca^{2+} outflow from the endoplasmic reticulum is mediated by an Ins 1,4,5 P_3-sensitive Ca^{2+} channel whilst in the sarcoplasmic reticulum a Ca^{2+} channel which interacts with the sarcolemmal voltage-operated Ca^{2+} channel probably mediates the release of Ca^{2+}.

The mitochondrial Ca^{2+} store acts as a sink for Ca^{2+} during prolonged increases in $[Ca^{2+}]_i$. Ca^{2+} flows into the mitochondrial matrix in response to an increase in $[Ca^{2+}]_i$. Within the matrix, Ca^{2+} is stored as a precipitate of calcium phosphate and as complexes with proteins. Ca^{2+} inflow to the mitochondrial matrix is associated with an increase in free Ca^{2+} in the matrix space and the activation of Ca^{2+}-responsive mitochondrial enzymes. The inflow process is facilitated by the Ca^{2+} uniporter which is an electrogenic transporter that uses energy provided by the electrochemical gradient across the mitochondrial inner membrane. Outflow to the cytoplasmic space is facilitated by an Na^+–Ca^{2+} or an H^+–Ca^{2+} exchange system.

Increases in $[Ca^{2+}]_i$ induced by agonists can be measured by a number of techniques. Use of intracellular fluorescent Ca^{2+} chelators, such as quin 2 and fura 2, has been most common. Most agonists cause a biphasic increase in $[Ca^{2+}]_i$ which consists of a transient spike of increased $[Ca^{2+}]_i$ followed by a plateau or oscillations in $[Ca^{2+}]_i$. This response is due to increased outflow of Ca^{2+} from the endoplasmic or sarcoplasmic reticulum and increased inflow of Ca^{2+} across the plasma membrane. Increased plasma-membrane Ca^{2+} inflow is responsible for the prolonged increase in $[Ca^{2+}]_i$. The increase in Ca^{2+} outflow from the endoplasmic reticulum is triggered by the binding of Ins 1,4,5 P_3 to the Ins 1,4,5 P_3-sensitive channel. The trigger for the release of Ca^{2+} from the sarcoplasmic reticulum is probably depolarization of the sarcolemma. Agonist-induced Ca^{2+} inflow across the plasma membrane is facilitated by voltage-operated Ca^{2+} channels and by receptor-activated Ca^{2+} inflow systems. The latter systems are not well understood.

The information conveyed by an agonist as an increase in $[Ca^{2+}]_i$ is transformed into intracellular responses by a number of Ca^{2+}-binding proteins called Ca^{2+}-modulated proteins. These can be divided into two groups: those which contain Ca^{2+}-binding domains called helix–loop–helix motifs and those which contain Ca^{2+}-binding sites with different structures. The chief members of the helix–loop–helix family are calmodulin, troponin C, and a group of Ca^{2+}-binding proteins called the S100 proteins. Each of the helix–loop–helix proteins has a low molecular weight and contains two or four Ca^{2+}-binding motifs. The function of these Ca^{2+}-modulated proteins is to confer Ca^{2+} responsiveness to a large number of enzymes and other proteins. These enzymes and proteins are oligomers which, in the presence of increased $[Ca^{2+}]_i$, consist of one or more catalytic subunits and a given type of Ca^{2+}-modulated helix–loop–helix protein.

Calmodulin is present in all cells and interacts with a wide variety of proteins called calmodulin-binding proteins. These include a number of different $(Ca^{2+} + $ calmodulin)-dependent protein kinases, enzymes involved in the metabolism of cyclic nucleotides, $(Ca^{2+} + Mg^{2+})ATPase$ Ca^{2+} transporters, and components of the cytoskeleton. In contrast with calmodulin, troponin C interacts only with tropomyosin present in heart and skeletal muscle. Each S100 protein confers Ca^{2+} responsiveness to one or more enzymes or proteins including those involved in altering the shape of the cytoskeleton.

Ca^{2+}-modulated proteins in which the Ca^{2+}-binding site is not the helix–loop–helix motif include protein kinase C, a group of Ca^{2+} and phospholipid binding proteins called the annexins, Ca^{2+}-activated ion channels, phospholipases

A_2 and D, and Ca^{2+}-responsive enzymes in the mitochondrial matrix. In most of these proteins, Ca^{2+} binds to an allosteric site which is on the same polypeptide chain as the catalytic or functional site.

References

Campbell, K. P., Leung, A. T., and Sharp, A. H. (1988). The biochemistry and molecular biology of the dihydropyridine-sensitive calcium channel. *Trends Neurosc.*, **11**, 425–30.

Carafoli, E. and Penniston, J. T. (1985). The calcium signal. *Sci. Am.*, **253**, 50–58.

Caroni, P. and Carafoli, E. (1981). The Ca^{2+}-pumping ATPase of heart sarcolemma. Characterisation, calmodulin dependence, and partial purification. *J. Biol. Chem.*, **256**, 3263–70.

Charest, R., Prpić, V., Exton, J. H., and Blackmore P .F. (1985). Stimulation of inositol trisphosphate formation in hepatocytes by vasopressin, adrenaline and angiotensin II and its relationship to changes in cytosolic free Ca^{2+}. *Biochem. J.*, **227**, 79–90.

Cheung, W. Y. (1970). Cyclic 3'5'-nucleotide phosphodiesterase. Demonstration of an activator. *Biochem. Biophys. Res Commun.*, **38**, 533 8.

Clarke, D. M., Loo, T. W., Inesi, G., and MacLennan, D.H. (1989). Location of high affinity Ca^{2+}-binding sites within the predicted transmembrane domain of the sarcoplasmic reticulum Ca^{2+}-ATP-ase. *Nature*, **339**, 476–8.

Connor, J. A., Cornwall, M. C., and Williams, G. H. (1987). Spatially resolved cytosolic calcium response to angiotensin II and potassium in rat glomerulosa cells measured by digital imaging techniques. *J. Biol. Chem.*, **262**, 2919–27.

Dabrowska, R., Sherry, J. M. F., Aromatorio, D. K., and Hartshorne, D. J. (1978). Modulator protein as a component of the myosin light chain kinase from chicken gizzard. *Biochemistry*, **17**, 253–8.

de Meis, L. (1981). *The sarcoplasmic reticulum*, p. 70. Wiley, New York.

DiPolo, R. and Beaugé, L. (1979). Physiological role of ATP-driven calcium pump in squid axon. *Nature*, **278**, 271–3.

Ebashi, S. and Kodama, A. (1965). A new protein

function promoting aggregation in tropomyosin. *J. Biochem.*, **58**, 107–8.

England, P. J. (1986). Intracellular calcium receptor mechanisms. *Br. Med. Bull.* **42**, 375–83.

Glossmann, H. and Ferry, D. R. (1983). Solubilization and partial purification of putative calcium channels labelled with [³H]-nimodipine. *Naunyn-Schmiedeberg's Arch. Pharmacol.*, **323**, 279–91.

Grynkiewicz, G., Poenie, M., and Tsien, R. Y. (1985). A new generation of Ca^{2+} indicators with greatly improved fluorescence properties. *J. Biol. Chem.* **260**, 3340–50.

Hamill, O. P., Marty, A., Neher, E., Sakmann, B., and Sigworth, F. J. (1981). Improved patch-clamp technique for high-resolution current recording from cells and cell-free membrane patches. *Pflug. Arch.*, **391**, 85–100.

Heilbrunn, L. V. (1940). The action of calcium on muscle protoplasm. *Physiol. Zool.* **13**, 88–94.

Heilbrunn, L. V. and Wiercinski, F.J. (1947). The action of various cations on muscle protoplasm. *J. Cell. Comp. Physiol.* **29**, 15–32.

Hodgkin, A. L. and Katz, B. (1949). The effect of sodium ions on the electrical activity of the giant axon of the squid. *J. Physiol.*, (London), **108**, 37–77.

Kakiuchi, S. and Yamazaki, R. (1970). Calcium dependent phosphodiesterase activity and its activating factor (PAF) from brain. Studies on cyclic 3′,5′-nucleotide phosphodiesterase (3). *Biochem. Biophys. Res. Commun.* **41**, 1104–10.

Klee, C. B., Newton, D. L., and Krinks, M. H. (1983). Versatility of calmodulin as a cytosolic regulator of cellular function. In *Affinity chromatography and biological recognition*, (ed. I. M. Chaiken, M. Wilchek, and I. Parikh), pp. 55–67. Academic Press, Orlando, Florida.

Kolesnick, R. N. and Gershengorn, M. C. (1985). Direct evidence that burst but not sustained secretion of prolactin stimulated by thyrotropin-releasing hormone is dependent on elevation of cytoplasmic calcium. *J. Biol. Chem.*, **260**, 5217–20.

Kowarski, D., Shuman, H., Somlyo, A. P., and Somlyo, A. V. (1985). Calcium release by noradrenaline from central sarcoplasmic reticulum in rabbit main pulmonary artery smooth muscle. *J. Physiol.*, **366**, 153–75.

Krstić, R. V. (1979). *Ultrastructure of the mammalian cell: an atlas*, pp. 96–7. Springer, Berlin.

Langer, G. A. (1978). The structure and function of the myocardial cell surface. *Am. J. Physiol.*, **235**, H461–8.

Lehninger, A. L., Carafoli, E., and Rossi, C. S. (1967). Energy-linked ion movements in mitochondrial systems. *Adv. Enzymol.* **29**, 259–320.

Levin, R. M. and Weiss, B. (1976) Mechanism by which pyschotropic drugs inhibit adenosine cyclic 3′,5′-monophosphate phosphodiesterase of brain. *Mol. Pharmacol.*, **12**, 581–9.

MacLennan, D. H. and Wong, P. T. S. (1971). Isolation of a calcium-sequestering protein from sarcoplasmic reticulum. *Proc. Natl Acad. Sci. USA*, **68**, 1231–5.

Niggli, V., Adunyah, E. S., Penniston, J. T., and Carafoli, E. (1981). Purified $(Ca^{2+} - Mg^{2+})$ATP-ase of the erythrocyte membrane. Reconstitution and effect of calmodulin and phospholipids. *J. Biol. Chem.*, **256**, 395–401.

Reuter, H. (1983). Calcium channel modulation by neurotransmitters, enzymes and drugs. *Nature*, **301**, 569–74.

Ringer, S. (1883). A further contribution regarding the influence of the different constituents of the blood on the contraction of the heart. *J. Physiol.* (London), **4**, 29–42.

Schatzmann, H. J. and Vincenzi, F. F. (1969). Calcium movements across the membrane of human red cells. *J. Physiol.* (London), **201**, 369–95.

Silver, R. A., Lamb, A. G., and Bolsover, S. R. (1990). Calcium hotspots caused by L-channel clustering promote morphological changes in neuronal growth cones. *Nature*, **343**, 751–4.

Stanfield, P. R. (1986). Voltage-dependent calcium channels of excitable membranes. *Br. Med. Bull.*, **42**, 359–67.

Szent-Györgyi, A.G., Szentkiralyi, E.M., and Kendrick-Jones, J. (1973). The light chains of scallop myosin as regulatory subunits. *J. Mol. Biol.* **74**, 179–203.

Tanabe, T., Takeshima, H., Mikami, A. Flockerzi, V., Takahashi, H., Kangawa, K. *et al.* (1987). Primary structure of the receptor for calcium channel blockers from skeletal muscle. *Nature*, **328**, 313–18.

Teo, T. S. and Wang, J. H. (1973). Mechanism of activation of a cyclic adenosine 3':5'-monophosphate phosphodiesterase from bovine heart by calcium ions. Identification of the protein activator as a Ca^{2+}-binding protein. *J. Biol. Chem.*, **248**, 5950–5.

Tsien, R. Y. (1980). New calcium indicators and buffers with high selectivity against magnesium and protons: design, synthesis and properties of prototype structures. *Biochemistry*, **19**, 2396–404.

Tsien, R. Y. (1981). A non-disruptive technique for loading calcium buffers and indicators into cells. *Nature* **290**, 527–8.

Vasington, F. D. and Murphy, J. V. (1962). Ca^{2+} uptake by rat kidney mitochondria and its dependence on respiration and phosphorylation. *J. Biol. Chem.*, **237**, 2670–7.

Williams, R. J. P. (1976). Calcium in Biological Systems. In *Symposium XXX, Society of Experimental Biology* (ed. C. J. Duncan), pp. 1–18. Cambridge University Press.

Woods, N. M., Cuthbertson, K. S. R. and Cobbold, P. H. (1987). Agonist-induced oscillations in cytoplasmic free calcium concentration in single rat hepatocytes. *Cell Calcium*, **8**, 79–100.

Zucker, R.S. and Fogelson, A. L. (1986). Relationship between transmitter release and presynaptic calcium influx when calcium enters through discrete channels. *Proc. Natl Acad. Sci. USA*, **83**, 3032–6.

Further reading

Borle, A. B. (1981). Control modulation and regulation of cell calcium. *Rev. Physiol. Biochem. Pharmacol.*, **90**, 13–153.

Campbell, A. K. (1986). Lewis Heilbrunn: pioneer of calcium as an intracellular regulator. *Cell Calcium*, **7**, 287–96.

Carafoli, E. (1987). Intracellular calcium homeostasis. *Ann. Rev. Biochem.* **56**, 395–433.

Carafoli, E. and Penniston, J. T. (1985). The calcium signal. *Sci. Am.*, **253**, 50–8.

Cohen, P. and Klee, C. B. (1988). *Calmodulin.* Elsevier, Amsterdam.

Evered, D. and Whelan, J. (1986). *Calcium and the cell*, Ciba Foundation Symposium 122. Wiley, New York.

Rasmussen, H. and Barrett, P. Q. (1984). Calcium messenger system: an integrated view. *Physiol. Rev.*, **64**, 938–84.

Thomas, M. V. (1982). Physical factors relating to the measurement of intracellular free Ca^{2+}. In *Techniques in calcium research* (M. V. Thomas), pp. 21–58. Academic Press, London.

Thompson, M. P. (1989). *Calcium binding proteins.* Vols. 1 and 2. CRC Press, Boca Raton.

Tsien, R. W. and Tsien, R. Y. (1990). Calcium channels, stores, and oscillations. *Ann. Rev. Cell Biol.*, **6**, 715–60.

8 *The intermediary metabolites*

8.1 Intermediary metabolites in intracellular communication

A number of intermediary metabolites regulate the activities of enzymes and proteins. These metabolites include substrates, products, co-enzymes, and allosteric modifiers. Each of these molecules binds to a specific site on the regulated enzyme or protein and alters the conformation and activity of the protein.

Certain intermediary metabolites play a variety of roles in intracellular communication. These include the co-ordination of flux through a given metabolic pathway, the co-ordination of metabolic flux through two or more pathways, as well as the provision in some special cases of the final link in the chain which connects receptors, intracellular messengers, and protein kinases to the regulation of a metabolic pathway. These functions of intermediary metabolites are not normally described as intracellular messenger functions. Nevertheless, some intermediary metabolites can be considered as intracellular messengers with a very restricted function. Members of this last group are fructose 2,6-bisphosphate, which functions in the regulation of glycolysis and gluconeogenesis, free fatty acids which regulate heat production in brown fat cells, NADPH and ATP which mediate insulin release in the β-cell of the pancreas, and pH_i which has been implicated in the control of cell growth.

This chapter will summarize the main identifiable contributions that intermediary metabolites make to the pathways of intracellular communication. After a brief discussion of the role of metabolites in the regulation of metabolic pathways, the actions of metabolites which have more specific functions as intracellular messengers will be described. These metabolites are fructose 2,6-bisphosphate, fatty acids, ATP and reduced pyridine nucleotides, and H^+ and Na^+.

8.2 Regulation of metabolic pathways

The fluxes through many metabolic pathways are controlled in part by metabolites which regulate the activities of specific enzymes or transport processes. These mechanisms of regulation (intrinsic mechanisms) supplement the regulation of the pathways by extracellular signals (extrinsic mechanisms). Some examples of the many pathways of metabolism which are known to be regulated by metabolites in an intrinsic manner are listed in Table 8.1.

Metabolites can control flux through a metabolic pathway by either feedback or feed-forward regulation. In feedback regulation an end product of a pathway inhibits one of the first enzymes in the pathway (Fig. 8.1). In feed-forward regulation, a metabolite formed at an early stage of the pathway activates an enzyme later in the pathway (Fig. 8.1). Feedback regulation was discovered in 1956 by Yates, Pardee, and Umbarger (Yates and Pardee 1956; Umbarger 1956). Yates and Pardee observed that in crude extracts of *E. coli*, cytidine nucleotides, which are end products of the pathway of pyrimidine

Table 8.1 *Examples of metabolic pathways which are subject to regulation by non-covalent modification of enzyme activity*

General area of metabolism	Specific pathway
Carbohydrate metabolism	Glycogen synthesis Glycogenolysis Gluconeogenesis Glycolysis Pentose phosphate pathway
Lipid metabolism	Interconversion of free fatty acids and triglyceride Fatty-acid synthesis Fatty-acid oxdiation Cholesterol synthesis
Nitrogen metabolism	Urea cycle
Energy metabolism	Citric acid cycle Oxidative phosphorylation
Specific biosynthetic pathways	Pyrimidine synthesis

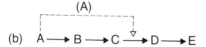

(a)

(b)

Fig. 8.1 A schematic representation of feedback or end-product inhibition (a) and feed-forward activation (b) in hypothetical metabolic pathways. A represents the initial substrate of the pathway, E the final product and B, C, and D represent intermediates. Inhibition and activation are represented by the broken lines and the symbols (I) and (A), respectively.

synthesis, inhibit the first enzyme of this pathway, aspartate transcarbamylase. Umbarger made a similar type of observation, also in crude extracts of *E. coli*. He found that isoleucine, an end product in the pathway for the synthesis of branched-chain amino acids, inhibits threonine dehydratase, the first enzyme of this pathway.

The role of metabolites in communicating between two different metabolic pathways can be best appreciated by the examination of an example. One of the most interesting is the regulation of the pathways of glycolysis and gluconeogenesis in the liver. In glycolysis, glucose is oxidized to pyruvate, which, in the presence of adequate oxygen, is oxidized further to CO_2 by pyruvate dehydrogenase and the enzymes of the citric acid cycle. Conversely, gluconeogenesis involves the synthesis of glucose from 3-carbon precursors such as pyruvate.

Some of the feedback-control mechanisms which govern flux through the glycolytic and gluconeogenic pathways are shown in Fig. 8.2. The rate of glycolysis is controlled, in part, by the concentrations of ATP and AMP. ATP inhibits both phosphofructokinase-1, which catalyses the conversion of fructose-6-phosphate to fructose 1,6-bisphosphate, and pyruvate kinase, which catalyses the conversion of phosphoenolpyruvate to pyruvate (Fig. 8.2). Inhibition of these reactions restricts the rate of glycolysis when sufficient ATP is present. AMP, the concentration of which probably increases when

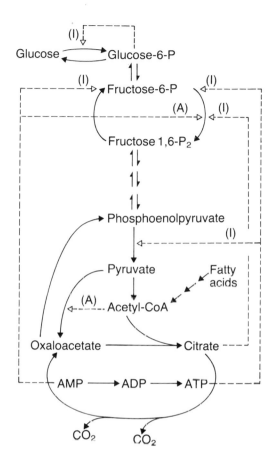

Fig. 8.2 A schematic representation of the regulation of the glycolytic and gluconeogenic pathways by the metabolites ATP, AMP, glucose-6-phosphate (glucose-6-P), citrate, and acetyl-CoA. Inhibition and activation are represented by the broken lines and the symbols (I) and (A), respectively.

there is a need for ATP and hence a need for increased flux through the glycolytic pathway, activates phosphofructokinase-1 and inhibits fructose bisphosphatase-1. The latter enzyme catalyses the hydrolysis of fructose 1,6-bisphosphate to fructose-6-phosphate.

Control of the glycolytic and gluconeogenic pathways by ATP and AMP is supplemented by a number of other mechanisms. Two of these involve glucose-6-phosphate and citrate. The initial step in the glycolytic pathway, the phos-

phorylation of glucose catalysed by hexokinase, is inhibited by its product, glucose-6-phosphate. Citrate, which like ATP, is formed when glycolytic flux is increased, inhibits phosphofructokinase-1.

During the shift from the fed to the fasted state, there is a switch in the direction of metabolism from glycolysis to gluconeogenesis in the liver. This is caused by an increase in the plasma concentration of glucagon and by changes in the concentrations of a number of other hormones. These inhibit glycolysis and activate gluconeogenesis. Target enzymes for the action of glucagon are phosphofructokinase-1, fructose bisphosphatase-1 (described later in the section on fructose 2,6-bisphosphate), pyruvate kinase, and pyruvate carboxylase, which catalyses the carboxylation of pyruvate to form oxaloacetate.

The actions of glucagon are aided by the inhibition by ATP of phosphofructokinase-1 and pyruvate kinase. The first enzyme in the pathway for the synthesis of glucose from pyruvate, pyruvate carboxylase, is activated by acetyl-CoA. This regulatory step links the increased rate of gluconeogenesis to an increased rate of fatty-acid oxidation since the need for gluconeogenesis during starvation is accompanied by the oxidation of fatty acids which, in turn, increases the concentration of acetyl-CoA.

Much of our information on metabolite regulation of glycolysis and gluconeogenesis and, indeed, other pathways has been derived from studies conducted with isolated enzymes. It is not always possible to be sure that the results of these experiments reflect the mechanism of regulation of the given enzyme in intact cells. This reservation should be borne in mind when considering the picture for the regulation of glycolysis and gluconeogenesis just described.

8.3   Fructose 2,6-bisphosphate

Fructose 2,6-bisphosphate links cyclic AMP-dependent protein kinase to the regulation of glycolysis and gluconeogenesis through its action on the enzymes phosphofructokinase-1 and fructose bisphosphatase-1. Regulation of the activity of these enzymes is the only known function of fructose 2,6-bisphosphate in animal cells.

The initial observation which led to the discovery of fructose 2,6-bisphosphate was made by four independent research groups (Castano *et al.* 1979; Clarke *et al.* 1979; Kagimoto and Uyeda 1979; Pilkis *et al.* 1979). Each group found that the kinetic properties of isolated phosphofructokinase-1 are altered after the incubation of hepatocytes with glucagon. In 1980, H. G. Hers and his colleagues observed that the alteration in kinetic properties disappeared upon gel filtration of phosphofructokinase-1 (Van Schaftingen *et al.* 1980). These workers obtained a low molecular weight fraction from liver which activated phosphofructo-

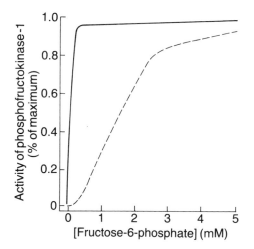

Fig. 8.3 Plots of the activity of phosphofructokinase-1 as a function of the concentration of fructose-6-phosphate in the presence of ATP and in the presence (full curve) and absence (broken curve) of 1μM fructose 2,6-bisphosphate. Fructose 2,6-bisphosphate activates phosphofructokinase-1 by increasing the affinity of the enzyme for fructose-6-phosphate. From Van Schaftingen *et al.* (1981).

kinase-1. The active component of this fraction was subsequently identified as fructose 2,6-bisphosphate. This unusual metabolite of glucose is not only present in liver but also in almost every animal tissue investigated.

Fructose 2,6-bisphosphate activates phosphofructokinase-1 in the presence of ATP by increasing the affinity of the enzyme for its substrate fructose-6-phosphate (Fig. 8.3). In contrast to its effects on phosphofructokinase-1, fructose 2,6-bisphosphate inhibits fructose bisphosphatase-1. Fructose 2,6-bisphosphate acts as an allosteric modifier of each of these enzymes. Its effects are synergistic with those of AMP.

How is fructose 2,6-bisphosphate formed and degraded? The reactions involved are similar to those which catalyse the formation and degradation of fructose 1,6-bisphosphate. The two catalytic activities involved, phosphofructokinase-2 and fructose bisphosphatase-2, both reside at separate catalytic sites on the same polypeptide chain. The bifunctional enzyme is composed of two identical subunits each with a molecular weight of 55 kDa. The reactions catalysed by these enzymes are shown in Fig. 8.4. The activities of phosphofructokinase-2 and fructose bisphosphatase-2 are regulated by cyclic AMP-dependent protein kinase. Phosphorylation of phosphofructokinase-2 leads to a decrease in enzyme activity whilst phosphorylation of fructose bisphosphatase-2 leads to an increase in enzyme activity (Fig. 8.4).

Fructose 2,6-bisphosphate allows glucagon to control hepatic glycolysis and gluconeogenesis at a critical regulatory step, the interconversion of fructose-6-phosphate and fructose 1,6-bisphosphate (Fig. 8.5). Not only are the actions of glucagon mediated by this pathway, but also those of other hormones which alter the intracellular concentration of cyclic AMP and hence the activity of cyclic AMP-dependent protein kinase. The activation of cyclic AMP-dependent

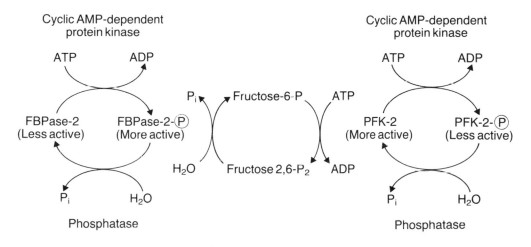

Fig. 8.4   The formation (phosphorylation) and degradation (dephosphorylation) of fructose 2,6-bisphosphate is catalysed by phosphofructokinase-2 (PFK-2) and fructose bisphosphatase-2 (FBPase-2). Phosphorylation of these enzymes by cyclic AMP-dependent protein kinase leads to a reduction in the activity of phosphofructokinase-2 and an increase in the activity of fructose bisphosphatase-2.

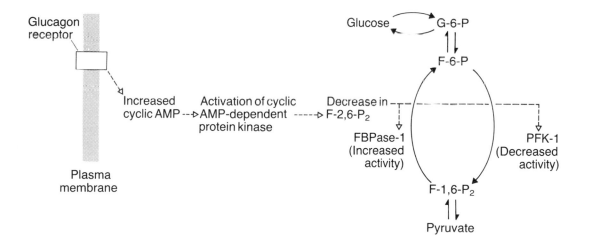

Fig. 8.5   The role of fructose 2,6-bisphosphate (F-2,6-P_2) in the regulation of glycolysis and gluconeogenesis by cyclic AMP-dependent protein kinase. Activation of cyclic AMP-dependent protein kinase leads to a decrease in the concentration of fructose 2,6-bisphosphate. This allows flux through fructose bisphosphatase-1 (FBPase-1) to increase (F-2,6-P_2 is an inhibitor of FBPase 1) and flux through phosphofructokinase-1 (PFK-1) to decrease (F-2,6-P_2 is an activator of PFK-1).

protein kinase leads to a decrease in fructose 2,6-bisphosphate which, in turn, promotes gluconeogenesis and inhibits glycolysis (Fig. 8.5).

In addition to regulation of the relative rates of glycolysis and gluconeogenesis in liver, fructose 2,6-bisphosphate probably has a broader role as a signal that can lead to an increase in flux through the glycolytic pathway under conditions in which the intracellular concentration of ATP, an inhibitor of the glycolytic pathway, is relatively high. Such an increase in glycolytic flux is required when the pathway of glycolysis supplies intermediates for anabolic reactions. A requirement for increased glycolysis in the presence of an adequate concentration of ATP can occur in many tissues, including skeletal muscle, adipose tissue, and liver. An example of this requirement for glycolysis is the provision of acetyl-CoA for lipogenesis. The formation of acetyl-CoA under these conditions requires the oxidation of glucose to pyruvate which is subsequently converted to acetyl-CoA.

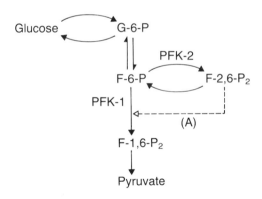

Fig. 8.6 Fructose 2,6-bisphosphate (F-2,6-P$_2$) activates the glycolytic pathway in the presence of ATP. The supply of glucose to a cell increases the formation of fructose 2,6-bisphosphate as well as that of fructose 1,6-bisphosphate (F-1,6-P$_2$) in the reactions catalysed by phosphofructokinases 2 and 1 (PFK-2 and PFK-1), respectively. Fructose 2,6-bisphosphate ensures adequate activity of the glycolytic pathway in the presence of ATP, an inhibitor of phosphofructokinase-1. Glucose-6-phosphate and fructose-6-phosphate are represented by G-6-P and F-6-P, respectively.

When glucose is metabolized in cells which contain phosphofructokinases 1 and 2, both fructose 1,6-bisphosphate and fructose 2,6-bisphosphate are formed (Fig. 8.6). The resulting increase in the concentration of fructose 2,6-bisphosphate activates phosphofructokinase-1 and hence probably contributes to activation of the glycolytic pathway (Fig. 8.6).

8.4 Fatty acids in brown fat cells

8.4.1 *Heat production in brown fat cells*
In brown fat cells, free fatty acids link the activation of triglyceride lipase by cyclic AMP-dependent protein kinase to a flow of H$^+$ through the mitochondrial inner membrane while also acting as a fuel for mitochondrial respiration. The increased flow of protons is not coupled to the generation of ATP but does lead to an increase in heat production.

The main physiological function of brown fat cells is thought to be the production of heat. The process of heat production by these types of cell is called non-shivering thermogenesis. This form of heat production is particularly important during the period of arousal from hibernation in hybernants, as a defence against hypothermia in most newborn mammals, and during the adaptation to cold in a large number of adult small mammals. A major signal for increased heat production in an animal is the release of the neurotransmitter noradrenalin from the sympathetic nervous system.

Brown fat cells contain very large numbers of mitochondria as shown in Fig. 8.7 which shows an electron micrograph of a brown fat cell. Indeed, each cell contains about 10 000 mitochondria which occupy about 30 per cent of the cell volume. These mitochondria exhibit two interesting properties. Firstly, in comparison with mitochondria from other types of cell the concentration of the ATP-synthetase is low. Secondly, when isolated by conventional meth-

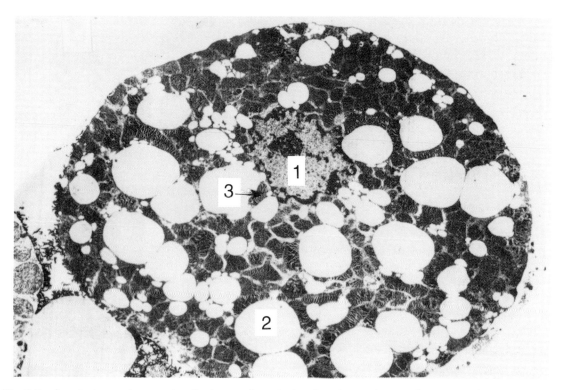

Fig. 8.7   An electron micrograph of a brown fat cell showing the nucleus at the centre of the cell (1), the large number of lipid droplets (2), and the large number of mitochondria (3). From Nedergaard and Lindberg (1982).

ods, brown fat cell mitochondria show a marked uncoupling of oxidative phosphorylation from respiration.

8.4.2   *Thermogenin*

The energy for heat production in brown fat cells is provided by the flow of protons through a protein called thermogenin, or uncoupling protein, which is located in the mitochondrial inner membrane (Fig. 8.8). This pathway of H^+ inflow to the mitochondrial matrix bypasses the H^+ translocating ATP-synthetase.

Thermogenin is a dimer composed of subunits of molecular weight of 32 kDa. The protein possesses a binding site for purine nucleotides and a binding site which accommodates fatty acids or fatty acyl-CoA molecules (Fig. 8.8). These binding sites are probably on the cytoplasmic face of the protein. Thermogenin allows the movement of H^+, OH^-, and chloride ions across the mitochondrial inner membrane, probably by creating a pore or channel for these ions. GTP, ATP, GDP, and ITP can bind to the purine nucleotide binding site. The combination of one of these molecules with this site inhibits the movement of H^+ or OH^- through the thermogenin channel. This inhibition is reversed by the binding of a fatty acid or fatty acyl-CoA molecule to the fatty-acid binding site. The affinity of this site for fatty acids or fatty acyl-CoA species is quite high, about 1 nM.

It was the ability of thermogenin to bind purine nucleotides which led to the discovery of this protein. In 1968, Hohorst and Rafael showed that the inclusion of GTP in incubations of isolated brown fat cell mitochondria markedly

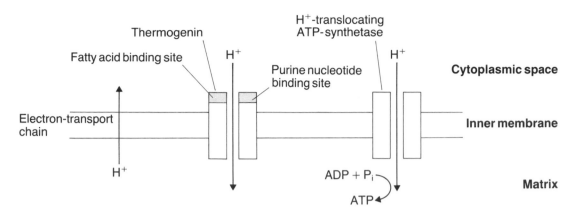

Fig. 8.8 The proton carrier thermogenin is located in the inner membrane of brown fat mitochondria. In the presence of free fatty acids or fatty acyl-CoA molecules, this protein facilitates the re-entry of H^+ to the matrix by-passing the proton-translocating ATP-synthetase.

improved the coupling of respiration to ATP synthesis. The action of GTP and other nucleotides was shown to be exerted at a site on the outside of mitochondria (Cannon *et al.* 1973). In 1974, Nicholls showed that the inner membrane of brown fat mitochondria contains a regulatable ion-translocation system which allows protons to re-enter the mitochondrial matrix without passing through the proton-translocating ATP-synthetase (Nicholls 1974). Two years later he identified a high-affinity binding site for purine nucleotides on the outer face of the mitochondrial inner membrane (Nicholls 1976). The purine nucleotide binding protein was labelled using the photoaffinity reagent [^{32}P]8-azido ATP, isolated, and shown to have a molecular weight of 32 kDa (Heaton *et al.* 1978). This protein, later called thermogenin (Cannon *et al.* 1981), was shown to be the proton-translocating system which 'short circuits' the ATP-synthetase.

8.4.3 *Fatty acids and the activation of thermogenin*

It is presently believed that the mechanism which activates the flow of protons through thermogenin involves the following steps, which are shown in Fig. 8.9. In the resting brown fat cell the presence of purine nucleotides and virtual absence of free fatty acids in the cytoplasmic space inhibits H^+ flow through thermogenin and maintains the mitochondria in a tightly coupled state. The binding of noradrenalin to its receptor on the plasma membrane leads to an increase in the concentration of cyclic AMP which activates cyclic AMP-dependent protein kinase. This, in turn, leads to the activation of triglyceride lipase and the generation of free fatty acids and glycerol.

The fatty acids formed in response to the activation of cyclic AMP-dependent protein kinase diffuse through the cytoplasmic space to the mitochondrial inner membrane where they are converted to fatty acyl-CoA derivatives. A small proportion of fatty acyl-CoAs probably bind to the fatty-acid binding site on thermogenin and allow the inflow of H^+ to the mitochondrial matrix through this pathway. The bulk of the fatty acyl-CoAs are oxidized in the β-oxidation pathway. These two actions of the fatty acyl-CoAs result in the generation of heat, although the mechanism by which heat is produced as a result of the increased flow of protons through thermogenin is not entirely clear. The production of heat by this mechanism is independent of the synthesis and hydrolysis of ATP.

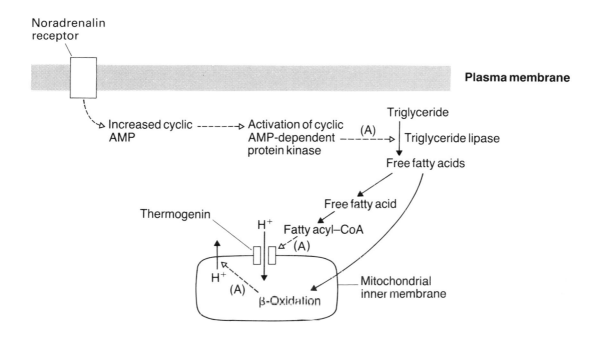

Fig. 8.9 Free fatty acids constitute the signal which links the action of noradrenalin in stimulating the hydrolysis of triglycerides to the production of heat by brown fat cells. The free fatty acids diffuse through the cytoplasmic space to the mitochondrial inner membrane where they are converted to the fatty acyl-CoA derivative. Fatty acyl-CoAs bind to thermogenin and stimulate the flow of H^+ to the mitochondrial matrix, by-passing the ATP-synthetase. Activation is represented by the symbol (A). The bulk of the fatty acyl-CoAs are oxidized to provide energy for the translocation of H^+ from the mitochondrial matrix to the cytoplasmic space.

A further control on heat production in brown fat cells is regulation of the amount of thermogenin present in the mitochondria. The intracellular concentration of thermogenin is increased in neonates but decreases in the post-natal period and increases during the adaptation of animals to a cold environment. These changes alter the capacity of brown fat cells to produce heat and hence the total heat produced in an animal by non-shivering thermogensis.

8.5 Nutrient-induced insulin secretion

In the β-cell of the pancreas, NADPH, ATP, and an ATP-sensitive K^+ channel are thought to link the initial metabolism of a nutrient such as glucose to the increase in $[Ca^{2+}]_i$ which is responsible for initiating the exocytosis of insu-

lin secretory granules. The main extracellular signals for increased insulin secretion are an increase in the concentration of glucose, arginine, or leucine in the blood. The action of these nutrients is stereospecific. For example, α-D-glucose is more potent than β-D-glucose in inducing insulin release.

Each nutrient which stimulates insulin secretion increases $[Ca^{2+}]_i$ in the β-cell. This, in turn, alters the activity of a number of enzymes and other proteins and causes the interaction of secretory granules with the plasma membrane and the release of insulin (Fig 8.10). The actions of glucose and amino acids in inducing insulin secretion are modified by hormones, for example glucagon and adrenalin (which acts at β-adrenergic receptors), and neurotransmitters, for example acetylcholine (which acts at muscarinic

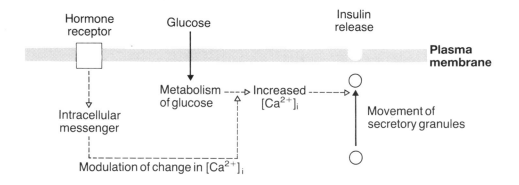

Fig. 8.10 Glucose, which induces the secretion of insulin by pancreatic β-cells, causes an increase in $[Ca^{2+}]_i$. This, in turn, induces the interaction of secretory granules with the plasma membrane and the release of insulin by exocytosis. The increase in $[Ca^{2+}]_i$ induced by glucose can be modified by hormones such as glucagon or adrenalin. The activation of protein kinase C by diacylglycerol may also be important in movement of the secretory granules.

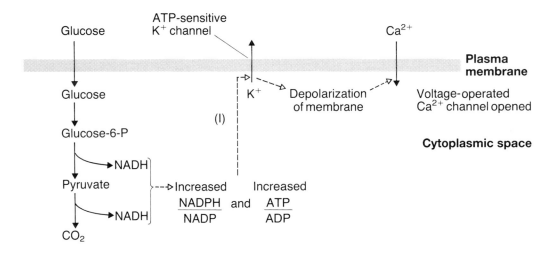

Fig. 8.11 A schematic description of the probable mechanism by which glucose induces the secretion of insulin. The metabolism of glucose by the β-cell leads to an inhibition (I) of K^+ inflow, depolarization of the plasma membrane and the opening of voltage-operated Ca^{2+} channels. The link between glucose metabolism and inhibition of K^+ inflow has not been clearly defined but is probably provided by increases in the ratios of NADPH/NADP and ATP/ADP.

receptors).

The question of how glucose and other nutrients induce the release of insulin has not yet been fully answered and remains one of the interesting questions in intracellular communication. A complete answer to this question would also help to define the mechanism by which nutrients induce the secretion of other hormones such as glucagon.

Over 20 years ago, when the question of how nutrients stimulate insulin release was first considered, two general hypotheses were formulated. One states that glucose interacts with a stereospecific receptor in a manner analogous to the interaction of a hormone with a plasma-membrane receptor; the other proposes that a metabolic product of glucose is the key signal which initiates insulin release. The body of knowledge presently available indicates that the second of these hypotheses, called the fuel hypothesis, is most likely to be the correct one.

The present version of the fuel hypothesis of glucose-induced insulin secretion is summarized in Fig. 8.11. It is proposed that the metabolism of glucose leads to increases in the ratios of NADPH/NADP and ATP/ADP. This increase in ATP inhibits K^+ outflow through ATP-sensitive K^+ channels in the plasma membrane. Inhibition of K^+ outflow causes depolarization of the membrane and opens voltage-operated Ca^{2+} channels. The events which follow inhibition of the K^+ channel and lead to activation of the voltage-operated Ca^{2+} channel are reasonably well established. However, the processes which link glucose metabolism to inhibition of the K^+ channel are less clearly defined.

The first rate-limiting step in the metabolism of glucose by the β-cell is the phosphorylation of glucose, catalysed by glucokinase. The relatively high apparent K_M (8 mM) of this enzyme for glucose governs the range of extracellular glucose concentrations to which the β-cell responds. Glucokinase and other enzymes of the glycolytic pathway are also responsible for determining the stereospecificity of the insulin-release system for glucose.

The metabolic effects of glucose may be amplified by inositol 1,4,5-trisphosphate and cyclic AMP. The initial increase in $[Ca^{2+}]_i$ caused by glucose may stimulate the formation of both inositol 1,4,5-trisphosphate and cyclic AMP. Inositol 1,4,5-trisphosphate probably amplifies the increase in intracellular free Ca^{2+} induced by the opening of voltage-operated Ca^{2+} channels by releasing Ca^{2+} from intracellular stores.

The mechanism by which leucine stimulates insulin secretion differs slightly from the action of glucose. Leucine is an allosteric activator of glutamate dehydrogenase. It is proposed that the binding of leucine to glutamate dehydrogenase stimulates flux through this reaction and increases the concentrations of NADH, NADPH, and ATP.

8.6   pH and the stimulation of DNA synthesis

8.6.1   *Increases in intracellular pH induced by growth factors*

A large number of experiments conducted over the past 10 years have led to the proposal that an increase in intracellular pH (pH_i) plays a permissive role in the process by which growth factors and other mitogens stimulate DNA synthesis during the transition of a cell from the G_0 phase to the S phase of the cell cycle. In 1982 Whitaker and Steinhardt observed that following the fertilization of sea-urchin eggs, pH_i rises rapidly. Later experiments showed that the increase in pH_i is caused by the activation of an Na^+–H^+ exchange system in the plasma membrane. The exchange of Na^+ for H^+ is catalysed by a glycoprotein with a molecular weight of 110 kDa which employs the inwardly directed Na^+ gradient to actively extrude H^+. The stoichiometry is one Na^+ exchanged for one H^+ so that the exchange process is electroneutral. A feature of the Na^+–H^+ exchange system is its inhibition by amiloride (Fig. 8.12) and a number of derivatives of this drug.

At about the same time as the observations of changes in pH_i in fertilized eggs, other experiments revealed that the actions of growth factors on fibroblasts and some other types of cell are also associated with changes in pH_i. In 1978, Smith and Rozengurt showed that growth factors activate Na^+–H^+ exchange in cultured cells. The stimulation of Na^+–H^+ exchange was later shown to be associated with an increase in pH_i (Schuldiner and Rozengurt 1982). The first continuous measurement of changes in pH_i induced by growth factors was made in 1983 by Moolenaar and his colleagues who used the fluorescent

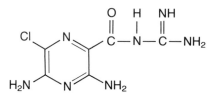

Fig. 8.12 The structure of amiloride (N-amidino-3,5-diamino-6-chloropyrazinecarboxamide), an inhibitor of the Na^+–H^+ exchange system.

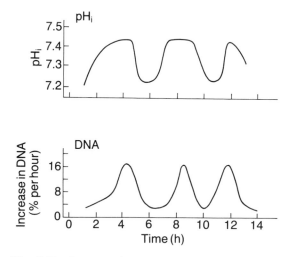

Fig. 8.13 Increases in pH_i correlate with increases in DNA synthesis during successive cell cycles of *Dictyostelium discordeum*. From Aerts *et al.* (1985).

dye bis-(carboxy-ethyl)-carboxyfluorescein (Moolenaar *et al.* 1983). In the following year, Moolenaar's group obtained evidence which indicated that one mechanism by which growth factors activate Na^+–H^+ exchange involves protein kinase C (Moolenaar *et al.* 1984). An effect of growth factors in increasing pH_i through the action of protein kinase C has now been shown for many growth factors in many types of cell.

Three other types of experiment have provided evidence which indicates that, at least in some types of cell, an increase in pH_i plays an important role in growth factor-induced stimulation of DNA synthesis. Firstly, it has been found that in a number of cells the increase in pH_i induced by growth factors is associated with increases in protein and DNA synthesis which occur as cells move from the growth-arrested G_0/G_1 phase of the cell cycle to the S phase. Elegant experiments have been performed to show a correlation between changes in pH_i and DNA synthesis during successive cell cycles (Fig. 8.13).

Secondly, in 1984 Pouyssegur and his colleagues developed a strategy which enabled them to isolate mutants of Chinese hamster lung fibroblasts in which the plasma membrane Na^+–H^+ exchange system is inoperative (Pouyssegur *et al.* 1984). In contrast to wild-type fibroblasts, which grow in an HCO_3^--free medium at a wide range of extracellular pH values (6.6–8.2), these mutants do not grow at neutral and acidic extracellular pH (below 7.2) but do grow at alkaline pH (8.0–8.3).

In the third set of experiments, amiloride analogues were used to inhibit Na^+–H^+ exchange. The ability of a series of amiloride analogues to inhibit this exchange system in Chinese hamster lung fibroblasts incubated in an HCO_3^--free medium correlated well with the ability of the same analogues to block the stimulation of DNA synthesis in G_0-arrested cells (L'Allemain *et al.* 1984).

Many of the observations which relate the action of growth factors to an increase in pH_i were made in cells incubated in an HCO_3^--free medium. This is a somewhat contrived and non-physiological condition, although the experimenters realized this. With this problem in mind, W. F. Boron and his colleagues conducted a series of experiments, the results of which suggested that the increase in pH_i induced by growth factors may not be such an important intracellular growth signal as suggested by the body of evidence accumulated over the past 10 years (Ganz *et al.* 1989).

Boron's group and others have shown that in a number of cell types there are, in addition to the Na^+–H^+ exchange system, two other exchange systems which contribute to the regulation of pH_i (Fig. 8.14). These both involve HCO_3^-. When cells are incubated in the presence of HCO_3^- (a more physiological environment) it is found that, in some cell types, growth factors stimulate the activity of all three H^+ and HCO_3^- exchange systems (Fig. 8.14) with a predominant effect on the HCO_3^- extrusion system. This results in a decrease, rather than an increase, in pH_i. Thus in some cases, the increase in pH_i observed following the action of growth factors on cells may be the result of the omission of HCO_3^- from the incubation medium.

8.6.2   *Activation of Na^+–H^+ exchange and the permissive action of pH_i*

The mechanisms by which growth factors activate Na^+–H^+ exchange and increase pH_i can be summarized in the following manner (Fig. 8.15). The activity of the amiloride-sensitive Na^+–H^+ exchange system is regulated, in part, by pH_i. Low values of pH_i (below about 7) activate the exchange system whereas values above about 7.4 inhibit exchange. Superimposed on this control mechanism are the actions of growth factors which lead to phosphorylation of the exchanger. This increases its affinity for H^+ and activates the Na^+–H^+ exchange system. There are two pathways for phosphorylation of the Na^+–H^+ exchange system. One is dependent on protein kinase C and one is independent of the activation of this protein kinase.

Stimulation of the activity of the Na^+–H^+ exchange system by growth factors leads to increases in pH_i and Na^+_i. The magnitude of the increase in pH_i is 0.1–0.3 pH units. A consequence of the increase in Na^+_i is activation of the $(Na^+ + K^+)$ATPase and an increase in K^+_i. It is considered that the change in pH_i, rather than the change in Na^+_i or K^+_i, is the key signal which influences cell growth.

The increase in pH_i induced by a mitogen probably works in conjunction with other intra-

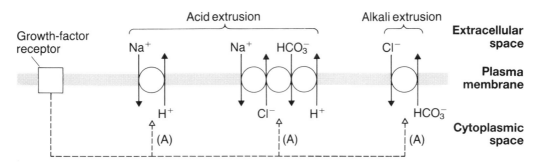

Fig. 8.14   A number of cell types possess two exchange systems which catalyse the extrusion of acid (H^+) and one which catalyses the extrusion of alkali (HCO_3^-). In cells incubated in a physiological medium (which contains HCO_3^-), growth factors stimulate (represented by A) alkali (HCO_3^-) extrusion as well as acid (H^+) extrusion. In some types of cell this leads to a decrease in pH_i.

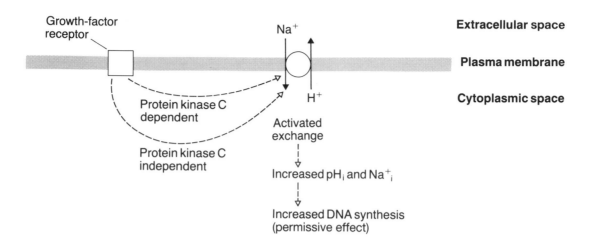

Fig. 8.15 The interaction of a growth factor with its receptor on a target cell often stimulates Na^+-H^+ exchange and H^+ extrusion. Under certain conditions, for example in cells incubated in a non-physiological medium which does not contain HCO_3^-, this leads to increases in pH_i and Na^+_i. Through a mechanism which is not yet understood, the increase in pH_i acts in a permissive manner to allow the stimulation of DNA synthesis. Growth-factor receptors are linked to the Na^+-H^+ exchange system either by a mechanism which involves protein kinase C or by a protein kinase C-independent mechanism.

cellular signals to allow the stimulation of DNA synthesis. The other signals involved include the actions of protein kinase C, (Ca^{2+} + calmodulin)-dependent protein kinases, cyclic AMP-dependent protein kinase, and the protein–tyrosine kinases, all of which probably ultimately lead to the phosphorylation of sequence-specific DNA-binding proteins.

A gap in the present knowledge of the permissive role of pH_i in the processes by which mitogens stimulate DNA synthesis and cell growth is the absence of information which explains how an increase in pH_i, which is such a general change in the intracellular environment, allows the stimulation of DNA synthesis. One possibility is that the increase in pH_i brings the pH of the nuclear space in the vicinity of DNA polymerase closer to the optimum pH of this enzyme, which is around pH 8. The increase in activity of this enzyme, and possibly in the activities of other enzymes, may facilitate or allow the activation of DNA synthesis.

8.7 Summary

A number of intermediary metabolites transfer information between sites within cells by modifying the activities of enzymes or other proteins in a non-covalent manner. Intermediary metabolites co-ordinate flux through metabolic pathways and perform certain specialized intracellular functions. Fructose 2,6-bisphosphate contributes to the regulation of glycolysis and gluconeogenesis by glucagon, free fatty acids probably regulate the movement of protons across the inner mitochondrial membrane in brown fat cells, ATP and reduced pyridine nucleotides provide part of the link between the metabolism of glucose or amino acids and insulin secretion in β-cells of the pancreas, and an increase in pH acts in a permissive fashion during the stimulation of DNA synthesis by mitogens.

Fructose 2,6-bisphosphate is an activator of phosphofructokinase-1 and an inhibitor of fructose bisphosphatase-1. It is formed from fruc-tose-1-phosphate in the reaction catalysed by phosphofructokinase-2, and is degraded to fruc-tose-1-phosphate by fructose bisphosphatase-2. In liver cells, these reactions are controlled by cyclic AMP-dependent protein kinase.

In brown fat cells, noradrenalin released from the sympathetic nervous system stimulates the hydrolysis of triglyceride and oxidation of the resulting free fatty acids. Free fatty acids link the signal delivered to the plasma membrane by noradrenalin to increased H^+ conductance across the mitochondrial inner membrane and subsequently to the generation of heat by the brown fat cell. Fatty acyl-CoAs bind with high affinity to thermogenin, a protein located in the mitochondrial inner membrane. The thermoge-nin–acyl-CoA complex facilitates the flow of H^+ from outside the mitochondrial inner membrane to the mitochondrial matrix by a pathway which is not coupled to the generation of ATP. The energy dissipated in this flow of H^+ is released as heat.

Glucose and certain amino acids are the main signals for the stimulation of insulin secretion in β-cells of the pancreas. Movement of the insu-lin secretory granules to the plasma membrane is initiated by an increase in free Ca^{2+} concen-tration in the cytoplasmic space. This increase is primarily due to the opening of voltage-oper-ated Ca^{2+} channels in the plasma membrane. An increase in the ratio NADPH/NADP and in the concentration of ATP, caused by the metabolism of glucose, probably inhibits an ATP-sensitive K^+ channel in the plasma membrane. This, in turn, induces depolarization of the membrane and the opening of voltage-operated Ca^{2+} chan-nels.

In some types of cell an increase in intracellu-lar pH (pH_i) plays a permissive role in the mecha-nism by which growth factors and other mitogens stimulate DNA synthesis. In these cells, growth factors increase the activity of an

Na^+–H^+ exchange system in the plasma mem-brane. This leads to an extrusion of H^+ and an increase in pH_i.

References

Aerts, R. J., Durston, A. J., and Moolenaar, W. H. (1985). Cytoplasmic pH and the regulation of the *Dictyostelium* cell cycle. *Cell*, **43**, 653–7.

Cannon, B., Nicholls, D. G., and Lindberg, O. (1973). Purine nucleotides and fatty acids in energy coupling of mitochondria from brown adipose tis-sue. In *Mechanisms in bioenergetics*, (ed. G. F. Azzone, L. Ernster, S. Papa, E. Quagliariello, and N. Siliprandi), pp. 357–63. Academic Press, New York.

Cannon, B., Nedergaard, J., and Sundin, U. (1981). Thermogenesis, brown fat and thermogenin. In *Survival in the cold* (ed. X. Y. Musacchia and L. Jansky), pp. 99–120. Elsevier North Holland, Amsterdam.

Castano, J. G., Nieto, A., and Feliu, J. E. (1979). Inactivation of phosphofructokinase by glucagon in rat hepatocytes. *J. Biol. Chem.*, **254**, 5576–9.

Clarke, S. D., Watkins, P. A., and Lane, M. D. (1979). Acute control of fatty acid synthesis by cyclic AMP in the chick liver cell: possible site of inhibition of citrate formation. *J. Lipid Res.*, **20**, 974–85.

Ganz, M. B., Boyarsky, G., Sterzel, R. B., and Boron, W. F. (1989). Arginine vasopressin enhances pH_i regulation in the presence of HCO_3^- by stimulating three acid–base transport systems. *Nature*, **337**, 648–51.

Heaton, G. M., Wagenvoord, R. J., Kemp, A. Jr, and Nicholls, D. G. (1978). Brown-adipose-tissue mitochondria: photoaffinity labelling of the regula-tory site of energy dissipation. *Eur. J. Biochem.*, **82**, 515–21.

Hohorst, H-J. and Rafael, J. (1968). Oxydative Phos-phorylierung durch Mitochondrien aus braunem Fettgewebe. *Hoppe Seylers Z. Physiol. Chem.*, **349**, 268–70.

Kagimoto, T. and Uyeda, K. (1979). Hormone-stimu-lated phosphorylation of liver phosphofructo kinase *in vivo*. *J. Biol. Chem.*, **254**, 5584–7.

L'Allemain, G., Franchi, A., Cragoe Jr, E., and

Pouyssegur, J. (1984). Blockade of the Na^+/H^+ antiport abolishes growth factor-induced DNA synthesis in fibroblasts. Structure–activity relationships in the amiloride series. *J. Biol. Chem.*, **259**, 4313–19.

Moolenaar, W. H., Tsien, R. Y., van der Saag, P. T., and de Laat, S. W. (1983). Na^+/H^+ exchange and cytoplasmic pH in the action of growth factors in human fibroblasts. *Nature*, **304**, 645–8.

Moolenaar, W. H., Tertoolen, L. G. J., and de Laat, S. W. (1984). Phorbol ester and diacylglycerol mimic growth factors in raising cytoplasmic pH. *Nature*, **312**, 371–4.

Nedergaard, J. and Lindberg, O. (1982). The brown fat cell. *Int. Rev. Cytol.*, **74**, 187–276.

Nicholls, D. G. (1974). Hamster brown-adipose-tissue mitochondria. The chloride permeability of the inner membrane under respiring conditions, the influence of purine nucleotides. *Eur. J. Biochem.*, **49**, 585–93.

Nicholls, D. G. (1976). Hamster brown-adipose-tissue mitochondria. Purine nucleotide control of the ion conductance of the inner membrane, the nature of the nucleotide binding site. *Eur. J. Biochem.*, **62**, 223–8.

Pilkis, S., Schlumpf, J., Pilkis, J., and Claus, T. H. (1979). Regulation of phosphofructokinase activity by glucagon in isolated rat hepatocytes. *Biochem. Biophys. Res. Commun.*, **88**, 960–7.

Pouysségur, J., Sardet, C., Franchi, A., L'Allemain, G., and Paris, S. (1984). A specific mutation abolishing Na^+/H^+ antiport activity in hamster fibroblasts precludes growth at neutral and acidic pH. *Proc. Natl Acad. Sci. USA*, **81**, 4833–7.

Schuldiner, S. and Rozengurt, E. (1982). Na^+/H^+ antiport in Swiss 3T3 cells: mitogenic stimulation leads to cytoplasmic alkalinization. *Proc. Natl Acad. Sci. USA*, **79**, 7778–82.

Smith, J. B. and Rozengurt, E. (1978). Lithium transport by fibroblastic mouse cells: characterisation and stimulation by serum and growth factors in quiescent cultures. *J. Cell. Physiol.*, **97**, 441–50.

Umbarger, H. E. (1956). Evidence for a negative feedback mechanism in the biosynthesis of isoleucine. *Science*, **123**, 848.

Van Schaftingen, E., Hue, L., and Hers, H.-G. (1980). Control of the fructose 6-phosphate/fructose 1,6-bisphosphate cycle in isolated hepatocytes by glucose and glucagon. Role of a low-molecular-weight stimulator of phosphofructokinase. *Biochem. J.*, **192**, 887–95.

Van Schaftingen, E., Jett, M-F., Hue, L., and Hers, H.-G. (1981). Control of liver 6-phosphofructokinase by fructose 2,6-bisphosphate and other effectors. *Proc. Natl Acad. Sci. USA*, **78**, 3483–6.

Whitaker, M. J. and Steinhardt, R. A. (1982). Ionic regulation of egg activation. *Quart. Rev. Biophys.*, **15**, 593–666.

Yates, R. A. and Pardee, A. B. (1956). Control of pyrimidine biosynthesis in *Escherichia coli* by a feedback mechanism. *J. Biol. Chem.*, **221**, 757–70.

Further reading

Hers, H.-G. and Van Schaftingen, E. (1982). Fructose 2,6-bisphosphate two years after its discovery. *Biochem. J.*, **206**, 1–12.

Madshus, I. H. (1988). Regulation of intracellular pH in eukaryotic cells. *Biochem. J.*, **250**, 1–8.

Nedergaard, J. and Lindberg, O. (1982). The brown fat cell. *Int. Rev. Cytol.*, **74**, 187–286.

Nicholls, D. G. and Rial, E. (1984). Brown fat mitochondria. *Trends Biochem. Sci.*, November 1984, 489–91.

Pouyssegur, J. (1985). The growth factor-activatable Na^+/H^+ exchange system: a genetic approach. *Trends Biochem. Sci.*, November 1985, 453–5.

9 *Metabolites of arachidonic acid*

9.1 Metabolites of arachidonic acid as extracellular and intracellular messengers

The chemical structure of arachidonic acid (all *cis*-5,8,11,14 eicosatetraenoic acid) is shown in Fig. 9.1. The main groups of oxygenated metabolites with biological function that are formed from this molecule are the prostaglandins (PGE_2, PGD_2, PGI_2, $PGF_{2\alpha}$), thromboxanes (TXA_2, TXB_2), hydroperoxyeicosatetraenoic acids (5-HPETE, 12-HPETE), leukotrienes (LTA_4, LTB_4, LTC_4, LTD_4, LTE_4), and lipoxins (LXA and LXB). These compounds are collect-

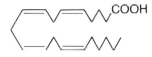

Fig. 9.1 The structure of arachidonic acid: all *cis*-5,8,11,14 eicosatetraenoic acid.

ively called the eicosanoids. The members of each group of arachidonic acid metabolites are formed from arachidonic acid through separate pathways which are shown in Fig. 9.2. Arachidonic acid can also be oxidized to epoxyeicosatrienoic acids and their di- and tri-hydroxylated forms by the actions of cytochrome P-450 epoxygenases. However, there is no evidence to indicate that epoxyeicosatrienoic acids are formed *in vivo*.

The scheme shown in Fig. 9.2 represents a highly simplified picture of the formation of arachidonic acid metabolites. The total number of metabolites which can be formed from arachidonic acid is daunting. The picture of metabolism is further complicated by the chemical instability of a number of the intermediates, many of which undergo non-enzymatic reactions.

The prostaglandins, thromboxanes, and leu-

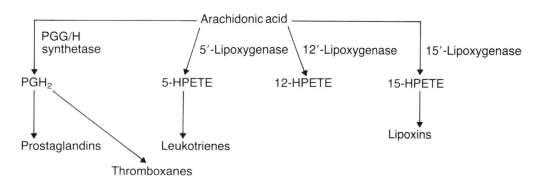

Fig. 9.2 The pathways for the biosynthesis of prostaglandins, thromboxanes, leukotrienes, lipoxins, and 12-HPETE. The enzyme which catalyses the first step in each pathway is shown. The other reactions in each pathway are represented by a single arrow.

kotrienes act as extracellular messengers. It is thought that arachidonic acid itself, 5-HPETE, 12-HPETE, and some leukotrienes may act as intracellular messengers in a manner analogous to cyclic AMP, Ca^{2+}, and inositol 1,4,5-trisphosphate. Under some conditions, the same molecule of arachidonic acid metabolite may act as both an extracellular messenger and an intracellular messenger.

The arachidonic acid metabolites differ from other extracellular messengers and intracellular messengers in several ways. Firstly, the number of compounds with messenger function which can be formed from arachidonic acid is very large. Secondly, since arachidonic acid metabolites are lipid soluble they pass through the plasma membrane and probably through other cellular membranes without the aid of a carrier protein and at a much greater rate than do most other extracellular and intracellular messengers. Hence a given arachidonic acid metabolite is not confined principally to either the intracellular or the extracellular space (Fig. 9.3). Thirdly, most arachidonic acid metabolites are degraded very rapidly by both enzymatic and non-enzymatic reactions.

Physiological actions of the major metabolites

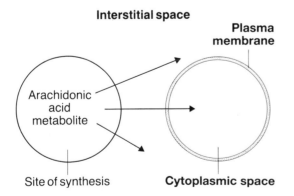

Interstitial space

Plasma membrane

Arachidonic acid metabolite

Site of synthesis   **Cytoplasmic space**

Fig. 9.3 Molecules of an arachidonic acid metabolite formed at an intracellular location can readily diffuse across the plasma membrane to the interstitial space and to the cytoplasmic space of neighbouring cells.

of arachidonic acid were first observed over fifty years ago. However, it has only been during the last 25 years that the structures of these molecules have been determined and their biological functions defined more clearly. In the mid 1930s, Euler (1934) and Goldblatt (1935) observed the presence in semen of compounds which exhibited vasodepressor action and which stimulated the contraction of smooth muscle. Almost 30 years later these compounds were isolated and shown to be PGE and PGF (Bergstrom and Sjovall 1957). The structures of PGE and PGF were elucidated in 1962 (Bergstrom *et al.* 1962; 1963). The endoperoxides from which these prostaglandins are derived were first isolated in 1973 (Hamberg and Samuelsson 1973; Nugteren and Halzelhof 1973). In the following three years thromboxane, first identified as a labile pro-aggregatory vasoconstrictor substance (Hamberg *et al.* 1975), and prostacyclin (Moncada *et al.* 1976) were discovered.

The first evidence for a physiological action of a leukotriene was obtained in 1938. This was the discovery of a factor, called slow-reacting substance, which is present in lung perfusates. This factor induces the contraction of smooth muscle (Feldberg and Kellaway 1938; Kellaway and Trethewie 1940). The structure of a major component, leukotriene C4, of slow-reacting substance was elucidated in 1979 (Murphy *et al* 1979; Hammarstrom *et al.* 1979).

The role of arachidonic acid metabolites in the process of inflammation has been of particular interest in clinical medicine. Arthritis and the response of tissues to allergens are both characterized by inflammation of certain tissues. The effected area becomes swollen, red, hot, and painful. These inflammatory responses are mediated by prostaglandins and leukotrienes as well as by other types of compound such as histamine, bradykinin, platelet-activating factor, and interleukin-1. Leukotrienes and prostaglandins, of which PGE_2 is probably the most important, cause dilatation of blood vessels in the inflamed area. LTB$_4$ acts to attract polymorphonuclear leucocytes by chemotaxis. Both prostaglandins and leukotrienes increase vascular permeability. The search for drugs which alleviate the symptoms of inflammation led to the discovery of aspirin and other non-steroid anti-inflammatory drugs, and to discovery of the anti-inflammatory actions of steroids.

In order to describe the role of arachidonic acid metabolites in the transmission of information within cells, it is first necessary to consider the reactions by which these metabolites are formed and degraded. Before the arachidonic acid can be converted to its metabolites it must be released from cellular phospholipids.

9.2 Release of arachidonic acid from phospholipids

The rate-limiting step in the formation of arachidonic acid metabolites is the release of the free fatty acid from phospholipids. Under physiological conditions, arachidonic acid is only released in response to an extracellular signal. In the absence of such a signal, the concentration of free arachidonic acid within the cell is substantially lower than the apparent K_M value for arachidonic acid of the enzymes which metabolize this fatty acid. The phospholipids which act as a source of arachidonic acid are located in the plasma membrane.

The amount of arachidonic acid released from phospholipids depends on the relative rates of hydrolysis of phospholipid and re-incorporation of arachidonic acid into phospholipid. These pathways are shown in Fig. 9.4. Re-incorporation involves the formation of arachidonyl-CoA in the reaction catalysed by arachidonyl-CoA synthetase, and the transfer of the arachidonic acid moiety to a lysophospholipid in the reaction catalysed by lysophosphoglycerate acyltransferase. The rate of re-incorporation of

arachidonic acid is controlled by the activity of lysophosphoglycerate acyltransferase. The acyltransferase pathway is poised to remove free arachidonic acid immediately it is formed. In response to an agonist which stimulates the hydrolysis of phospholipid to form arachidonic acid, metabolic flux through the acyltransferase pathway increases. However, flux through this pathway is lower than the flux of phospholipid hydrolysis so that the intracellular concentration of arachidonic acid is increased while an agonist is present, thus making arachidonic acid available for conversion to it metabolites.

There are two main pathways for the release of arachidonic acid from phospholipids. In one,

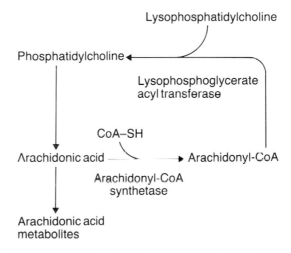

Fig. 9.4 The intracellular concentration of arachidonic acid present at any given time is determined by the balance of the reactions which catalyse the hydrolysis of phospholipids, such as phosphatidylcholine, to yield free arachidonic acid and the activities of arachidonyl-CoA synthetase and lysophosphoglycerate acyltransferase which catalyse the re-incorporation of arachidonic acid into phospholipids. Although the scheme shows phosphatidylcholine as the source of arachidonic acid, the metabolism of phosphatidylinositol and phosphatidylethanolamine is described by a similar scheme. Under normal conditions, the hydrolysis of phospholipid is enhanced only by the action of an agonist on a cell. Increased flux through this pathway leads to an increase in the concentration of free arachidonic acid which is converted to arachidonic acid metabolites.

the ester bond at position 2 of the phospholipid is hydrolysed to release free arachidonic acid and a lysophospholipid. This reaction is catalysed by phospholipase A_2 (Fig. 9.5). The major substrates for this enzyme are phosphatidylcholine, phosphatidylethanolamine, phosphoinositides, phosphatidylserine, and phosphatidic acid. The other pathway involves phospholipase C, which catalyses the formation of diacylglyerol from phosphatidylcholine or phosphoinositides with the release of phosphorylcholine or an inositol polyphosphate. The hydrolysis of phosphatidylcholine by this pathway is shown in Fig. 9.5. The resulting diacylglycerol is cleaved by diacylglycerol and monoacylglycerol lipases to release arachidonic acid as well as stearic acid and glycerol. In some types of cell, both the phospholipase A_2 and phospholipase C pathways are active, while in other types of cell one of these pathways is predominant.

Arachidonic acid can also be released from plasmalogens in a reaction catalysed by phos-

pholipase A_2 (Fig. 9.5). Plasmalogens are glycerophospholipids in which the hydroxyl group of carbon 1 of the glycerol backbone is linked to a hydrocarbon chain through a vinyl ether bond rather than an ester bond. Most plasmalogens contain ethanolamine esterified to the phosphate group.

Receptors which stimulate the release of arachidonic acid are probably directly coupled to phospholipase A_2 or phospholipase C by GTP-binding regulatory proteins (G proteins). The nature and mechanism of action of G proteins are described in Chapter 3. Some of the G proteins which couple with phospholipase A_2 are sensitive to inhibition by pertussis toxin. Two examples are the G proteins involved in the coupling of α-adrenergic agonists to phospholipase A_2 in thyroid cells, and in coupling the absorption of light to phospholipase A_2 in rod outer segments of the bovine retina.

The interaction of an agonist with an appropriate receptor determines whether phospholi-

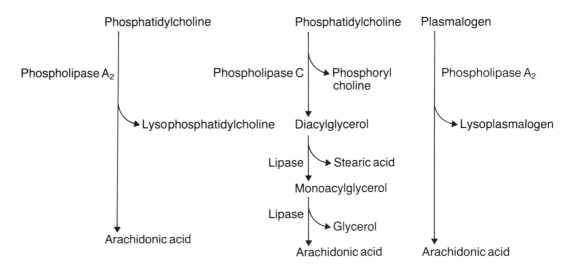

Fig. 9.5 The pathways for the release of arachidonic acid from phospholipids and plasmalogens. In addition to phosphatidylcholine, other phospholipids including phosphatidylethanolamine, the phosphoinositides, phosphatidylserine and phosphatidic acid, are hydrolysed by phospholipase A_2 with the release of arachidonic acid. Moreover phospholipases C can hydrolyse phosphatidylethanolamine and phosphoinositides as well as phosphatidylcholine to release diacylglycerol which can subsequently be hydrolysed by lipases to release arachidonic acid.

pase C or phospholipase A_2 is switched on or off. When switched on, the activity of phospholipase A_2 is also controlled by proteins called lipocortins which are inhibitors of this enzyme. Lipocortins have molecular weights ranging from 15 to 40 kDa and are located at the plasma membrane. The lipocortins are members of the calpactin family of Ca^{2+}- and phospholipid-binding proteins which are described in the section on Ca^{2+}-binding proteins in Chapter 7. The inhibition of phospholipase A_2 by lipocortins may involve either direct interaction of the lipocortin with the enzyme or interaction of the lipocortin with phospholipid substrates.

The synthesis of lipocortins is induced by glucocorticoids. This means that in the presence of elevated concentrations of glucocorticoids the activity of phospholipase A_2 is diminished. This leads to a decrease in the intracellular concentration of arachidonic acid released in response to an agonist and is the mechanism by which glucocorticoids exhibit an anti-inflammatory action. In addition to regulation by induction of enzyme synthesis, the action of lipocortins is also controlled by phosphorylation.

9.3   Formation of metabolites of arachidonic acid

When the concentration of arachidonic acid in a given cell is increased the nature of the arachidonic acid metabolites formed depends on the enzymes present within that cell. Not all the enzymes of arachidonic acid metabolism are present in any one cell type. For example, TXA_2 is the predominant metabolite formed in platelets, PGI_2 in smooth muscle and vascular endothelial cells, leukotrienes in eosinophils and neutrophils, PGE_2 in kidney collecting-tubule cells, and $PGF_{2\alpha}$ in the uterine endometrium.

Once free arachidonic acid is formed in a given cell there is a cascade of metabolic events which yields all potential enzymatic and non-enzymatic

products which can be formed by the enzyme complement of that cell type. The key enzymes which determine the pathway by which arachidonic acid is metabolized in a given cell are PGG_2/H_2 synthetase, the first enzyme in the pathway for the formation of prostaglandins and thromboxanes; 5-lipoxygenase, the first enzyme in the pathway which leads to leukotriene synthesis; 12-lipoxygenase, which forms 12-HPETE; and 15- and 5-lipoxygenases which are required for the formation of lipoxins. The presence or absence of any one of these enzymes determines the mix of arachidonic acid metabolites formed in a given cell.

The enzymes which metabolize arachidonic acid are associated with intracellular membranes such as the endoplasmic reticulum, or are present at locations in the cytoplasmic space other than the plasma membrane and endoplasmic reticulum. This means that arachidonic acid metabolites are formed in the interior of the cell, in contrast to the majority of other intracellular messengers which are formed at the plasma membrane.

The conversion of arachidonic acid to PGH_2 involves two enzyme-catalysed reactions. These are the synthesis of PGG_2 in the reaction catalysed by cyclo-oxygenase and the conversion of PGG_2 to PGH_2 in the reaction catalysed by peroxidase (Fig. 9.6). Both these enzyme activities reside on the same enzyme. This enzyme is called PGG_2/H_2 synthetase (prostaglandin endoperoxide synthetase) or fatty-acid cyclo-oxygenase. Subsequent enzyme-catalysed reactions convert PGH_2 to PGE_2, PGD_2, PGI_2, $PGF_{2\alpha}$ and TXA_2. A number of additional metabolites, including 6-keto $PGF_{1\alpha}$ and TXB_2, are formed by non-enzymatic reactions (Fig. 9.6).

The first enzyme in the pathway for the formation of prostaglandins and thromboxanes, PGG_2/H_2 synthetase, is inhibited by acetylsalicylic acid (aspirin), indomethacin, and a number of other drugs. These compounds are members

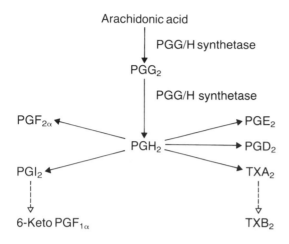

Fig. 9.6 The key intermediate in the formation of prostaglandins and thromboxanes is PGH_2. This is formed from arachidonic acid in the two reactions catalysed by PGG_2/H_2 synthetase. These are the formation of PGG_2, catalysed by the cyclo-oxygenase component of PGG_2/H_2 synthetase, and the conversion of PGG_2 to PGH_2, catalysed by the peroxidase component of this enzyme. The numerous sequential steps in the conversion of PGH_2 to prostaglandins and TXA_2 are represented by a single arrow. Solid lines represent enzyme-catalysed pathways and broken lines non-enzymatic reactions.

of a family of drugs called the non-steroidal anti-inflammatory drugs. There are a large number of these drugs which inhibit PGG_2/H_2 synthetase. Some non-steroidal anti-inflammatory drugs inhibit other reactions in the prostaglandin and thromboxane biosynthetic pathways. Aspirin and indomethacin inhibit the formation of PGG_2 from arachidonic acid, the reaction catalysed by the cyclo-oxygenase activity of PGG_2/H_2 synthetase, but do not inhibit the conversion of PGG_2 to PGH_2, the reaction catalysed by the peroxidase activity of PGG_2/H_2 synthetase. The interaction of acetylsalicylic acid with PGG_2/H_2 synthetase results in acylation of a serine residue on the enzyme. This covalent modification leads to non-reversible inhibition of the reaction catalysed by the cyclo-oxygenase catalytic site.

The enzyme 5'-lipoxygenase catalyses the first

reaction in the pathway for the formation of leukotrienes (Fig. 9.7). This is the conversion of arachidonic acid to 5-HPETE, which is then converted to the highly unstable 5,6-epoxide, LTA_4, by a dehydratase. LTA_4 is either hydrolysed to LTB_4 or reacts with glutathione to form LTC_4, the 5-hydroxy-6-glutathionyl derivative of LTA_4. The addition of glutathione is catalysed by glutathione-S-transferase. LTC_4 is metabolized successively by γ-glutamyl transpeptidase and cysteinyl-glycine dipeptidase to form LTD_4 and LTE_4 (Fig. 9.7).

The formation of lipoxins A and B probably involves the successive actions of 15'-lipoxygenase and 5'-lipoxygenase and subsequent oxidation reactions. These are shown in Fig. 9.8.

Once formed, the biologically active metabolites of arachidonic acid are very rapidly converted to inactive metabolites by both non-enzymatic and enzyme-catalysed reactions. The initial step in the degradation of prostaglandins and thromboxanes is oxidation of the 15-hydroxyl group. This is catalysed by a variety of 15-hydroxyprostaglandin dehydrogenases. Leukotriene degradation is initiated by hydroxy-

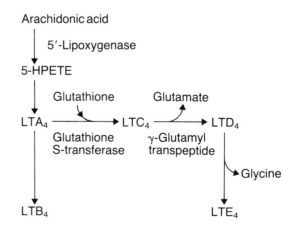

Fig. 9.7 Formation of the leukotrienes involves first the conversion of arachidonic acid to 5-HPETE and LTA_4, the precursor of the other leukotrienes. The first step in the conversion of LTA_4 to LTC_4, LTD_4, and LTE_4 is the addition of glutathione to LTA_4.

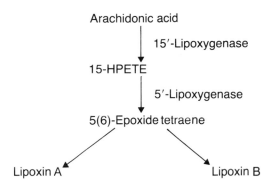

Fig. 9.8 The initial step in the formation of lipoxins A and B involves the synthesis of 15-HPETE in the reaction catalysed by 15'-lipoxygenase. 15-HPETE is probably converted to lipoxins A and B via the intermediate 5(6)-expoxide tetraene.

lation of the carbon atom at position 19 or 20. As a result of these reactions, many metabolites of arachidonic acid have very short half-lives. For example, at 37 °C the half-life of TXA_2 is 30 s while that of PGI_2 is 5 min.

9.4 Arachidonic acid metabolites as extracellular messengers

The arachidonic acid metabolites which act as extracellular messengers are the prostaglandins, thromboxanes, and leukotrienes. These compounds convey information between cells over short distances. In this respect they are similar to many growth factors but differ from most hormones. However, in contrast to growth factors which, as their names suggest, stimulate cell proliferation or the growth of differentiated cells, arachidonic acid metabolites often act as signals which initiate specialized cell functions such as a change in shape or movement.

Arachidonic acid metabolites have been detected in many animal tissues and in the medium of a variety of cell types incubated *in vitro*. Moreover, many cells respond to arachidonic acid metabolites. However, it has not always been possible to clearly identify the cell type

from which a given arachidonic acid metabolite is released and the cell type on which this metabolite acts. A number of the situations in which the nature of the cell that generates the arachidonic acid metabolite and the nature of the target cell upon which this metabolite acts are reasonably clearly defined are listed in Table 9.1.

Arachidonic acid metabolites that act as extracellular messengers are formed following the combination of an agonist with its receptor on an initiating cell. This leads to the release of arachidonic acid and the formation of an arachidonic acid metabolite (Fig. 9.9). The arachidonic acid metabolites readily diffuse out of the initiating cell through the plasma membrane into the surrounding space where they bind to receptors on the plasma membrane of a second cell, the target cell. Receptors for PGE_2, $PGF_{2\alpha}$, PGI_2, TXA_2, LTB_4, and LTD_4 have so far been identified. The interaction of an arachidonic acid metabolite with its plasma-membrane receptor induces a response in the target cell through the activation of G proteins and effector enzymes, the generation of intracellular messengers, and the activation of protein kinases (Fig. 9.9).

The duration and intensity of signals carried by arachidonic acid between cells depends, in part, on the rate of degradation of the metabolites. As described earlier, most biologically active arachidonic acid metabolites are unstable and have half-lives of the order of minutes.

In addition to the transfer of information between different cells, arachidonic acid metabolites can also bind to receptors on the cell in which they are formed. This usually leads to an amplification of the signal originally carried to the initiating cell by the agonist. This action of an arachidonic acid metabolite is called an autocoid function.

Two of the most clearly defined examples of the actions of arachidonic acid metabolites as extracellular messengers are the roles of TXA_2 and PGI_2 in regulation of the aggregation of

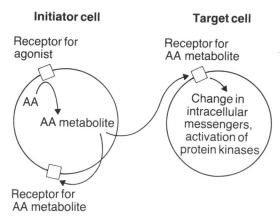

Initiator cell   **Target cell**

Fig. 9.9 A general scheme for the action of an arachidonic acid metabolite (AA metabolite) as an intercellular messenger. The combination of an agonist with a cell (the initiator cell) leads to the formation of the arachidonic acid metabolite which diffuses out of the cytoplasmic space to the interstitial space. Some molecules of arachidonic acid metabolite bind to receptors on a neighbouring cell (the target cell) and induce a response in that cell. Receptors for the arachidonic acid metabolite are coupled to the generation of an intracellular messenger through membrane and intracellular signal transducing systems. Molecules of the arachidonic acid metabolite can also act on the initiator cell to amplify the signal carried to that cell by the original agonist. This is known as an autocoid function.

platelets. TXA_2 is produced by blood platelets in response to thrombin. There are two immediate intracellular consequences of the combination of thrombin with the thrombin receptor on the platelet plasma membrane. The first is activation of the intracellular messenger system which induces an aggregation response in that platelet. The second is the release of arachidonic acid and the formation of TXA_2 which diffuses out of the initiating platelet and binds to TXA_2 receptors on nearby platelets (Fig. 9.10). This, in turn, leads to the formation of the intracellular messengers diacylglycerol and inositol 1,4,5-trisphosphate, an increase in $[Ca^{2+}]_i$, activation of protein kinase C and $(Ca^{2+} + calmodulin)$-dependent protein kinase, and aggregation of the target platelet.

Since a small number of thrombin molecules induce the formation of a relatively large number of TXA_2 molecules which can interact with many nearby platelets, TXA_2 acts to amplify the signal initially carried by thrombin (Fig. 9.11). TXA_2 can also interact with TXA_2 receptors on the platelet in which it was synthesized. This ampli-

Table 9.1   *Examples of the actions of metabolites of arachidonic acid as extracellular messengers*

Arachidonic acid metabolite	Cell type from which metabolite is released	Target cell type	Response of target cell
PGE_2	Endothelial cells in microvessels of the aorta	Smooth muscle (vascular)	Contraction
	Renal collecting tubule	Renal, thick ascending limb and renal collecting tubule	Attenuation of water reabsorption and NaCl reabsorption in response to vasopressin
PGD_2	Platelets	Platelets	Inhibition of aggregation
TXA_2	Platelets	Platelets	Aggregation
PGI_2	Smooth-muscle endothelium	Platelets	Inhibition of aggregation
LTB_4	Neutrophils	Polymorphonuclear leucoytes	Chemokinetic Chemotactic Degranulation Emigration
LTC_4, LTD_4, LTE_4	Mast cells Eosinophils Macrophages	Smooth muscle (respiratory, vasculature, intestinal)	Contraction

Initiator platelet   **Target platelet**

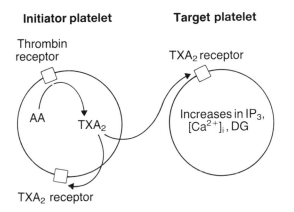

Fig. 9.10 The action of thromboxane A$_2$ (TXA$_2$) as an intercellular messenger in platelets. TXA$_2$ is formed from arachidonic acid (AA) in response to the combination of an agonist, such as thrombin, with its receptor. TXA$_2$ binds to TXA$_2$ receptors present on neighbouring platelets and on the initiator platelet. This leads to the generation of inositol 1,4,5-trisphosphate (IP$_3$) and diacylglycerol (DG), an increase in [Ca^{2+}]$_i$, the activation of (Ca^{2+} + calmodulin)-dependent protein kinase and protein kinase C, and platelet aggregation.

fies the effect of thrombin on this platelet (Fig. 9.10).

The action of PGI$_2$ on platelets is an example of an arachidonic acid metabolite acting as an intercellular messenger between different cell types. PGI$_2$ is synthesized by endothelial cells and diffuses to platelets where it binds to the PGI$_2$ receptor on the platelet plasma membrane (Fig. 9.12). This receptor is coupled to adenylate cyclase through the oligomeric GTP-binding protein G$_s$ so that the binding of PGI$_2$ to its receptor leads to the activation of adenylate cyclase and to an increase in the concentration of cyclic AMP. Subsequent activation of cyclic AMP-dependent protein kinase leads to inhibition of platelet aggregation.

9.5 Arachidonic acid metabolites as intracellular messengers

During the past twenty years there have been numerous suggestions that arachidonic acid

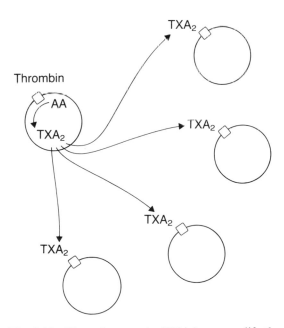

Fig. 9.11 Thromboxane A$_2$ (TXA$_2$) can amplify the signal carried by thrombin or another agonist to platelets by binding to TXA$_2$ receptors on many neighbouring platelets.

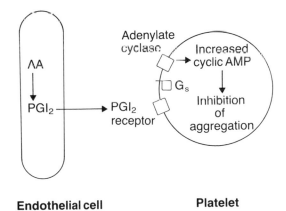

Endothelial cell   **Platelet**

Fig. 9.12 Prostacyclin (PGI$_2$), which is formed from arachidonic acid (AA) in endothelial cells, inhibits platelet aggregation. PGI$_2$ binds to a receptor on the plasma membrane of platelets. Subsequent activation of adenylate cyclase through the G protein G$_s$ leads to an increase in cyclic AMP concentration, activation of cyclic AMP-dependent protein kinase, and the inhibition of aggregation induced by another agonist such as thrombin.

metabolites may act as intracellular messengers in the same way as the cyclic nucleotides and inositol 1,4,5-trisphosphate. The general idea is that an arachidonic acid metabolite is formed as a result of the combination of an agonist with a plasma-membrane receptor on a target cell. This arachidonic acid metabolite then acts at a site within the cytoplasmic space of that same cell (Fig. 9.13). This idea has been difficult to test and the results are equivocal.

A number of possible actions of arachidonic acid metabolites as intracellular messengers have been identified. These include the opening of certain types of K^+ channels, the activation of protein kinase C, the activation of guanylate cyclase, and the release of Ca^{2+} from the endoplasmic reticulum.

An example of the possible role of arachidonic acid metabolites in opening K^+ channels is the action of acetylcholine on myocardial atrial cells. The combination of this neurotransmitter with a muscarinic acetylcholine receptor in atrial cells opens a subgroup of K^+ channels called the muscarinic acetylcholine-responsive K^+ channels. This action of acetylcholine is associated with the activation of phospholipase A_2 and the formation of a variety of metabolites of arachidonic acid. The application of 5-

HPETE, LTB_4, LTC_4, or LTA_4 to the plasma membranes of atrial cells increases the opening of muscarinic acetylcholine-responsive K^+ channels. For example, Fig. 9.14 shows that 5-HPETE increases the flow of K^+ through the sarcolemma of an atrial cell whereas 5-HETE has no effect. These observations have led to

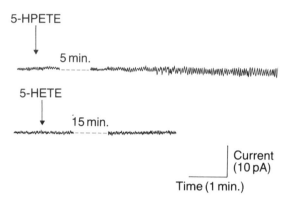

Fig. 9.14 An experiment which suggests that the arachidonic acid metabolite 5-HPETE may play a role as an intracellular messenger by activating K^+ channels. These channels are called muscarinic acetylcholine K^+ channels because they are activated by the combination of acetylcholine with muscarinic receptors. The opening of muscarinic acetylcholine K^+ channels was measured in atrial cells as the current carried by K^+ ions which flow through these channels in a whole cell patch-clamp experiment. 5-HPETE, but not 5-HETE, induces an increase in current. From Kim *et al.* (1989).

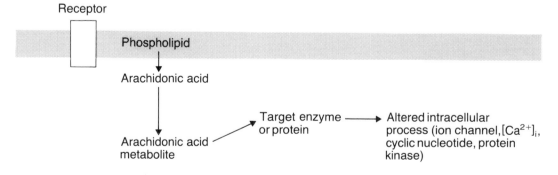

Fig. 9.13 A general scheme for the proposed role of an arachidonic acid metabolite as an intracellular messenger. It is proposed that once formed in response to an extracellular agonist the arachidonic acid metabolite diffuses through the cytoplasmic space and subsequently binds to an allosteric site on a target enzyme (for example, protein kinase C) or protein (for example an ion channel). Although this is an attractive idea, there is little convincing evidence to support the proposal.

the proposal that in atrial cells, 5-HPETE, LTB$_4$, LTC$_4$, or LTA$_4$ link the combination of acetyl-choline with muscarinic acetylcholine receptors to the opening of the subgroup of K$^+$ channels which are controlled by the muscarinic acetyl-choline receptors. A similar role for another ara-chidonic acid metabolite, 12-HPETE, has been proposed as the mechanism by which certain peptide neurotransmitters open K$^+$ channels in a sensory neuron.

Protein kinase C and guanylate cyclase are activated by arachidonic acid and by a number of arachidonic acid metabolites. Arachidonic acid itself, but not its metabolites, releases Ca^{2+} from the endoplasmic reticulum. It is not yet clear whether the effects of arachidonic acid and its metabolites on K$^+$ channels, protein kinase C, guanylate cyclase, and Ca^{2+} release from the endoplasmic reticulum represent true physio-logical actions of these compounds as intracellu-lar messengers.

9.6   Summary

The major groups of arachidonic acid metab-olites (eicosanoids) with biological functions are the prostaglandins, thromboxanes, hydroper-oxy-eicosatetraenoic acids, leukotrienes, and lipoxins. These are formed by the enzyme cata-lysed oxidation of arachidonic acid. These lipid-soluble metabolites can readily pass through the plasma membrane and intracellular membranes without the requirement for a specific carrier protein. The prostaglandins, thromboxanes, and leukotrienes act as extracellular messengers over short distances. Arachidonic acid itself, 5-HPETE, 12-HPETE, and the leukotrienes may function as intracellular messengers, although this has not been shown conclusively. Some ara-chidonic acid metabolites may act as both an extracellular messenger and an intracellular messenger.

Arachidonic acid is released from phospholi-pids in response to the combination of an agonist with its receptor on the plasma membrane. This induces the hydrolysis of phospholipids in the plasma membrane and releases free arachidonic acid which is subsequently metabolized to oxy-genated metabolites of arachidonic acid. The release of arachidonic acid from phospholipids, such as phosphatidylcholine, is the rate-limiting step in the formation of arachidonic acid metab-olites. Arachidonic acid is released from phos-pholipids in the reaction catalysed by phospholipase A$_2$, which forms a lysophospho-lipid as well as arachidonic acid, and by phospholipase C, which catalyses the formation of diacylglycerol. This is subsequently hydro-lysed to yield arachidonic acid and monoacylgly-cerol in the reaction catalysed by diacylglycerol lipase. Free arachidonic acid is rapidly re-esteri-fied to form phospholipids. In the presence of an appropriate agonist, the rate of phospholipid hydrolysis is greater than the rate of arachidonic acid re-esterification so that the concentration of free arachidonic acid, and hence the concen-trations of arachidonic acid metabolites, increase.

Oxygenation of arachidonic acid occurs whenever the intracellular concentration of ara-chidonic acid is increased above the basal value. The nature of the metabolites formed by a given cell depends on the enzymes of the arachidonic acid metabolic pathways which are present in that cell type. The key enzymes involved in this metabolism are PGG$_2$/H$_2$ synthetase, the first enzyme in the pathway for the formation of pros-taglandins and thromboxanes, 5'-lipoxygenase, the first enzyme in the pathway which leads to leukotriene synthesis, 12'-lipoxygenase, which forms 12-HPETE, and 15'- and 5'-lipoxygenases which are required for the formation of lipoxins.

The prostaglandins, thromboxanes, and leu-kotrienes act as extracellular messengers. The action of any one of these compounds as an extracellular messenger involves its formation in one cell, its diffusion to the extracellular space, and its subsequent binding to a receptor on the plasma membrane of a neighbouring target cell. The receptor–arachidonic acid metabolite complex then induces a specific response in the target cell through one or more pathways of intracellular communication, for example those which involve cyclic AMP, inositol 1,4,5-trisphosphate, or diacylglycerol.

It has been difficult to show conclusively that metabolites of arachidonic acid act as intracellular messengers in a manner analogous to cyclic AMP, Ca^{2+}, and inositol 1,4,5-trisphosphate. Examples of the likely actions of arachidonic acid metabolites as intracellular messengers are the activation of K^+ channels in heart atrial cells and in sensory neurons, the activation of protein kinase C and guanylate cyclase by arachidonic acid, 5- and 12-HPETE, and certain leukotrienes, and the release of Ca^{2+} from the endoplasmic reticulum induced by arachidonic acid.

References

Bergström, S. and Sjövall, J. (1957). The isolation of prostaglandin. *Acta Chem. Scand.*, **11**, 1086.

Bergstrom, S., Dressler, F., Krabisch, L., Ryhage, R., and Sjovall, J. (1962). The isolation and structure of a smooth muscle stimulating factor in normal sheep and pig lungs. *Arkiv. fur Kemi.*, **20**, 63–6.

Bergstrom, S., Ryhage, R. Samuelsson, B., and Sjovall, J. (1963). The structures of prostaglandin E_1, $F_{1\alpha}$, and $F_{1\beta}$. *J. Biol. Chem.*, **238**, 3555–64.

Euler, U. S. von (1934). Zur Kenntnis der pharmakologischen Wirkungen von Nativsekreten und Extrakten mannlicher accessorischer Geschlechtsdrusen. *Arch. Exptl. Pathol. Pharmakol.*, **175**, 78–84.

Feldberg, W. and Kellaway, C. H. (1938). Liberation of histamine and formation of lysocithin-like substances by cobra venom. *J. Physiol.*, **94**, 187–226.

Goldblatt, M. W. (1935). Properties of human seminal plasma. *J. Physiol. (London)*, **84**, 208–18.

Hamberg, M. and Samuelsson, B. (1973). Detection and isolation of an endoperoxide intermediate in prostaglandin synthesis. *Proc. Natl Acad. Sci. USA*, **70**, 899–903.

Hamberg, M., Svensson, J., and Samuelsson, B. (1975). Thromboxanes: a new group of biologically active compounds derived from prostaglandin endoperoxides. *Proc. Natl Acad. Sci. USA*, **72**, 2994–8.

Hammarström, S., Murphy, R. C., Samuelsson, B. Clark, D. A., Mioskowski, C. *et al.* (1979). Structure of leukotriene C. Identification of the amino acid part. *Biochem. Biophys. Res. Commun.*, **91**, 1266–72.

Kellaway, C. H. and Trethewie, E. R. (1940). The liberation of a slow-reacting smooth muscle-stimulating substance in anaphylaxis. *Quart. J. Exp. Physiol. Cogn. Med. Sci.*, **30**, 121–45.

Kim, D., Lewis, D. L., Graziadei, L., Neer, E. J., Bar-Sagi, D., and Clapham, D. E. (1989). G-protein βγ-subunits activate the cardiac muscarinic K^+-channel via phospholipase A_2. *Nature*, **337**, 557–60.

Moncada, S., Gryglewski, R., Bunting, S., and Vane, J. R. (1976). An enzyme isolated from arteries transforms prostaglandin endoperoxides to an unstable substance that inhibits platelet aggregation. *Nature*, **263**, 663–5.

Murphy, R. C., Hammarström, S., and Samuelsson, B. (1979). Leukotriene C: a slow-reacting substance from murine mastocytoma cells. *Proc. Natl Acad. Sci. USA*, **76**, 4275–9.

Nugteren, D. H. and Halzelhof, E. (1973). Isolation and properties of intermediates in prostaglandin biosynthesis. *Biochim. Biophys. Acta*, **326**, 448–61.

Further reading

Johnson, M., Carey, F., and McMillan, R. M. (1983). Alternative pathways of arachidonate metabolism: prostaglandins, thromboxane and leukotrienes. *Essays in Biochemistry*, **19**, 40–141.

Irvine, R. F. (1982). How is the level of free arachidonic acid controlled in mammalian cells? *Biochem. J.*, **204**, 3–16.

Samuelsson, B. and Funk, C. D. (1989). Enzymes involved in the biosynthesis of leukotriene B4. *J. Biol. Chem.*, **264**, 19469–72.

Smith, W. L. (1989). The eicosanoids and their biochemical mechanisms of action. *Biochem. J.*, **259**, 315–24.

10 *Sequence-specific DNA-binding proteins*

10.1 The roles of sequence-specific DNA-binding proteins in intracellular communication

The mechanisms by which information is transferred from plasma-membrane receptors to enzymes in the cytoplasmic space, and between different sites in the cytoplasmic space, have been discussed in the preceding chapters. An equally important component of intracellular communication is the transfer of information from the cytoplasmic space to specific genes in the nucleus, and between different genes within the nucleus. The transfer of this information is achieved by sequence-specific DNA-binding proteins. This term will be abbreviated here to DNA-binding proteins.

Extracelluar signals which increase the rate of transcription of a gene do so by increasing the frequency of initiation of transcription by RNA polymerase II. The main types of extracelluar signals which stimulate gene transcription in this way are morphogens, growth factors and other mitogens, and steroid and thyroid hormones. Morphogens and growth factors induce cell differentiation during embryogenesis, growth factors can alter the pathway of differentiation in differentiating cells, growth factors and other mitogens can induce cell proliferation, and steroid and thyroid hormones activate specialized cell functions. Some of the DNA-binding proteins that are involved in these pathways are listed in Table 10.1. The DNA-binding proteins fall into two groups. These are the sequence-specific transcription factors which

mediate changes in cell proliferation and cell differentiation, and DNA-binding receptor proteins which mediate the actions of steroid and thyroid hormones.

The final step in the intracellular action of an extracelluar signal which leads to a stimulation of gene transcription is generally the activation of a DNA-binding protein (Fig. 10.1). The activated DNA-binding protein then binds to the promoter region of a second gene, stimulates the transcription of that gene and consequently

Table 10.1 *The main groups of DNA-binding proteins which function in the transfer of information from extracellular signals to stimulate the transcription of specific genes*

Process governed by extracellular signal	DNA-binding protein
Cell differentiation	Homeotic proteins Retinoic acid binding proteins *fos* protein DNA-binding proteins specific to a given cell type (e.g. *myo* D_1 in myoblasts)
Cell proliferation	*jun* proteins Serum-response factor cAMP response element binding protein Transcription factors which bind to histone gene promoters
Responses to steroid and thyroid hormones	Steroid hormone-receptor proteins Thyroid hormone-receptor proteins

increases the concentration of the protein encoded by the second gene. The second gene may encode another DNA-binding protein, which stimulates the transcription of other genes, or may encode an enzyme or other protein with a cytoplasmic function (Fig. 10.1).

DNA-binding proteins are called *trans*-acting factors because they allow one gene to affect the activity of another gene. The regions of the DNA with which DNA-binding proteins interact are termed *cis*-acting elements since these regions modify the function of base sequences within the same gene. The activities of some DNA-binding proteins, such as the *jun* proteins,

are modified directly by cytoplasmic signalling pathways whilst the activities of others, for example the *fos* and c-*myc* proteins, change in response to the action of another DNA-binding protein.

The aims of this chapter are to consider the nature and functions of each of the different types of DNA-binding proteins in turn. The DNA-binding proteins have been grouped into those involved in cell differentiation, the control of cell proliferation, and the receptors for steroid hormones, thyroid hormones, and retinoic acid. Before these proteins are considered, some general principles which govern the roles of

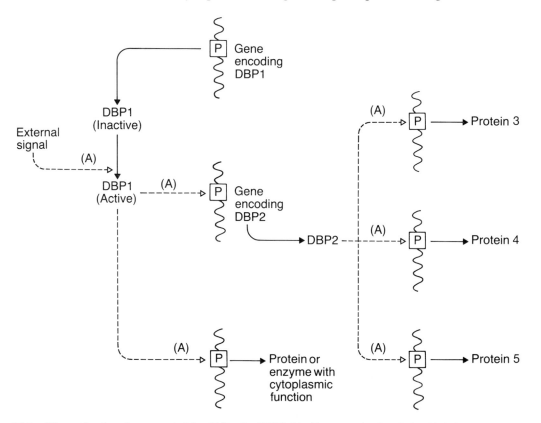

Fig. 10.1 The activation (represented by (A)) of a DNA-binding protein (DBP1) which is one of a number of DNA-binding proteins that are activated by an extracellular signal which stimulates the transcription of one or more genes. The active DNA-binding protein binds to the promoter region (P) of a second gene and increases the transcription of that gene. The second gene may encode another DNA-binding protein (DBP2), which stimulates the transcription of another set of genes to yield proteins 3, 4, and 5, or it may encode an enzyme or other protein with a cytoplasmic function. DBP1 itself is encoded by a specific gene.

DNA-binding proteins in the stimulation of gene transcription will be described.

10.2   Modulation of gene transcription by sequence-specific DNA-binding proteins

10.2.1   *Sequence-specific DNA-binding proteins and the initiation of transcription*

Initiation of the transcription of a given gene requires RNA polymerase II, a set of DNA-binding proteins called general initiation factors, and may also require one or more sequence-specific DNA-binding proteins which are also called sequence-specific transcription factors. The general initiation factors and sequence-specific transcription factors are sometimes called promoters. In eukaryotic cells, there are four general initiation factors, BTF1 (also called TFIID), BTF2, BTF3, and STF. These DNA-binding proteins are required for the initiation of transcription of all genes and are constitutively expressed in each cell. Some other transcription factors, such as Sp-1, are also constitutively expressed. These stimulate the transcription of defined sets of genes. The sequence-specific transcription factors modulate the rate of transcription of certain genes. The activity or concentration of these sequence-specific transcription factors is regulated by extracelluar signals.

The general initiation factors and many sequence-specific transcription factors bind to the promoter region of the gene. The promoter controls expression of the gene and is located in the vicinity of the transcription start site, usually on the 5′ side of this site (Fig. 10.2). The promoter region consists of a group of

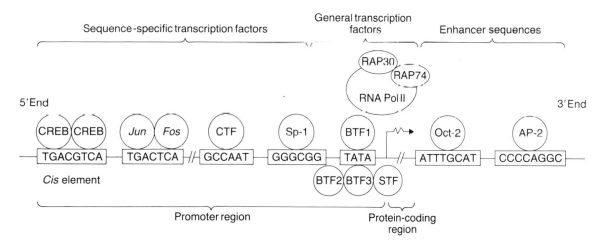

Fig. 10.2   The promoter region of a eukaryotic gene is a group of *cis* elements each of which binds a general initiation factor or a sequence-specific transcription factor. The *cis* elements are located in the vicinity of the transcription start site, often on the 5′ side of this site. The general transcription factors include BTF1, BTF2, BTF3, and STF. Examples of sequence-specific transcription factors are the cyclic AMP response-element-binding protein (CREB), CTF (NF-1), the *jun* protein, and the *fos* protein. Enhancer sequences, such as Oct-2 and AP-2, are often located on the 5′ side of the transcriptional start site some distance from this site, and sometimes at the 3′ side of the transcriptional start site (shown) some distance from the promoter region. The scheme shows the approximate interactions of the general initiation factors with the TATA box and RNA polymerase II (Pol II) since a complete description of the nature of the initiation complex is not yet available. Adapted from Mitchell and Tjian (1989).

transcriptional control modules called *cis* elements. Each module is 7–20 base pairs in length and contains one or more recognition sites for transcription factors. One module, often the TATA box, determines the start site for RNA synthesis. One or more other modules, for example the base sequences GGGCGG (the GC box) and CCAAT, regulate the frequency of initiation of transcription. These modules are often located 30–110 base pairs upstream of the transcription start site.

Some of the *cis* elements which control the initiation of gene transcription have been called enhancer elements. These were originally distinguished from promoter elements by the observation that each enhancer element is located at a large distance (up to 1000 nucleotide base pairs) from the promoter region, and can be either upstream or downstream from the transcription start site. A good example of an enhancer element is the glucocorticoid response element to which the glucocorticoid–glucocorticoid receptor complex binds.

Enhancer sequences act by affecting the activity of the nearest promoter. In the absence of a promoter sequence, an enhancer sequence cannot increase the frequency of initiation of transcription. In some situations, the activity of an enhancer sequence is strongly influenced by the nature of the nucleotide base sequences which lie between the enhancer and the promoter and protein-coding regions and the relative position of the enhancer sequence on the DNA alpha helix. Differences in the nature of these intervening sequences may partly explain why the action of any particular enhancer element depends on the cell type and on the physiological environment of that cell. The distinction between the terms 'promoter element' and 'enhancer element' is largely an operational one which is related to the distance over which the signal must be conveyed. However, the mechanisms of action of transcription factors which

bind to promoter and enhancer *cis* elements is probably qualitatively similar.

The presence of *cis* element modules in the promoter region of a gene allows that gene to be regulated by a diverse set of signals. It is probable that during the activation of transcription several sequence-specific transcription factors bind to the promoter region of the gene at any one time. This may allow a large number of genes in the nucleus to be controlled by a limited number of sequence-specific transcription factors.

10.2.2 *Structure of sequence-specific DNA-binding proteins*

Sequence-specific DNA-binding proteins have molecular weights in the range 35–80 kDa. At least four functional domains have been identified within each of these proteins. These are a DNA-binding domain, a transcriptional activation domain, a dimerization domain, and, for those proteins which interact with cytoplasmic

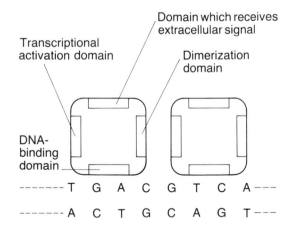

Fig. 10.3 Most sequence-specific DNA-binding proteins bind as dimers to specific palindromic base sequences on the DNA. Each subunit of the dimer possesses a DNA-binding domain, a transcriptional activation domain, a dimerization domain and may possess a domain with which a cytoplasmic signal, for example a protein kinase or a steroid or thyroid hormone, interacts.

or extracelluar signals, a domain which can interact with this signal (Fig. 10.3).

Most sequence-specific DNA-binding proteins bind to *cis* elements as homodimers or heterodimers (Fig. 10.3). The base sequences to which they bind are palindromic. Palindromes are base sequences which read the same in both directions. An example is the base sequence of the cyclic AMP response element (CRE) which is shown in Fig. 10.3. The palindromic base sequence is probably recognized by a dimeric DNA-binding domain with two-fold symmetry. Each component of the dimer binds to an identical base sequence.

10.2.3   *Structure of the DNA-binding domain*

The role of the DNA-binding domain is to recognize the specific gene or genes to which the DNA-binding protein binds, and to bring the protein into the correct position so that it can interact with other components of the initiation complex to give a functional transcriptional initiation complex. Four characteristic motifs which constitute different types of DNA-binding domains have so far been identified. These are the helix–turn–helix–motif (Fig. 10.4), a cluster of zinc fingers (Figs 10.5 and 10.6), the leucine zipper motif (Fig. 10.8) and the helix–loop–helix motif which is present in the myogenin and *myo* D

proteins which contribute to determining the state of differentiation of muscle cells. The majority of sequence-specific transcription fac-

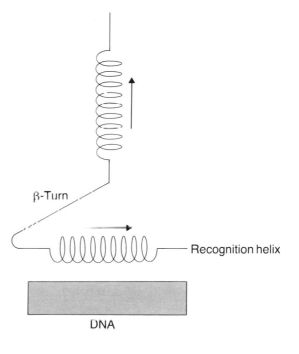

Fig. 10.4   The helix–turn–helix motif in the DNA-binding domain of a sequence-specific DNA-binding protein. Amino-acid residues in only one helix, the recognition helix, make specific contacts with bases in the DNA. The directions of the helices are indicated by the arrows.

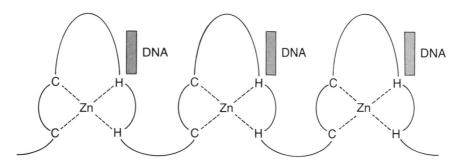

Fig. 10.5   A series of three cys2/his2 zinc finger motifs in the DNA-binding domain of a sequence-specific DNA-binding protein. Each zinc finger is composed of about 30 amino acids, including two invariant cysteine (C) and two invariant histidine (H) residues. The cysteine and histidine residues form co-ordinate bonds with Zn^{2+}. Part of the loop (the finger) formed between cysteine and histidine binds to the DNA.

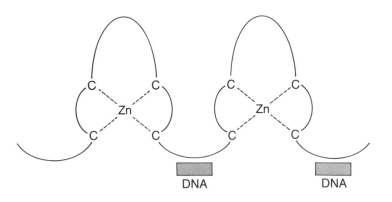

Fig. 10.6 Two cys2/cys2 zinc finger motifs in the DNA-binding domain of a sequence-specific DNA-binding protein. In these structures, each Zn atom is co-ordinately linked to four cysteine residues. The site of interaction with DNA is thought to occur at a region outside the zinc finger.

tors possess one of these motifs in the DNA-binding domain. There are probably other DNA-binding motifs that have not yet been characterized. Some amino acids within each characteristic DNA-binding motif may interact directly with the DNA. However, the most important function of the motifs is probably to determine the overall topology of the DNA-binding domain.

The helix–turn–helix motif was first identified in two DNA-binding repressor proteins of lambda phage, the Cro protein and the lambda repressor protein (CI), and in the cyclic AMP receptor protein of *E. coli*. Subsequently it was found that DNA-binding proteins encoded by a number of the homeotic genes possess a form of the helix–turn–helix structure which is slightly different from that of the bacterial proteins. (The term homeotic gene is defined in Section 10.3.2.) In the helix–turn–helix motif, two α-helices are separated by a tight β-turn. One helix, called the recognition helix, makes direct contact with bases exposed in the major groove of target DNA (Fig. 10.4). The other helix lies across the major groove and makes non-specific contacts with bases.

There are two forms of the zinc finger motif. In one, called the cys2/his2 zinc finger, Zn^{2+} is

co-ordinated to two cysteine and two histidine residues (Fig. 10.5) while in the other, called the cys2/cys2 zinc finger, Zn^{2+} is co-ordinated to four cysteine residues (Fig. 10.6). The cys2/his2 zinc finger motif was first identified in a transcription factor, TFIIIA, isolated from *Xenopus laevis* (Miller *et al.* 1985). This form of the zinc finger motif has also been found in a number of proteins encoded by non-homeotic genes which encode DNA-binding proteins that control development in *Drosophila* and in mice, and in several yeast DNA-binding proteins. TFIIIA has a molecular weight of 40 kDa and contains about 10 moles of Zn per mole of protein. Within the amino-acid sequence of the protein there are nine repetitive zinc-binding domains each of which is 30 amino acids in length. Each zinc-binding domain contains two invariant histidine and two invariant cysteine residues. The remainder of the amino-acid sequence of the binding domain is enriched in residues which can interact with base sequences in the DNA. The tetrahedral chelation of Zn^{2+} by histidine and cysteine forms the loop which composes the zinc finger (Fig. 10.5).

The nine zinc fingers of TFIIIA bind to a region of DNA which is 50 nucleotide bases in length. The distance between the contact points formed by two zinc fingers is five nucleotide bases. This is half a turn of the double helix. It is proposed that the backbone of the TFIIIA protein lies on only one side of the double helix so that successive zinc fingers lie on alternate sides of the major axis of the helix (Fig. 10.7). At the site of contact with the zinc finger the DNA is enriched in guanine residues.

The number of zinc fingers in other DNA-binding proteins which possess the cys2/his2 zinc finger motif differs from one protein to another. For example, the proteins encoded by the *Drosophila melanogaster Kr* gene, the *Drosophila snail* gene, and the mouse MKR1 gene have four, five, and seven fingers, respectively. The protein encoded by the *Drosophila hunchback* gene has two clusters of zinc fingers, one composed of four and the other of two fingers. The specific interaction of a DNA-binding protein which possesses a zinc finger motif with DNA probably depends on the binding of the cluster of zinc fingers to the appropriate *cis* element of the promoter of a target gene rather than on the precise interaction of individual zinc fingers with adjacent nucleotides.

The cys2/cys2 zinc finger structure (Fig. 10.6) is found in the DNA-binding domain of steroid hormone receptors. This type of zinc finger motif was discovered in the yeast transcriptional factor GAL4. The DNA-binding domain of steroid hormone receptors contains two cys2/cys2 zinc fingers.

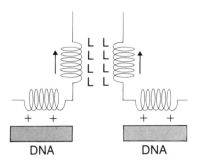

Fig. 10.8. The leucine zipper motif is one of the substructures responsible for the dimerization of DNA-binding proteins. Hydrophobic bonds formed between a line of four leucine residues in each α-helix hold the two proteins together. A positively charged region adjacent to the leucine α-helix binds to the DNA. The arrows indicate the directions of the helices.

The leucine zipper motif (Fig. 10.8) was discovered in a rat liver-enhancer-binding protein called C/EBP. This motif is present in the yeast transcriptional activator GCN4 and in the *jun*, *fos*, and *myc* proteins. The binding of each of these proteins to DNA is dependent on the formation of a dimer with either a molecule of the same protein or a molecule of a different protein. For example, the *jun* protein can bind to the AP-1 site as a *jun* homodimer or as a *jun–fos* heterodimer. The dimers are held together by the leucine zipper which does not, itself, interact with DNA.

Each DNA-binding protein which possess a leucine zipper motif contains a highly conserved

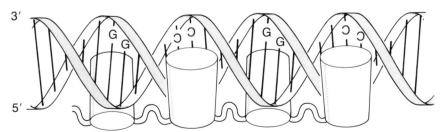

Fig. 10.7 A model for the interaction between DNA and a cluster of cys2/his2 zinc fingers in the DNA-binding domain of transcription factor TFIIIA from *Xenopus laevis*. The backbone of the sequence-specific DNA-binding protein lies on one side of the double helix. Successive zinc fingers are proposed to lie on alternate sides of the major axis of the helix. From Fairall *et al.* (1986).

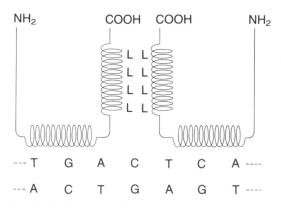

Fig. 10.9 Subunits of the *jun* homodimer are held together by the hydrophobic bonds of a leucine zipper. Each *jun* protein binds to one half of the palindromic base sequence in the *cis* element of the DNA.

stretch of 30 amino acids, which includes a substantial number of positively charged residues. This is followed by an α-helical region which contains four leucine residues spaced at intervals of seven amino acids. This results in a leucine residue at every second turn of the helix at about the same rotational position so that a line of four leucine residues is formed along one side of the helix. This region of the helix forms stable hydrophobic bonds with a similar helix on the second component of the dimer (Fig. 10.8). The positively charged region of the polypeptide chain adjacent to the leucine zipper binds to the DNA (Fig. 10.8). An example of the action of a leucine zipper is the formation of *jun* dimers which bind to a consensus sequence at the AP-1 binding site (Fig. 10.9).

10.2.4   *Formation of the active transcription initiation complex*

Formation of the active complex between the DNA, RNA polymerase II, and transcription factors is probably initiated by the binding of general initiation factor BTF1 to the TATA box. This allows binding of the other general initiation factors, sequence-specific transcription factors, and RNA polymerase II. It is not yet clear how sequence-specific transcription factors

increase the rate of transcription of a gene simply by binding to *cis* elements scattered in various parts of the promoter region of the gene. However, it seems that the interaction between different transcription factor proteins is as important as the interaction of each transcription factor with the appropriate *cis* element in the DNA. Each transcription factor which forms part of the transcription initiation complex must be able to interact with a *cis* element of the DNA and with binding sites on other transcription factors which are tethered to their corresponding *cis* elements in the promoter region. The formation of the correct initiation complex may involve a looping of the DNA so that the components of the initiation complex interact appropriately (Fig. 10.10).

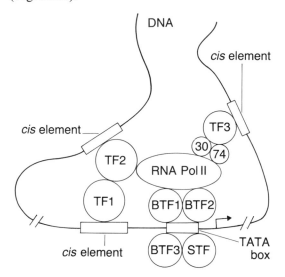

Fig. 10.10 Formation of a transcription initiation complex between general initiation factors (BTF1, BTF2, BTF3, and STF), the proteins RAP30 (30) and RAP74 (74), RNA polymerase II (RNA Pol II), and sequence-specific initiation factors (designated TF1, TF2, and TF3) probably involves folding or looping of the DNA. This allows specific protein–protein interactions between the various transcription factors. Both protein–protein interaction and folding of the DNA are required for formation of the initiation complex. The locations of the initiation factors are approximate as the nature of the initiation complex has not yet been fully elucidated.

The transcriptional activation domains of sequence-specific transcription factors probably allow these proteins to interact with components of the general transcription apparatus, including BTF1 and the transcription factors to which RNA polymerase II binds. The transcriptional activation domains of sequence-specific DNA-binding proteins consist of regions of 30–100 amino acids which are separate from the DNA-binding domain. A DNA-binding protein may often possess more than one transcription-activation domain. Three types of transcriptional activation domains have been identified. These are acidic (negatively charged) α-helices, regions rich in glutamate residues, and regions rich in proline residues. Acidic α-helices are found in glucocorticoid receptors, in transcription factors, such as *jun*, which bind to AP-1 sites, and in yeast GAL4. Glutamate-enriched regions are found in Sp-1, some homeotic proteins, *jun*, AP-2, and in serum response factor (SRF), while proline-rich regions are found in CTF/NF-1.

10.3 Cell differentiation

10.3.1 *Embryogenesis and differentiation*

The embryonic development of an animal involves the establishment from progenitor stem cells of differentiated cells which serve specific functions, for example myocardial muscle cells, liver parenchymal cells, or cells of the central nervous system. Maintenance of a differentiated cell type requires the expression of a specific set of genes which is unique for that cell type. These genes specify enzymes and other proteins required for the maintenance of cell structure, specific cell functions, and intracellular and extracelluar signalling. In a particular differentiated cell type, expression of a particular gene which is specific for that cell type is governed in part by the binding of a number of ubiquitous transcription factors and the binding of a limited number of sequence-specific transcription fac-tors to the promoter region of that gene.

In general the process of embryonic differentiation in *Drosophila* and probably other animals is directed by morphogens, such as retinoic acid, growth factors, and the *bicoid* and *nanos* proteins. These extracellular agents, which are secreted by certain cells, form concentration gradients in the embryo. The growth and differentiation of any one cell in the early embryonic stage is determined by the nature and concentration of the morphogens present at that spatial location of the embryo. The composition and concentration of morphogens change as a function of time.

Each morphogen acts on those target cells which possess specific receptors for that morphogen. Within each target cell, the action of a morphogen induces a rapid onset of the transcription of a specific set of genes, called the primary response genes, and a slow onset of the transcription of another specific set of genes, called the secondary response genes. Initiation of the transcription of primary response genes does not require the machinery of protein synthesis, although protein synthesis is required for the formation of new protein encoded by the mRNA formed in transcription of the primary response genes. Initiation of the transcription of secondary response genes does require machinery of protein synthesis.

The mechanisms by which morphogens increase the transcription of specific genes are not yet fully understood. However, the general picture is something like this. Morphogens probably modify the activity of a number of different sequence-specific transcription factors, each of which stimulates the transcription of one or more primary response genes (Fig. 10.11). A number of the primary response proteins are, themselves, sequence-specific transcription factors which bind to the promoter regions of other genes and increase the transcription of these secondary response genes (Fig. 10.11).

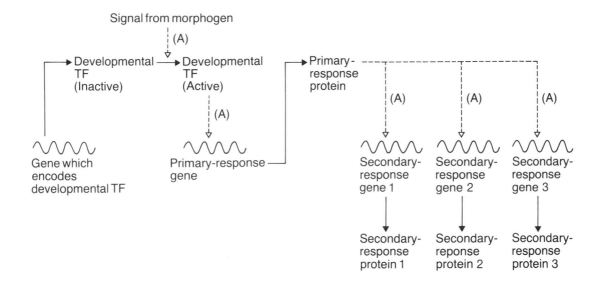

Fig. 10.11 The probable mechanism of action of morphogens. Each morphogen activates (represented by (A)) a sequence-specific transcription factor (represented as 'developmental TF') which increases the rate of transcription of one or more genes, called the primary-response genes. Many of the proteins encoded by these primary-response genes are, themselves, sequence-specific transcription factors, which activate the transcription of other sets of genes, the secondary-response genes. Activation of the transcription of primary-response genes does not require the machinery of protein synthesis whereas this is required for activation of the transcription of secondary-response genes.

Only a small number of the sequence-specific transcription factors that are affected by morphogens and growth factors during embryogenesis have so far been identified. An important group of these proteins are the homeotic proteins, the properties of which are described in the next section. Other DNA-binding proteins known to be involved in development and differentiation are: myogenin, the *myo* D1 protein, and the *myd* protein which, together with other DNA-binding proteins, contribute to the specification of differentiated muscle cells; the *glass* protein which has a zinc finger DNA-binding domain and contributes to specification of a neuronal cell type in *Drosophila*; the *fos* protein which is present in all cells; and LF-B1/HNF-1, a sequence-specific transcription factor found only in the liver.

10.3.2   *The homeotic proteins*

Considerable information on the role of sequence-specific DNA-binding proteins in embryogenesis has been provided by a group of mutations which affect development in *Drosophila melanogaster*, an insect that has been most useful in a genetic approach to the elucidation of the processes which control development. The genes detected by these mutations fall into three groups. These are the maternal-effect genes, which specify the spatial co-ordinates of the egg, the segmentation genes, which specify the number and polarity of body segments, and the homeotic genes, which specify the identity of each body segment.

The term homeosis was proposed by Bateson (1894) to describe the replacement of one structure in a body segment of *Drosophila* by a homologous structure from another segment. For example, mutation or over-expression of the *Antennapedia* (*Antp*) gene leads to the replacement of the antenna by a pair of middle legs (Fig. 10.12). In *Drosophila* there are two main clusters of homeotic genes, the antennapedia complex, ANT-C, which includes the genes *Antp*, *fushi tarazu* (*Ftz*), *deformed* (*Dfd*), and sex combs reduced (*Scr*), and the biothorax complex, BX-C, which includes the genes *Ubx*, *infra-abdominal*-2, *infra-abdominal*-7, and *Zerknullt* (*zen*). Another example of a *Drosophila* homeobox gene is *engrailed* (*en*). Since their discovery in *Drosophila*, homeotic genes have been

detected in the cells of a number of other animals. So far, over 80 homeotic genes have been identified. These include at least nine genes (designated *xhox*) from the frog *Xenopus laevis*, 20 genes (designated *Hox*) from the mouse, and 21 human genes (designated *huhox*). Human homeotic genes include the Oct 1, Oct 2, and Pit-1/GHF-1 genes.

The homeotic genes contain a highly conserved base sequence called the homeobox. This sequence is 180 base pairs in length and is located near the intron–exon boundary in the exon nearest the 3' end of each homeotic gene. The homeobox sequence was first discovered in studies of the *Antp* gene. A search of the ability of *Antp* cDNA to hybridize with other regions of DNA revealed several hybridization complexes. Two of these were subsequently shown to be part of the *ftz* and *ubx* genes (McGinnis *et al.* 1984; Scott and Weiner 1984). The region responsible for this hybridization was called the homeobox. Many homeotic genes were first identified through the presence of the homeobox region.

The proteins encoded by the homeotic genes have molecular weights which range from 40 to 60 kDA. The sequence of amino acids encoded by the homeobox region is called the homeodomain. This contains a helix-turn-helix DNA-binding motif (Fig. 10.13). About 30 per cent of the amino acids present in the homeodomain are the basic amino acids arginine and lysine. The amino terminus of homeotic proteins is conserved between different proteins. A variable region and a conserved 5-amino-acid sequence called the homeopeptide lies between the amino terminus and the homeodomain. A short domain at the carboxy terminus is often acidic.

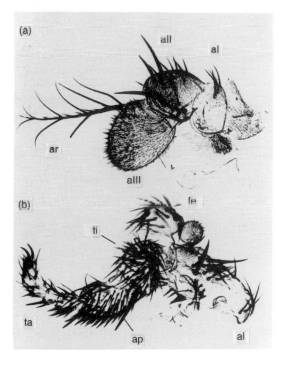

Fig. 10.12 The antenna of a normal *Drosophila melanogaster* fly (a) and an antenna which has been transformed into a middle leg in a transformed fly (b) in which an additional *Antennapedia* (*Antp*) gene has been expressed. Expression of the additional *Antp* gene was induced by a heat-inducible promoter. The abbreviations are: a l, a ll, and a lll, the first, second, and third antennal segments; ar, arista; ta, tarsus; ti, tibia; fe, femur, and ap, apical bristle. From Schneuwly *et al.* (1987).

Experiments conducted with *Drosophila* have shown that a particular homeotic protein is only transcribed in certain types of cell. This has been demonstrated by the use of antibodies to the homeotic protein and by *in situ* mRNA hybridization. One of the most striking examples of

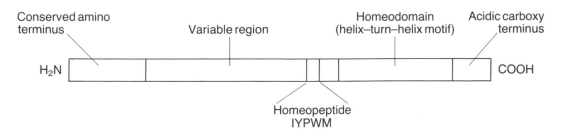

Fig. 10.13 A schematic representation of the structure of a homeotic protein. At the amino terminus is a conserved sequence of amino acids alongside a variable region. Near the homeodomain, which contains the helix–turn–helix DNA-binding domain, is a conserved peptide called the homeopeptide. The carboxy terminus of the molecule is acidic.

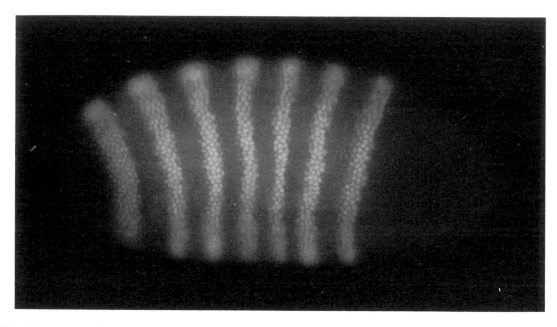

Fig. 10.14 The embryo of *Drosophila* at the blastoderm stage stained to reveal those cells that contain the *ftz* protein. A pattern of seven stripes, which represents the spatial pattern of expression of the *ftz* gene, is observed. The *ftz* protein was detected using an antibody to this protein and a fluorescence detection system. The anterior of the embryo is on the left and the dorsal surface is on the top. From Gehring (1987).

the spatial distribution of the expression of a homeotic gene is the pattern of stripes observed for the segmentation gene *fushi tarazu (ftz)* in the blastoderm embryo (Fig. 10.14). Experiments of the type described in Fig. 10.14 show that each embryonic cell contains a unique combination of homeotic proteins. One of the functions of these proteins in *Drosophila* is

sub-division of the embryo along the anterio–posterior axis into fields of cells with different developmental potential.

The transcription of the genes which encode homeotic proteins is probably regulated by morphogens such as retinoic acid, peptide growth factors, and the *Drosophila bicoid* and *nanos* proteins. Some homeotic genes, for example those in the mouse *Hox* 3 complex, are controlled by a single master promoter.

Through its action as a sequence-specific transcription factor, each homeotic protein probably activates the transcription of a battery of other genes, many of which are other homeotic genes. Several different homeotic proteins may compete for the same *cis* element on a given promoter. Examples of homeotic proteins which control homeotic genes are the *eve* and *ftz* proteins, which bind to the promoter region of the *engrailed* gene, and the *caudal* and *ftz* proteins, which bind to the promoter regions of the *Kr* and *Hb* genes. Examples of homeotic proteins which control the transcription of other types of genes are the Oct 2 and Pit-1/GHF-1 proteins in mammals. The Oct 2 protein, which is present in lymphoid tissue, binds to the promoters of many genes, the functions of which are not yet known. The Pit-1/GHF-1 protein, which is present only in pituitary cells, binds to the promoters of the genes which encode growth hormone and prolactin.

10.3.3 *Differentiation of blood cells*
The processes involved in the formation of mature blood cells have been studied in considerable detail. These processes are an example of cell differentiation in an adult animal. There are eight main types of mature blood cells, for example erthyrocytes, neutrophils, and lymphocytes. Mature blood cells originate from haemopoietic stem cells. The process of stem cell differentiation involves two stages, the formation of committed progenitor cells and the formation of morphologically identifiable immature cells. The processes of differentiation and commitment are regulated by the haemopoietic growth factors of which the colony stimulating factors and the interleukins are two of the most important groups. Each of these growth factors probably directs the actions of a number of sequence-specific transcription fac-

tors, although most of these have not yet been identified. Two that have been partially characterized are GF-1 and the *myb* protein. GF-1 regulates the synthesis of β-globin. The *myb* protein is a phosphorylated protein and is the normal form of the protein encoded by the *myb* oncogene.

10.3.4 *Phenotypic changes in nerve cells*
A number of external stimuli induce an altered state of differentiation of nerve cells or a change in cell phenotype, such as that associated with the development of memory. These changes require alterations in gene expression. The stimuli which induce these changes include natural stimuli such as nerve growth factor (NGF), which induces neuronal differentiation, other neurotrophic factors, neurotransmitters, and artificial stimuli, such as experimentally induced depolarization of the plasma membrane, agents which stimulate Ca^{2+} inflow through voltage-operated Ca^{2+} channels, and drugs such as the convulsent pentylenetetrazole. The action of each of these stimuli is associated with the transient induction of the transcription of a number of primary response genes which are also called the immediately early genes. These genes include *fos*, *jun*, and c-*myc*, which encode sequence-specific transcription factors, and a gene called NGF1B, which encodes a DNA-binding receptor protein for an unknown agonist. The transient increases in transcription of the *fos* and c-*myc* genes which occur in response to the action of NGF on a cultured neuronal cell line are shown in Fig. 10.15. The maximal increase in transcription of the *fos* gene occurs within about 5 min. following the addition of NGF whereas maximal increase in c-*myc* transcription occurs after a much longer period of time.

The rate of transcription of primary response genes like *fos*, *jun*, and c-*myc* in nerve cells is probably increased as a result of the activation, by an external signal such as NGF, of one or

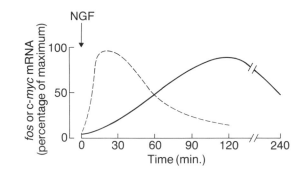

Fig. 10.15 An example of the increased transcription of genes which encode sequence-specific transcription factors during changes in the state of differentiation of a nerve cell induced by a growth factor. NGF induces transient increases in the rates of synthesis of c-*myc* (full curve) and *fos* (broken curve) mRNA in cultured rat pheochromocytoma (PC12) cells, a neuronal cell line. The increase in c-*myc* mRNA synthesis is maximal at 120 min. while the increase in *fos* mRNA synthesis is maximal at about 15 min. Adapted from Greenberg *et al.* (1985).

more sequence-specific transcription factors. The activated transcription factor binds to a *cis* element on the promoter site of each primary response gene. The *fos, jun*, and c-*myc* proteins probably activate the transcription of a number of other genes, the secondary response genes, by binding to *cis* elements in the promoters of these genes.

10.4　Regulation of cell proliferation

10.4.1　*Steps of the cell cycle and regulation of progression through the cycle*

Cells in a differentiating or differentiated tissue can exist in one of three states. These are active division, a resting state called the G_0 state, and a state in which the cells are programmed to die and will not divide again. Cells in G_0 state do not divide but can be stimulated to divide by extracellular signals.

　　The process by which cells grow and divide is called the cell cycle. The major steps in this cycle are the G_1 (G represents gap), S (DNA

synthesis), G_2 and M (cell division) phases (Fig. 10.16). G_1 is the phase in which cell differentiation is initiated. The cell cycle can be viewed as a linear sequence of events in which each event is required to take place before the next event can occur. This ensures that a cell does not divide before the DNA has been replicated, the subcel-

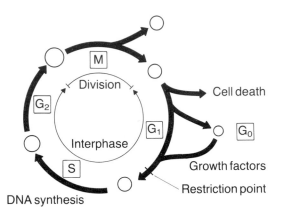

Fig. 10.16 The main phases in the cell cycle are G_1 (enzyme synthesis), S (DNA synthesis), G_2 (late interphase), and M (cell division). (The term 'G' represents gap.) In the absence of growth factors, cells at the beginning of G_1 phase become quiescent and cease to grow. This state is described as the G_0 state. Cells in the G_0 state have the potential to divide if stimulated by growth factors. Some cells are programmed to die, and never divide again after mitosis.

lular organelles duplicated, and the cell has grown to a critical size. There is probably some overlap between the phases of the cell cycle. For example, reactions that are part of the G_1 phase (the preparation for S phase) may begin in the G_2 phase of the previous cycle, and reactions that are part of the G_2 phase may begin in the preceding S phase.

　　Three important transition points in the cell cycle have been identified. These are passage through a point late in G_1 phase, named the restriction point or Start, which commits the cell to initiating DNA synthesis, entry into mitosis, and exit from mitosis. When the restriction point is reached, the cell is committed to progress through the cell cycle. Progression through the cell cycle after the restriction point does not depend on the presence of extracellular signals. At a point in the cycle before the restriction point is reached, cells will remain quiescent (in the G_0 state) as long as extracellular signals which stimulate cell division are absent.

Each of the three transitions in the cell cycle is probably regulated by a protein kinase, named p34 kinase, which is encoded by the *cdc* 2 gene. p34 kinase was originally identified as mitosis-inducing protein kinase. This protein kinase, which is also discussed in Chapter 4, Section 4.7, has also been called maturation promoting factor. The p34 kinase may regulate gene transcription by, for example, the phosphorylation of RNA polymerase II. The activity of the p34 kinase is controlled by the reversible phosphorylation of a tyrosine and a threonine residue on the p34 polypeptide chain and by its interaction with proteins called cyclins and a protein called p13^{suc-1}. There are probably also other important controls of p34 kinase activity which have not been elucidated.

The cyclins which interact with the p34 kinase are G_1 phase-specific cyclin and mitosis-specific cyclin. The concentration of each of these cyclins changes during the cell cycle as a result of the synthesis and degradation of the cyclin protein. Proteolysis of cyclins may ensure that the cell cycle progresses only in one direction. The concentration of G_1 phase-specific cyclin increases in G_1 phase while the concentration of mitosis-specific cyclin increases during mitosis. The protease which degrades cyclins is regulated by reversible phosphorylation. Phosphate addition is catalysed by the protein kinase p39^{mos}. An abnormal counterpart of the p39^{mos} protein is encoded by the *mos* oncogene, a species-specific oncogene.

The progression of a cell through the cell cycle requires an increased rate of transcription of a subset of genes. These encode enzymes and regulatory proteins required for growth and division. Increased transcription of the genes is initiated by mitogens.

10.4.2 *Genes transcribed in response to the action of mitogens*

Entry to the cell cycle may occur soon after a previous mitosis or meiosis, or after a period of time spent in the G_0 state. A cell in a quiescent state (G_0 state) will only move to the G_1 phase in the presence of a mitogen (Fig. 10.16). A mitogen is also required to continue the proliferation of a cell that has reached the G_1 phase after mitosis. In the absence of a mitogen such a cell will move to the quiescent (G_0) state. Extracellular signals which stimulate cell division include growth factors, hormones, intercellular contact, and some morphogens. In tumour cells, the requirement for these extracellular signals is bypassed by the constitutive action of proteins encoded by oncogenes. These oncogenic proteins are described in Chapter 11.

Each mitogen induces the transcription of a number of genes. As in the case of the action of morphogens on target cells, the mRNAs and proteins specified by these genes can be divided into two groups. These are the immediate early mRNAs and proteins, which are encoded by the primary response genes and appear rapidly, and the late mRNAs and proteins, which are encoded by the secondary response genes and appear after some period of time. Formation of the immediate early mRNAs does not require the synthesis of new protein, in contrast to the formation of late mRNAs. About 100 immediate early proteins are formed in response to mitogens. These proteins include sequence-specific transcription factors encoded by the c-*myc*, *fos*, *fra*-1, *fos*-B, *egr*-1, *KROX* 20, *jun*, *jun* B, and *jun* D genes, the DNA-binding receptor protein encoded by the NGF 1B gene, cyclins encoded by the JE, TCA3, TIS7 and NS1 genes, and a number of proteins, the function of which is not yet known. The late proteins synthesized in response to mitogens include enzymes and proteins required for cell growth and division.

10.4.3 *Sequence-specific DNA-binding proteins activated by mitogens*

How do mitogens switch a cell from the quiescent G_0 state to enter the G_1 phase of the cell cycle? This is probably achieved by the activation of sequence-specific transcription factors, which in turn, are responsible for increasing the transcription of immediate early genes and, subsequently, the transcription of late genes. The combination of a mitogen with a plasma-membrane receptor activates transcription factors through a pathway which involves intracel-

lular messengers and protein kinases (Fig. 10.17). The final step in this pathway is probably the phosphorylation of a sequence-specific transcription factor and modification of the activity of this factor.

A number of transcription factors, the activities of which are modified by mitogens, have been identified. Four of these, together with the *cis* element to which they bind, are listed in Table 10.2. These transcription factors probably represent only a small proportion of the total number of sequence-specific transcription factors regulated by mitogens.

Protein kinase C and cyclic AMP-dependent protein kinase modify the activities of more than one sequence-specific transcription factor. The main target for protein kinase C seems to be the *jun* protein. As described earlier, in its active

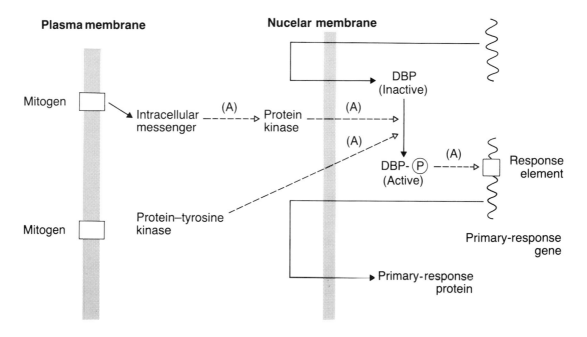

Fig. 10.17 Mitogens, such as growth factors, which bind to plasma-membrane receptors alter gene transcription by the phosphorylation of a sequence-specific DNA-binding protein (DBP), for example the *jun* protein, the cyclic AMP response element binding protein or the serum response factor. The activated sequence-specific transcription factor binds to a *cis* element, called a response element, in the promoter region of another gene, a primary response gene, and induces the transcription of the primary response gene. The symbol (A) represents activation.

Table 10.2 *Sequence-specific transcription factors which are responsive to mitogens*

Transcription factor	Molecular weight (kDa)	*cis* Element bound by transcription factor	Base sequence of binding site on DNA (5'–3')	Example of signal which activates transcription factor
c-*jun* protein	36	AP-1	TGAC	Tetradecanoyl phorbol acetate
AP-2 protein	48	AP-2	CCCAGGC	Tetradecanoyl phorbol acetate Cyclic AMP
Cyclic AMP-response element binding protein (CREB)	43	Cyclic AMP-response element (CRE)	TGACGTCA	Cyclic AMP
Serum response factor (SRF)	52	Serum response element (SRE)	GATGTCCATA-TTAGGACATC	Serum, EGF, tetradecanoyl phorbol acetate, insulin

form the *jun* protein forms a dimer with the *fos* protein or with another of the proteins which can bind to the AP-1 site in the promoter region of target genes. The main target for cyclic AMP-dependent protein kinase is the cyclic AMP response element binding protein (CREB). Phosphorylation of this protein by cyclic AMP-dependent protein kinase induces dimerization of CREB, binding of the dimer to the CRE *cis* element of target genes and the stimulation of transcription of these genes. The *jun–fos* hetero-dimers and CREB homodimers are held together by leucine zipper motifs. The serum response element (SRE), the binding site for serum response factor (SRF), is located in the promoter region of genes which are targets for SRF, about 300 base pairs before the start codon, ATG. One of the target genes for SRF is the *fos* gene.

10.4.4 *Mitogen-induced transcription of the* myc, fos, *and* jun *genes*

Changes in the mRNA and proteins encoded by three of the immediate early genes transcribed in response to the action of mitogens have been studied in some detail. These genes are the c-*myc*, *fos*, and *jun* genes. It was possible to obtain considerable knowledge of the products of these genes because the genes were originally identified as oncogenes.

Expression of the c-*myc*, *fos*, and *jun* genes is transient. For example, increased transcription of the c-*jun* protein occurs during transition from the G_0 state to the G_1 phase of the cell cycle and is rapid in onset. Another example is the c-*myc* gene. A number of mitogenic stimuli, including platelet-derived growth factor, concanavalin A, and the tumour promoter tetradecanoyl phorbol acetate, induce a 30 to 40-fold increase in c-*myc* mRNA and protein in quiescent cells (Fig. 10.18). This increase is associated with the transition from the G_0 state to the G_1 phase of the cell cycle. After the cell has entered the cell cycle the concentration of c-*myc* mRNA remains elevated at a value about 10-fold higher than that present in quiescent cells and undergoes no further change in the concentration during the rest of the cell cycle.

The concentrations of the c-*myc*, *fos*, and *jun* proteins are controlled not only by their rates of synthesis but also by the rates of degradation of the proteins and the mRNA which encodes the proteins. The half-lives of these protein and

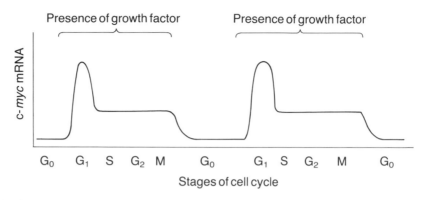

Fig. 10.18 An increased rate of transcription of the c-*myc* gene is associated with the entry of a cell to the cell cycle. The c-*myc* gene is normally transcribed at a low rate. The interaction of a mitogenic stimulus such as platelet-derived growth factor (PDGF) with a cell causes an increase of about 10-fold in c-*myc* mRNA during the period in which the cell moves from the G_0 state to the G_1 phase. During subsequent steps of the cell cycle the concentration of c-*myc* mRNA decreases but remains above the value in the G_0 state. A second cycle of growth, and hence of increased c-*myc* mRNA synthesis, requires a second exposure of the cell to the mitogen.

mRNA species are short. Control of the degradation of c-*myc* RNA is probably exerted by the region at the 5' end of the mRNA encoded by untranslated exon 1 of the c-*myc* gene. Removal of this regulatory region of the mRNA leads to a marked decrease in the rate of c-*myc* mRNA degradation and to increases in the concentrations of c-*myc* mRNA and protein. The *fos* protein is extensively phosphorylated. Changes in the degree of phosphorylation may also contribute to regulation of the activity of this protein.

The molecular weight of the protein encoded by c-*myc* is 58 kDa. Two regions of the polypeptide chain near the amino terminus and one region at the carboxy terminus have been shown to be essential for the cellular functions of the c-*myc* protein. Antibodies to the mature c-*myc* protein have been used to show that in cells in which the c-*myc* gene is transcribed at a high rate the c-*myc* protein moves to the nucleus after its synthesis in the cytoplasmic space. The residues between amino-acid 320 and amino-acid 335 at the carboxy terminus of the c-*myc* protein represent a signal sequence which is required for translocation of the protein to the nucleus.

Two other *myc* genes, designated N-*myc* and L-*myc*, have been identified. The proteins encoded by these genes are composed of between 370 and 470 amino-acid residues. There are a number of regions of homology between the c-*myc*, N-*myc*, and L-*myc* proteins. Expression of c-*myc* is maintained at a low level in most types of cell and does not change substantially during development. However, the N-*myc* and L-*myc* genes are only expressed in certain tissues, and are transcribed at the highest rates during development of the embryo.

10.4.5 *Sequence-specific DNA binding proteins which stimulate histone gene transcription*

So far, two types of sequence-specific transcription factors have been described in relation to the cell cycle. These are the DNA-binding proteins which are activated by mitogens and the DNA-binding proteins which are encoded by immediate early genes. Other sequence-specific transcription factors probably co-ordinate the transcription of sets of genes during the cell cycle. Only a few examples of genes controlled in this manner are known. One of these is the set of genes which encode the histone proteins.

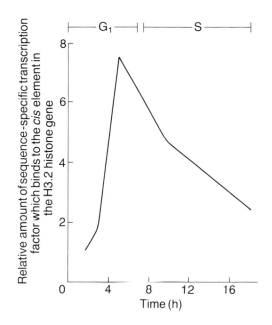

Fig. 10.19 The concentration of the sequence-specific transcription factor which binds to a *cis* element in the promoter region of the H3.2 histone gene increases during late G_1 and early S phases of the cell cycle. The concentration of the transcription factor was measured by its ability to form a complex with DNA which contains the H3.2 histone gene. From Artishevsky *et al.* (1987).

Table 10.3   *The members of the major families of hormones and morphogens which bind to sequence-specific DNA-binding receptor proteins*

Family	Members of family
Steroid hormones	Glucocorticoids
	Mineralocorticoids (aldosterone)
	Progestins
	Oestrogens
	Androgens (testosterone)
Vitamin D	Dihydrocholecalciferol (vitamin D)
Ecdysteroids (insects)	Ecdysone
Thyroid hormones	Triiodothyronine
	Thyroxine
Retinoids	Retinol
	Retinoic acid

Transcription of all five sub-types of histone gene is increased at the time of increased DNA synthesis. This is probably due to increases in the concentrations of sequence-specific transcription factors which act at *cis* elements in the promoter regions of histone genes. These transcription factors include OTF-1, which stimulates the transcription of the histone H2b gene, and H4T f-1 and H4T f-2 which stimulate transcription of the histone H4 gene. The concentration of these transcription factors, and the concentrations of transcription factors which bind to the promoters of other histone genes, change during the cell cycle (Fig. 10.19).

10.5   DNA-binding receptor proteins

10.5.1   *Nature of DNA-binding receptor proteins*

The steroid hormones, vitamin D (dihydroxycholecalciferol), thyroid hormones, and retinoids are the main families of agonists which bind to sequence-specific DNA-binding receptor proteins (Table 10.3). In the present description of the nature and mechanism of action of the sequence-specific DNA-binding receptor proteins the term 'DNA-binding receptor' will be used to describe these proteins. There are at least two forms of the thyroid hormone receptor. These are encoded by the c-*erb* Aα and c-*erb* Aβ genes and are the normal counterparts of the *erb* A oncogene, the properties of which are described in Chapter 11.

The first DNA-binding receptor protein to be discovered was the receptor for oestrogen. Early studies on the actions of oestrogens had suggested the presence of an oestrogen receptor in oestrogen target tissues. The idea of a receptor was strengthened by the work of Jensen and Jacobson who in 1962 showed that [³H]oestradiol is taken up by target tissues for oestrogens, the uterus, and vagina, but not by non-target tissues. In 1964, Talwar *et al.* obtained a protein fraction from rat uterus which bound oestrogen and, in the absence of oestrogen, inhibited RNA polymerase. Two years later the oestrogen receptor protein was isolated from rat uterus by Toft and Gorski (1966). The primary amino-acid sequence of the oestrogen receptor was determined by Green *et al.* in 1986.

Each hormone–DNA-binding receptor or morphogen–DNA-binding receptor complex induces an increase in the rate of transcription of a specific set of genes. In the case of glucocorticoids, the term 'glucocorticoid domain' has been used by Ivarie and O'Farrell (1978) to describe the genes which are responsive to these hormones. The genes affected by a hormone or morphogen represent only a small fraction of the total number of transcribed genes in an animal cell. Stimulation of the transcription of these genes induces a pleotropic response in the target cell and allows the cell to carry out a particular specialized function. The genes affected by a given hormone depend on the nature of the hormone and the cell type (Table 10.4). As described earlier, morphogens stimulate the transcription of genes which probably chiefly encode sequence-specific transcription factors.

Hormones or morphogens which act through DNA-binding receptor proteins only affect transcriptionally active genes. The rate of tran-scription, which may be very low in the absence of hormone or morphogen, is increased substantially in the presence of hormone or morphogen. The response of a particular cell type to a hormone or morphogen is determined by the structure of the chromatin, the particular genes which are being transcribed in the absence of the hormone or morphogen, the interaction of other hormone–DNA-binding receptor complexes with the DNA in that same cell, and the actions of other sequence specific DNA-binding proteins within the nucleus.

10.5.2 *Steps in the action of DNA-binding receptor proteins*

The central steps in the process by which the interaction of steroid hormone with a DNA-binding receptor protein in the cytoplasmic space of a target cell leads to an increase in gene transcription in the nucleus were first proposed by Jensen and Gorski and their colleagues (Jensen *et al.* 1968; Gorski *et al.* 1968). They developed a two-step model in which the first step is the formation of the hormone–DNA-binding receptor complex in the cytoplasmic space and the second step is the movement of the hormone–DNA-binding receptor complex to the nucleus and the interaction of this complex with the DNA.

Table 10.4 *Examples of genes activated by hormones which bind to DNA-binding receptor proteins*

Hormone	Target cell type	Gene transcribed at a greater rate
Glucocorticoid	Liver	Phosphoenolypyruvate carboxykinase Tyrosine aminotransferase
	Anterior pituitary	Growth hormone
Oestradiol	Uterus	Vitellgenin
Progesterone	Uterus	Ovalbumin Transferrin Ovomucoid Lysosome Uteroglobin
Thyroid hormone	Anterior pituitary	Growth hormone

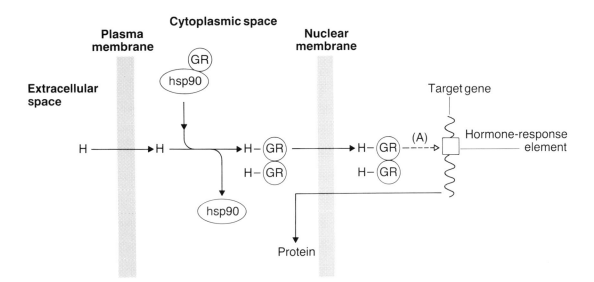

Fig. 10.20   A schematic description of the mechanism by which glucocorticoids stimulate the transcription of target genes. In the absence of glucocorticoid, the glucocorticoid DNA-binding receptor protein is located in the cytoplasmic space as a complex with heat-shock protein 90 (hsp90). Following an increase in glucocorticoid concentration in the extracellular fluid, the hormone diffuses across the plasma membrane to the cytoplasmic space. Within this space the hormone binds to the glucocorticoid receptor (GR), displaces hsp90, and induces dimerization of GR. The resulting complex of hormone and GR moves towards the nuclear membrane and through a pore in this membrane. Within the nucleus the glucocorticoid–GR complex binds to the hormone-response element of a target gene. This leads to stimulation of the transcription of the gene and synthesis of the proteins encoded by the gene. Although only one target gene is shown, each glucocorticoid–GR complex binds to a number of target genes.

The mechanism by which glucocorticoids stimulate gene transcription has been studied in great detail. As it is presently understood the process can be described as follows. In the absence of hormone, the glucocorticoid DNA-binding receptor (GR) is located in the cytoplasmic space in association with a protein called heat-shock protein 90, hsp90 (Fig. 10.20). When the concentration of glucocorticoid in the extracellular medium is increased, the hormone moves across the plasma membrane into the cytoplasmic space where it binds to the GR and induces dissociation of the GR–hsp90 complex and dimerization of the GR. The hsp90 protein probably acts to retain GR in a particular conformation (see Chapter 2, Section 2.6) in the cytoplasmic space by preventing the formation of GR dimers in the absence of glucocorticoid.

Formation of the hormone–GR complex involves the combination of one molecule of hormone with one molecule of GR protein. There are probably several thousand copies of GR present in each cell. The concentration of GR is regulated by a number of mechanisms, including glucocorticoids themselves and cyclic AMP-dependent protein kinase. The GR has a high affinity (K_d of about 5 nM) for glucocorticoids. The binding of the hormone induces a temperature-dependent conformational change in GR. This change has been detected as a decrease in net negative charge, a change in chromatographic behaviour of the GR protein, and altered accessibility of GR to antibodies against this protein.

Formation of the hormone–GR complex unmasks a nuclear localization signal in GR.

This allows the glucocorticoid–GR complex to move to the nuclear membrane and through a nuclear pore to the nucleus. Within the nucleus, the glucocorticoid–GR complex interacts with specific sites on the DNA and induces an increase in the transcription of specific genes. The isolation from cultured mouse lymphoma and human lymphoblastic leukaemia cells of spontaneous mutants (Table 10.5) in which the

Table 10.5 *Spontaneous mutants of cultured animal and human cells in which a given step is defective in the pathway by which the DNA-binding steroid-hormone receptor protein acts to stimulate gene transcription*

Mutant	Phenotype
r^-	Deficient in interaction with hormone
nt^-	Deficient in transfer to nucleus
nt^i	Exhibit increased rate of transfer of hormone–receptor complex to nucleus
act^l	Hormone–DNA-binding receptor–DNA complex is unusually labile (activation labile)

action of glucocorticoid is impaired has helped to confirm the existence of the pathway shown in Fig. 10.20.

The mechanisms by which other steroid hormones, vitamin D, the thyroid hormones, and the retinoids stimulate DNA synthesis are generally similar to the mechanism for glucocorticoid action. The domain in the regulatory region of genes to which each of these hormone–receptor complexes binds is called the hormone-response element. Three classes of hormone-response elements have so far been discerned. These are the oestrogen response elements, the glucocorticoid response elements, and the thyroid hormone-response elements.

10.5.3 *Structure of DNA-binding receptor proteins*

Elucidation of the primary amino-acid

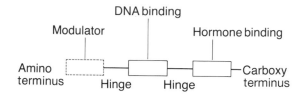

Fig. 10.21 A schematic representation of the functional domains identified in DNA-binding receptor proteins. The three domains are separated by sequences of amino-acid residues called flexible hinge regions. The hormone-binding domain at the carboxy terminus probably also contains a nuclear localization signal sequence, a transcriptional activation domain, and a motif which permits the formation of dimers of the DNA-binding receptor protein.

sequences of the DNA-binding receptor proteins has revealed the presence of three functional domains (Fig. 10.21). These are the DNA-binding domain, which is located in the centre of the polypeptide chain, the hormone-binding domain located at the carboxy terminus, and a modulator domain located at the amino terminus. Although all DNA-binding receptor proteins have the same general structure, there is considerable variation in the length of the polypeptide chains of individual proteins (Fig. 10.22). Comparison of the structures of different DNA-binding receptor proteins reveals a high degree of homology in the domains which bind DNA and hormones. Indeed, it was this homology that helped to identify the DNA-binding and hormone-binding domains. Most divergence in the structures of different DNA-binding receptor proteins is observed in the modulator domain at the amino terminal region of each protein.

As described earlier, the DNA-binding domain, which is enriched in cysteine residues, contains two cys2/cys2 zinc fingers. Each zinc finger is encoded by a separate exon. The role of the DNA-binding domain in the action of the hormone–receptor complex has been verified by the construction of mutant forms of the receptor in which the DNA-binding domain is

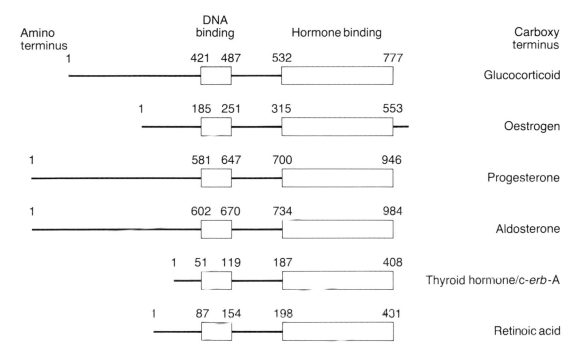

Fig. 10.22 A schematic representation of the primary structures and functional domains of a number of DNA-binding receptor proteins. The amino acid sequences of the DNA-binding domains have been aligned vertically.

deleted. The mutant proteins are unable to bind DNA and are unable to induce gene transcription.

The carboxy terminus of each DNA-binding receptor protein possesses several other substructures in addition to the hormone-binding domain. These other substructures include amino-acid residues which signal the nuclear localization of the DNA-binding receptor protein, a transcriptional activation domain, and a substructure which allows dimerization of the receptor.

A modulator domain is present in some, but not all, DNA-binding receptor proteins. Although the functions of this domain have not yet been clearly defined, some experiments indicate that it may assist in permitting the receptor to distinguish between specific and non-specific binding sites on DNA. The amino-acid sequences which link the modulator, DNA-

binding, and hormone-binding domains have considerable flexibility and are termed hinge regions (Fig. 10.21).

The construction of chimeric receptor DNA-binding proteins has provided a powerful experimental approach for evaluation of the role of the DNA-binding domain in recognizing the hormone-response element in the promoter region of target DNA. These experiments have also shown that this interaction does not depend on the nature of the hormone-binding domain which is attached to the DNA-binding domain. For example, Evans and his colleagues (Giguere *et al.* 1987) have constructed a chimeric receptor which consists of the DNA-binding domain (which binds to the glucocorticoid response element) of the glucocorticoid receptor and the hormone-binding domain of the retinoic acid receptor (Fig. 10.23). The functions of this chimeric receptor, the normal glucocorticoid recep-

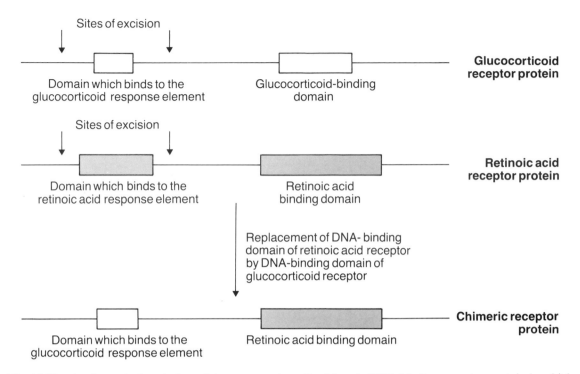

Fig. 10.23 A schematic description of the construction of a chimeric DNA-binding receptor protein in which the DNA-binding domain (which binds to the retinoic acid response element) of the retinoic acid receptor protein is replaced by the DNA-binding domain (which binds to the glucocorticoid response element) from the glucocorticoid receptor.

tor, and the normal retinoic acid receptor were tested by transfecting cultured CV-1 cells separately with the gene encoding each of these receptor constructs. The CV-1 cells employed in this experiment contained a glucocorticoid-response element linked to a reporter gene, bacterial chloramphenicol acyltransferase (CAT). Glucocorticoid induced the transcription of CAT in cells to which the glucocorticoid receptor was introduced but did not affect CAT transcription in cells to which the retinoic acid receptor was introduced. However, retinoic acid but not glucocorticoid induced CAT transcription in cells to which the chimeric receptor was introduced.

10.5.4 *Interaction of DNA-binding receptor proteins with DNA in chromatin*

The hormone–DNA-binding receptor complex binds to specific regions of DNA in the chromatin. This interaction has been most clearly shown for the action of ecdysone using fluorescently labelled antibodies raised against the hormone or against the ecdysone receptor protein, or by electron microscopy. These techniques have shown, for example, that complexes between ecdysone, the ecdysone receptor, and polytene chromosomes of *Drosophila* are formed in specific regions of the chromosome. These regions correspond with loci at which chromosomal puffs are induced by ecdysone (Fig. 10.24). The presence of these chromosomal puffs indicates regions of enhanced gene transcription.

The binding of hormone–receptor complexes to chromatin alters the structure of the chromatin at the site of interaction. Changes in chromatin structure have been detected using the

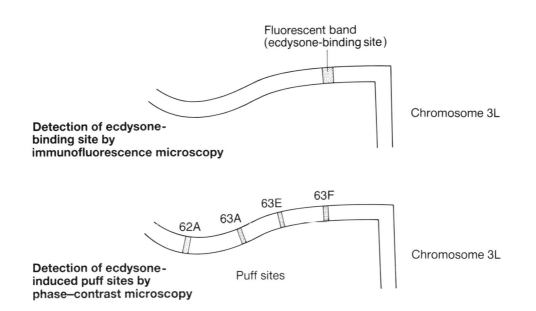

Fig. 10.24 Localization of an ecdysone binding site in the distal part of the chromosome 3L of *Drosophila melanogaster* during the growth period between the third and fourth moult (ecdysis) (the third instar). The location of the binding site for ecdysone corresponds with that of ecdysone-induced chromosome puff 63F. Other chromosome puffs are designated 62A, 63A, and 63E. Ecdysone binding sites in polytene chromosomes were detected using rabbit anti-ecdysone antiserum, fluorescein isothionate-coupled goat ant–rabbit immunoglobulins, and immunofluorescence microscopy. From Gronemeyer and Pongs (1980).

enzyme DNAase 1. Sites at which hormone-induced gene transcription occurs are revealed as regions or domains of increased sensitivity to DNAase. Within these domains are smaller sectors of DNA, termed hypersensitive sites, which are much more sensitive to hydrolysis by DNAase. The binding of hormone–receptor complexes to chromatin alters the number and distribution of both the domains and the hypersensitive sites that are sensitive to the action of DNAase. The mechanism by which hormone–receptor complexes alter chromatin structure is not fully understood. It may involve the introduction of negative supercoils in the DNA.

10.5.5 *Location of the hormone-response elements in specific genes*

Much has been learned about the interaction of DNA-binding receptor proteins with DNA and about the subsequent induction of gene transcription by studying the regulation of a few well-defined hormone-sensitive genes. These include the genes which encode mouse mammary tumour virus (MMTV), the metallothionein gene, and the lysozyme gene, which are all induced by glucocorticoids; the ovalbumin gene and gene p52, which are induced by oestrogen; the uteroglobin gene, which is induced by progesterone; and the C3 gene of prostate cells which is induced by androgens.

One of the most common models for studies of the action of DNA-binding receptor proteins is the MMTV genome. This inducible gene system was discovered accidently when it was observed that glucocorticoids stimulate the formation of MMTV in cultures of mouse mammary carcinoma cells (McGrath 1971). The genome of the mouse mammary tumour virus contains a single strand of RNA. Replication of the virus requires the formation of a DNA intermediate, called the provirus, which is synthesized by a reverse transcriptase encoded by the viral RNA. In the normal life cycle of MMTV, the proviral DNA becomes integrated at random locations into the chromosome of the host cell to form a stable genetic element which behaves in the same manner as the genes which encode other proteins such as tyrosine aminotransferase or albumin. The MMTV genome is then transcribed and the resulting mRNA is translated to form proteins which make up the complete virus.

During synthesis of the MMTV proviral DNA by the reverse transcriptase, sequences at the 5' and 3' ends of the viral RNA are duplicated. The duplicated sequences are called long terminal-repeat sequences (LTR sequences). These sequences are integrated into the host cell DNA along with the viral genome. The long terminal-repeat sequences contain at least one glucocorticoid-response element (Fig. 10.25). This is responsible for the observed ability of glucocorticoids to stimulate transcription of the integrated MMTV by up to 100-fold. The MMTV glucocorticoid-response elements may have been derived from cellular genes during evolution of the virus. This may have conferred a selective

advantage on the virus.

The results of experiments conducted with hormone-sensitive genes like the MMTV gene have shown that the sites on the DNA to which a given hormone–receptor complex binds are located in the vicinity of each of the genes regulated by that hormone–receptor complex. This is indicated by the results of two types of experiment. In the first, glucocorticoid-sensitive genes, such as the MMTV and metallothionein IIA genes, have been transferred from one genomic environment to another. Provided that sufficient nucleotide bases on both the 5' and 3' ends of the gene are transferred with the gene, the glucocorticoid sensitivity is also transferred.

In the second type of experiment, genes which are not responsive to glucocorticoids have been made responsive to the action of these hormones by incorporation of the genes into chimeric DNA molecules. The chimeric DNA consists of the promoter and protein-coding region of the unresponsive gene under test linked to the regulatory region of a glucocorticoid-responsive gene such as the LTR sequence of the MMTV gene (Fig. 10.26). The regulatory region of the glucocorticoid-responsive gene must include the DNA sequences which bind glucocorticoid–

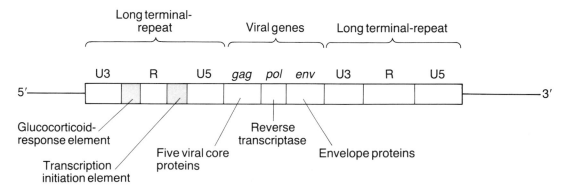

Fig. 10.25 The structure of the MMTV proviral DNA. The proviral DNA is synthesized from the single-stranded RNA which encodes the viral genome by the reverse transcriptase encoded by the *pol* gene of the virus itself. During synthesis of the proviral DNA, sequences at the 5' and 3' ends of the viral genome are duplicated. These sequences are called long terminal-repeat sequences. They contain the promoter region of the viral genome and at least one glucocorticoid response element.

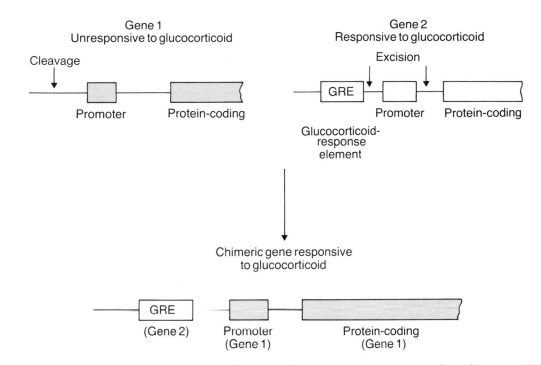

Fig. 10.26 The insertion of a glucocorticoid-response element in the regulatory region of a gene which is normally unresponsive to glucocorticoids renders the gene responsive to glucocorticoids. The chimeric gene is formed by the excision of a glucocorticoid-response element (GRE) from a glucocorticoid-responsive gene (gene 2) and its insertion in the promoter and protein-coding region of a gene that is not responsive to glucocorticoids (gene 1).

DNA-binding receptor proteins. Genes which are normally unresponsive to glucocorticoids but which are transcribed in a glucocorticoid-dependent fashion when linked to the MMTV LTR sequences include the genes for thymidylate kinase and dihydrofolate reductase, and *ras* oncogenes.

Gene transfer experiments have also been used to show that the action of the glucocorticoid regulatory sequences present in the MMTV LTR does not depend specifically on the presence of the MMTV promoter. For example the thymidine kinase gene can be made responsive to glucocorticoids by placing the MMTV LTR sequence from which the promoter region has been removed upstream of the thymidine kinase promoter in the thymidine kinase gene.

The position of the hormone-responsive el-

ement within the regulatory domain of hormone-responsive genes has been determined using the techniques of deletion mutation and DNAase I footprinting. In the latter technique, crude or partially purified nuclear extracts are incubated with the DNA-binding receptor protein under investigation and the enzyme DNAase I. This enzyme hydrolyses all DNA which is not bound to a protein. The base-sequence of the remaining DNA can then be determined. The relationship between the glucocorticoid response element and the transcription initiation site in the regulatory domain of the MMTV gene, determined using these techniques, is shown in Fig. 10.27.

In hormone-responsive genes, the hormone-response element is usually located within a few hundred base pairs at the 5′ region of the tran-

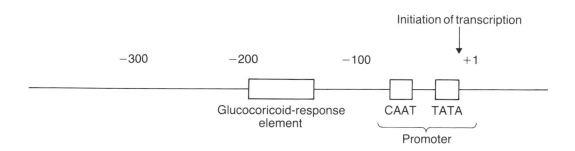

Fig. 10.27 The location of the glucocorticoid response element within the MMTV long terminal-repeat sequence. The core promoter is the minimal region of the long terminal-repeat sequence required for basal levels of transcription. The position of the glucocorticoid-response element has been determined using the techniques of deletion analysis and DNAase I footprinting.

scription start site and is distinct from the core promoter region. However, the distance between the hormone-response element and the promoter element of a gene can be varied considerably and still allow a gene to respond to hormones. Experimental constructs of the steroid-response element in which the distance between the hormone-response element and the promoter is decreased, or is increased by up to 1000 nucleotide bases, or in which the steroid-response element is placed on the 3′ side of the promoter, are also responsive to steroid hormones. These properties of the steroid-response element are characteristic of those of a *cis* element which acts as an enhancer element.

The sequences of nucleotide bases in the hormone-response elements have been identified using the DNAase footprinting technique and base sequence analysis. This has shown that the palindromic consensus sequences which bind DNA are GGTCA*nnn*TGACC (*n* represents any base) in the oestrogen-response element, GAA-CA*nnn*TGTTC in the glucocorticoid-response elements, and GGTCATGACC in the thyroid hormone-response elements. Some hormone-response elements contain multiple copies of the consensus sequence. A given consensus sequence binds to a DNA-binding receptor protein homodimer through the zinc finger motifs of the two DNA-binding domains.

Although it is known that hormone–receptor complexes bind to specific sites on DNA as just described, it is not yet clear how the hormone–receptor complex is directed towards these sites. In experimental systems, hormone–receptor complexes bind to many regions of isolated DNA, not only to those domains thought to contain specific-binding sequences. Additional proteins may be required to direct the hormone–receptor complex within the intact nucleus so that it interacts with specific base sequences. The importance of these protein–protein interactions in the formation of initiation complexes was described earlier in Section 10.2.4.

10.6 Summary

The final step in the action of a number of extracellular signals on a target cell is stimulation of the transcription of a specific set of genes. Extracellular signals which use this general pathway are morphogens and growth factors in the regulation of embryonic development, growth factors in the regulation of the differentiation of cells in an adult animal, mitogens in the stimulation of cell growth and proliferation, and steroid and thyroid hormones in the stimulation of specific cell functions. Each of these agents acts by either directly or indirectly modifying the activity of one or more sequence-specific DNA-binding proteins (DNA-binding proteins). These include various types of sequence-specific transcription factors and the DNA-binding receptor proteins which are receptors for steroid and thyroid hormones and retinoids. Binding of the active form of a sequence-specific DNA-binding protein or a DNA-binding receptor protein to a specific base sequence in the promoter region of a target gene increases the frequency of initiation of transcription of that gene. The product of the target gene may be another DNA-binding protein, which stimulates the transcription of another set of genes, or may be an enzyme or other protein with another cellular function.

The initiation of the transcription of a gene by RNA polymerase II involves the binding to the promoter region of the gene of several DNA-binding proteins, called general initiation factors, one or more sequence-specific transcription factors, which are specific for a small number of genes, and RNA polymerase II which interacts with one or more of the general initiation factors. The sequence-specific transcription factors and general initiation factors bind to *cis* elements in the promoter region of the gene. Some of the *cis* elements to which DNA-binding receptor proteins and some other sequence-specific transcription factors bind are called enhancer elements.

Most sequence-specific transcription factors and DNA-binding receptor proteins bind to base sequences in DNA as homodimers or heterodimers. Each of these DNA-binding proteins possesses a DNA-binding domain, a dimerization domain, a transcriptional activation domain, and a domain which is either phosphorylated or which interacts with a hormone or morphogen. One of several motifs, each with a distinct primary and secondary structure, are present in most DNA-binding domains. These are the helix–turn–helix motif, a cluster of zinc fingers, and a group of positively charged residues that are adjacent to a leucine zipper structure. The leucine zipper structure is responsible for the association of the dimers in some DNA-binding proteins.

The ability of a sequence-specific transcription factor or DNA-binding receptor protein to activate transcription depends on its role as a component of the initiation complex which is formed between the relevant sequence-specific DNA-binding proteins, general initiation factors, RNA polymerase II, and the DNA. Formation of the active initiation complex probably depends on precise interactions between the transcription activation domains of the various DNA-binding proteins and may involve looping of the DNA to which the DNA-binding proteins are attached.

During embryonic development in *Drosophila melanogaster* and, most likely, in other animals the differentiation of cells is regulated by concentration gradients of morphogens within the embryo. Morphogens probably alter the activities of subsets of DNA-binding proteins which, in turn, regulate the transcription of specific sets of genes. An important group of these DNA-binding proteins are the homeotic proteins. These were discovered in *Drosophila* and are recognized as a family by the presence of a conserved sequence of bases, called the homeobox, in the gene which encodes each protein. The homeobox encodes a helix–turn helix DNA-binding motif. In addition to the homeotic proteins, a number of other DNA-binding proteins which regulate cell development have been described. These induce the differentiation of specific cell types, for example muscle cells or blood cells. Another example of the role of DNA-binding proteins in development are the phenotypic changes induced in nerve cells by a variety of external stimuli. These changes are associated with increases in the concentration of the DNA-binding proteins encoded by the *fos* and c-*myc* genes.

The transition of a differentiated cell from the resting G_0 state to the G_1 phase of the cell cycle requires the presence of appropriate mitogens (growth factors). These external signals activate sequence-specific transcription factors, including the *jun* protein, the cyclic AMP response element binding protein, and the serum response factor, through the actions of mobile intracellular messengers and the protein kinases. The activated sequence-specific transcription factors stimulate the transcription of a set of genes called the primary response genes. These include genes which encode the *fos* and c-*myc* proteins, a number of other DNA-binding proteins, and the cyclins, which are involved in regulation of the cell cycle through modification of the action of p34 kinase.

The DNA-binding receptor proteins which are receptors for the steroid and thyroid hormones, vitamin D, and the retinoids differ from other sequence-specific DNA-binding proteins in that they also contain a stereospecific binding site for the hormone or retinoid. In the absence of hormone, the glucocorticoid receptor is located in the cytoplasmic space as a complex with heat-shock protein 90. An increase in the extracellular concentration of glucocorticoid leads to an increase in the concentration of glucocorticoid in the cytoplasmic space as a result of diffusion of the hormone across the plasma membrane. This leads to the binding of glucocorticoid to the glucocorticoid receptor. The resulting complex moves across the nuclear membrane and binds to the promoter regions of target genes. This interaction involves two zinc fingers of the DNA-binding domain of the receptor protein and a *cis* element of the DNA called the hormone-response element. The *cis* element acts as an enhancer element which stimulates transcription of the target gene.

References

Artishevsky, A., Wooden, S., Sharma, A., Resendez, E., and Lee, A. S. (1987). Cell-cycle regulatory sequences in a hamster histone promoter and their interactions with cellular factors. *Nature*, **328**, 823–7.

Bateson, W. (1984). *Materials for the study of variation treated with especial regards to discontinuity in the origin of species.* Macmillan, London.

Fairall, L., Rhodes, D., and Klug, A. (1986). Mapping of the sites of protection on a 55 RNA gene by the *Xenopus* transcription factor III A. A model for the interaction, *J. Mol. Biol.,* **192**, 577–91.

Gehring, W. J. (1987) Homeo boxes in the study of development. *Science*, **236**, 1245–52.

Giguere, V., Ong, E. S., Segui, P., and Evans, R. M. (1987). Identification of a receptor for the morphogen retinoic acid. *Nature*, **330**, 624–9.

Gorski, J., Toft, D., Shyamala, G., Smith, D., and Notides, A. (1968). Hormone receptors: studies on the interaction of estrogen with the uterus. *Recent Prog. Hormone Res.*, **24**, 45–80.

Greenberg, M. E., Greene, L. A., and Ziff, E. B. (1985). Nerve growth factor and epidermal growth factor induce rapid transient changes in proto-oncogene transcription in PC12 cells. *J. Biol. Chem.*, **260**, 14101–10

Green S., Walter, P., Kumar, V., Krust, A., Bornert, J.-M., Argos, P., and Chambon, P. (1986). Human oestrogen receptor cDNA: sequence, expression and homology to v-*erb*-A. *Nature*, **320**, 134–9

Gronemeyer, H. and Pongs, O. (1980). Localization of ecdysterone on polytene chromosomes of *Drosophila melanogaster*. *Proc. Natl Acad. Sci. USA*, **77**, 2108–12.

Ivarie, R. D., and O'Farrell, P. H. (1978). The glucocorticoid domain: steroid-mediated changes in the rate of synthesis of rat hepatoma proteins. *Cell*, **13**, 41–55

Jensen, E. V. and Jacobson, H. I. (1962). Basic guides to the mechanism of estrogen action. *Recent Prog. Hormone Res.*, **18**, 387.

Jensen, E. V., Suzuki, T., Kawashima, T., Stumpf, W. E., Jungblut, P. W., and DeSombre, E. R. (1968). A two-step mechanism for the interaction of estradiol with rat uterus. *Proc. Natl Acad. Sci. USA*, **59**, 632–8.

McGrath, C. M. (1971). Replication of mammary tumor virus in tumor cell cultures: dependence on hormone-induced cellular organisation. *J. Natl Cancer Inst.*, **47**, 455–67.

McGinnis, W., Levine, M. S., Hafen, E., Kuroiwa, A., and Gehring, W. J. (1984). A conserved DNA sequence in homoeotic genes of the *Drosophila*, Antennapedia and bithorax complexes. *Nature*, **308**, 428–33.

Miller, J., McLachlan, A. D. and Klug, A. (1985). Repetitive zinc-binding domains in the protein transcription factor IIIA from *Xenopus* oocytes. *EMBO J.*, **4**, 1609–14.

Mitchell, P. J. and Tjian, R. (1989). Transcriptional regulation in mammalian cells by sequence-specific DNA-binding proteins. *Science*, **245**, 371–8.

Schneuwly, S., Klemenz, R., and Gehring, W. J. (1987). Redesigning the body plan of *Drosophila* by ectopic expression of the homoeotic gene *Antennapedia*. *Nature*, **325**, 816–18.

Scott, M. P. and Weiner, A. J. (1984) Structural relationships among genes that control development: sequence homology between the Antennapedia, Ultrabiothorax, and fushi tarazu loci of *Drosophila*. *Proc. Natl Acad. Sci. USA*, **81**, 4115–19.

Talwar, G. P., Segal, S. J., Evans, A., and Davidson, O. W. (1964). The binding of estradiol in the uterus: a mechanism for depression of RNA synthesis. *Proc. Natl Acad. Sci. USA*, **52**, 1059–66.

Toft, D. and Gorski, J. (1966). A receptor molecule for estrogens: isolation from the rat uterus and preliminary characterisation. *Proc. Natl Acad. Sci. USA*, **55**, 1574–81.

Further reading

Alberts, B., Bray, D., Lewis, J., Raff, M., Roberts, K., and Watson, J. D. (1989). *Molecular biology of the cell* (2nd edn), Chs 10, 16, and 17. Garland, New York.

Beato, M. (1989). Gene regulation by steroid hormones. *Cell*, **56**, 335–44.

Cross, F., Roberts, J., and Weintraub, H. (1989). Simple and complex cell cycles. *Ann. Rev. Cell Biol.*, **5**, 341–95.

Gehring, W. J. and Hiromi, Y. (1986). Homoeotic genes and the homoeobox. *Ann. Rev. Genetics*, **20**, 147–73.

Johnson, P. F. and McKnight, S. L. (1989). Eukaryotic transcriptional regulatory proteins. *Ann. Rev. Biochem.*, **58**, 799–839.

Murray, A. W. (1989). The cell cycle as a cdc2 cycle. *Nature*, **342**, 14–15.

Pardee, A. B. (1989). G_1 events and regulation of cell proliferation. *Science*, **246**, 603–8.

Ransone, L. J. and Verma, I. M. (1990). Nuclear proto-oncogenes *fos* and *jun*. *Ann. Rev. Cell Biol.*, **6**, 539–57.

Ringold, G. M. (1985). Steroid hormone regulation of gene expression. *Ann. Rev. Pharmacol. Toxicol.*, **25**, 529–66.

Weintraub, H., Davis, R., Tapscott, S., Thayer, M., Krause, M., Benezra, R. *et al.* (1991). The *myo* D gene family: nodal point during specification of the muscle cell lineage. *Science*, **251**, 761–6.

Whitelaw, E. (1989). The role of DNA-binding proteins in differentiation and transformation. *J. Cell Sci.*, **94**, 169–73.

Wright, C. V. E., Cho, K. W. Y., Oliver, G., and De Robertis, E. M. (1989). Vertebrate homoeodomain proteins: families of region-specific transcription factors. *Trends Biochem. Sci.*, **14**, 52–6.

Yamamoto, K. R. (1985). Steroid receptor regulated transcription of specific genes and gene networks. *Ann. Rev. Genetics*, **19**, 209–52.

11 *The oncogenes*

11.1 Oncogenes and tumour suppressor genes in the development of knowledge of intracellular communication

The proteins encoded by the normal counterparts of oncogenes play key roles in the processes of intracellular communication. Identification of the oncogenes has made an invaluable contribution to the development of knowledge of intracellular communication since characterization of these genes has led to the discovery of a number of important pathways of intracellular communication and of some of the proteins which play key roles in these pathways. The very existence of transformed cells and tumours in animals and the severity of the consequences which can arise from defects in one or more of the critical steps of intracellular communication also emphasizes the importance of many of the pathways through which information is transferred within cells.

In the preceding chapters, the structures and functions of the proteins encoded by the normal counterparts of the oncogenes have been described. In this chapter, the structures of the oncogenic proteins will be described together with a summary of how the activities of these proteins differ from those of the normal proteins.

In order to understand the nature of oncogenes, it is useful to first consider the complex process by which animal tumours develop, some of the steps in the discovery of oncogenes, how an oncogene is defined, and how a normal gene is converted to an oncogene. Another group of genes called the tumour suppressor genes, the nature and function of which are less clearly defined, also encode proteins which play key roles in the processes of intracellular communication. The properties of these genes, in so far as they are known, will also be described.

11.2 Steps in the process of tumorigenesis

11.2.1 *Development of tumours in animals*
In the current model of tumorigenesis it is proposed that the conversion of a normal cell to one which is fully tumorigenic involves mutations in at least two genes, each of which is the normal counterpart of an oncogene. Each of these genes encodes a protein which plays a critical role in regulation of the cell cycle. One of these proteins is thought to function in the nucleus and the other in the cytoplasmic space.

In experimental systems, tumorigenic cells can be formed by the transfection of normal cells with a combination of mutant *ras* and *myc* genes. These encode cytoplasmic and nuclear proteins, respectively. This observation suggests that mutations in both a *ras* and a *myc* gene will cause an animal tumour. However, few animal tumours contain mutant forms of both *ras* and *myc* genes. It is therefore thought that a tumorigenic cell is generated by at least one mutation in *ras* or another gene which encodes a critical cytoplasmic protein, and at least one mutation in a *myc*-like gene which encodes a nuclear protein. While there is sound evidence to support this model it is undoubtedly an oversimplification of the true picture. For example, mutations in more than two different genes are required for the generation of many tumorigenic cells. Moreover, a number of tumours probably arise as a result of a mutation in one or more tumour suppressor genes.

In descriptions of experimental animal models of the process of tumorigenesis, such as the generation of tumours in mouse skin by the application of a carcinogen, the process of tumorigenesis has been divided into three separate steps. These are initiation, promotion, and progression. Initiation involves a mutation, induced by the carcinogen, in a gene which is probably the normal counterpart of an oncogene such as *ras*. The application of an exogenous promoter permits the formation of one or more clones of cells. Each cell in these clones bears the original mutation. In these experimental systems certain phorbol esters can act as excellent promoters.

Progression is thought to involve a second genetic change which is of very low probability but which occurs in at least one of the large number of cells that have undergone the first genetic change and are growing in a clone induced by the promoter. The second genetic change is probably a mutation in a gene which encodes a nuclear protein. The resulting cells which carry both mutations express all the properties of tumorigenic cells and grow to form a tumour. As described earlier, a similar sequence of events, involving mutations in at least two normal counterparts of oncogenes, is thought to underlie the formation of tumours in humans and animals under normal environmental conditions. However, in this case the mechanisms of promotion most likely differ from the artificial promoters used in experimental animal models.

Each of the steps in the process of tumorigenesis can be considered as a barrier through which the cell must pass if it is to become a tumorigenic cell. These barriers are composed of the normal intracellular and extracellular mechanisms which tightly control cell growth. The intracellular mechanisms probably include the actions of the products of tumour suppressor genes whilst the extracellular controls include the actions of inhibitory growth factors secreted by neighbouring cells.

11.2.2 *Transformation of established cultured cell lines*

In an established cell line such as Rat 1 cells or NIH-3T3 fibroblasts, which express an immortalized phenotype, transfection of cells with a single mutant gene, such as the *ras* oncogene, results in transformed and tumorigenic cells. The term 'transformed cell' is used to describe a cell cultured *in vitro* which, as a result of the introduction of an oncogene to its complement of DNA, has gained the abnormal phenotypic properties, such as loss of contact inhibition, that are characteristic of cells in animal tumours.

It is thought that a single mutant gene can transform cultured cells *in vitro* because the established cell line already contains mutant forms of one or more genes, such as those of the *myc* gene family, which encode nuclear proteins. Indeed, NIH-3T3 cells have been used to test the ability of mutant DNA and potential carcinogens to induce a tumorigenic cell.

Transformed cells differ from their non-transformed precursors in three major ways. Firstly, transformed cells are morphologically different, being typically round and refractile. In a culture of normal cells, transformed cells are often recognized as foci. These are disorganized clusters of the transformed cells. The morphological changes in transformed cells reflect alterations in the structure of the cytoskeleton. Secondly, transformed cells proliferate in the absence of exogenous mitogenic stimuli. This constitutive proliferation is thought to result from the presence of an oncogene which encodes an abnormal growth factor, an abnormal plasma-membrane receptor for a growth factor, or an altered component of one of the pathways of intracellular signalling. The third difference is the ability of the transformed cell to grow without a requirement for attachment to a substrate. This is called anchorage-independent growth. This trait is associated with an alteration in the composition of the extracellular matrix.

11.3   The discovery of oncogenes

11.3.1   *Identification of viral and human tumour oncogenes*

Oncogenes were discovered as components of the genome of certain retroviruses. Retroviruses, such as the Rous sarcoma virus or murine sarcoma virus, can induce tumours in experimental animals and can transform an established cultured cell line, such as NIH-3T3 fibroblasts, from a normal to a tumorigenic state. When

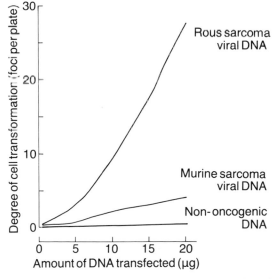

Fig. 11.1 Transformation of NIH-3T3 cultured fibroblasts by DNA from cells transformed by the Rous sarcoma virus or from the murine sarcoma virus induces the growth of cells in foci. Viral-derived DNA was introduced to fibroblasts by exposing the cells to a calcium phosphate precipitate of the DNA. From Copeland *et al.* 1979.

transfected into an established cultured cell line, the RNA isolated from these retroviruses can also induce cell transformation. An example of this is shown in Fig. 11.1 in which the presence of transformed cells is detected by the development of foci on the plates of cultured cells, and transformation has been induced by RNA from the Rous sarcoma virus or the murine sarcoma virus. One of the striking observations about the ability of retroviruses to transform an established cultured cell line was the small size of the viral genome in comparison with the large size of the genome of the transfected animal cell.

It was possible to isolate from the viral genome the gene responsible for transformation of the recipient animal cell. In each retrovirus a single gene, for example *src* or *ras*, was found to be responsible for cell transformation. These genes, which clearly have powerful and wide-ranging effects on the animal cell into which they are transfected, were called viral oncogenes.

Analysis of the properties of the viral oncogenes enabled a further major discovery to be made. In 1976, Stehelin, Varmus, Bishop, and Vogt showed that the *src* oncogene, present in the Rous sarcoma virus, is derived from a gene which is present in normal animal cells. Subsequently it was found that many retroviral oncogenes have counterparts in animal cells. These normal counterparts of viral oncogenes are sometimes called proto-oncogenes.

Another major discovery was made during the period 1978–1985. This was based on the observation that the DNA obtained from human tumour cells could also cause cell transformation when transfected into NIH-3T3 fibroblasts or another established cell line. The experiments showed that one or more specific genes which are present in human tumour cells can induce cell transformation. One of these genes, the *ras* oncogene, which is responsible for the ability of DNA from EJ bladder carcinoma to induce cell transformation, was identified and shown to be of non-viral origin (Shih *et al.* 1979; Shih *et al.* 1981; Krontiris and Cooper 1981; Perucho *et al.* 1981). In 1983, normal counterparts of *ras* oncogenes were detected in normal mammalian cells (Balmain and Pragnell 1983; Sukumar *et al.* 1983; Eva and Aaronson 1983).

Work from many other laboratories showed that there are a number of genes of non-viral origin which are present in human tumour cells and which are capable of transfecting established cell lines. These genes have also been called oncogenes, and their normal counterparts have been called proto-oncogenes. Other experiments showed that, for a number of retroviral oncogenes, there are oncogene counterparts of non-viral origin present in the DNA of human tumours.

11.3.2 *Evolution of knowledge of the function of oncogenes*

The emergence of the idea that only a small number of oncogenes are required to transform a normal animal cell to a tumorigenic cell raised the question of how the abnormal products encoded by these oncogenes could have such a profound effect on a cell. Important discoveries which suggested a partial answer to this question were made between 1978 and 1980. These were the observations that the protein encoded by the *src* oncogene has a protein–tyrosine kinase catalytic site (Collett and Erikson 1978; Hunter and Sefton 1980; Oppermann *et al.* 1979). Not long after this, other workers found that certain plasma-membrane receptors, including those for insulin and EGF, also possess a protein–tyrosine kinase catalytic site on the cytoplasmic domain.

As described in Chapters 1 and 4, it is proposed that, through the phosphorylation of target proteins, the receptor protein–tyrosine kinase provides the mechanism by which signals are transmitted from the receptor to the intracellular enzymes and proteins. This led to the idea that the *src* oncogene protein exerts its effects

on the cell through the phosphorylation of target proteins in a manner analogous to the action of the protein–tyrosine kinase receptors. The idea that the *src* oncogene encodes a protein–tyrosine kinase was confirmed when the amino-acid sequence of the *src* protein was elucidated (Czernilofsky *et al.* 1980; 1983; Schwartz *et al.* 1983; Takeya *et al.* 1982) and found to have considerable homology with receptor protein–tyrosine kinases.

Studies of the *ras* oncogene protein also helped to formulate general ideas about the way in which oncogene proteins function. The proteins encoded by the *ras* genes were first characterized in 1979 by Scolnick and his colleagues (Scolnick *et al.* 1979). The amino-acid sequences of the *ras* proteins were elucidated in 1983 (Capon *et al.* 1983; Fasano *et al.* 1983; McGrath *et al.* 1983; Shimizu *et al.* 1983; Taparowsky *et al.* 1983). These sequences showed considerable homology with the α subunit of the plasma membrane oligomeric GTP-binding regulatory proteins, suggesting that the products of the *ras* genes might be involved in transmembrane signal transduction. Indeed, as described later, while the normal *ras* proteins exhibit GTPase activity, this is significantly depressed in oncogenic *ras* proteins.

While the structures and catalytic properties of the proteins encoded by the *src* and *ras* genes were being elucidated, the properties of the protein products encoded by many of the known oncogenes were described. These are outlined in the next section and categorized according to their proposed mode of action.

11.4   The nature of oncogenes and their normal counterparts

At least 50 oncogenes and their normal counterparts have so far been identified. These can be distinguished by their amino-acid sequences, predicted secondary and tertiary structures,

Table 11.1 *A classification of the normal counterparts of oncogenes by their cellular functions and enzymatic properties*

Gene	Cellular function of gene product
sis *int*-2	Growth factor or morphogen
erb-B *fms*	Plasma-membrane receptors with protein–tyrosine kinase catalytic site
src *abl* *fps/fes*	Protein–tyrosine kinases without transmembrane regions and extracellular domains
mos *raf* (*mil*)	Protein–serine (threonine) kinases
mas	Receptor linked to generation of an intracellular messenger
ras *orf*	Monomeric GTP-binding proteins
gsp	$G_{\alpha s}$, the α-subunit of the oligomeric GTP-binding regulatory protein, G_s
myc *myb* *fos*	Sequence-specific DNA-binding proteins
erb-A	DNA-binding receptor protein

catalytic activities, location within the cell, proposed function, and by some other properties. On this basis, the normal counterparts of the oncogenes can be classified into several groups (Table 11.1). There are a large number of oncogene proteins with protein–tyrosine kinase activity. Only those that have been reasonably well characterized are included in Table 11.1.

As described earlier, many oncogenes are found in transforming retroviruses. A retroviral oncogene is that portion of the viral RNA which is responsible for transformation of the infected cell when incorporated as reverse transcriptase DNA into the host genome. Oncogenes which have been identified in retroviruses are derived from normal counterparts present in animal cells. At some stage in the past, the normal gene was incorporated into the viral genome (Fig. 11.2). For example, the *src* oncogene was acquired from the chicken genome by a retrovirus which has become, in the process, the Rous sarcoma virus.

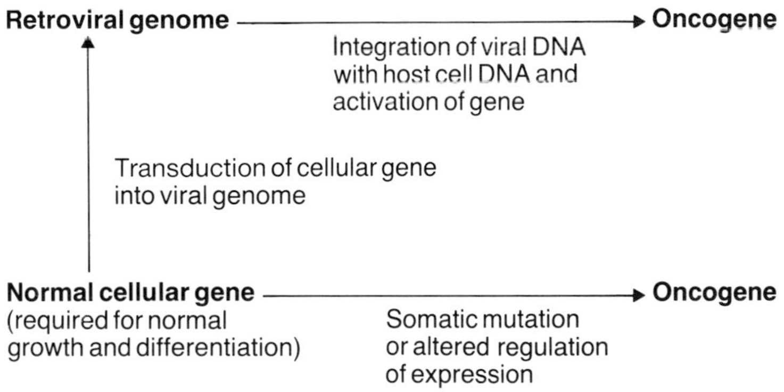

Retroviral genome ──────────────► **Oncogene**

Integration of viral DNA
with host cell DNA and
activation of gene

Transduction of cellular gene
into viral genome

Normal cellular gene ──────────────► **Oncogene**
(required for normal
growth and differentiation)   Somatic mutation
or altered regulation
of expression

Fig. 11.2 Activation of a normal gene to its oncogene counterpart by transduction into the genome of a retrovirus or by somatic mutation. The formation of a retroviral oncogene involves transfer of the normal gene from the genome of an animal cell to the genome of a virus and mutation or rearrangement (activation) of the gene. The viral oncogene can transform a host animal cell if the oncogene is integrated with host cell DNA following infection of the host by the retrovirus. The activation of a normal gene to an oncogene in the absence of a retrovirus involves somatic mutation of the gene or rearrangement of the regulatory elements of the gene.

Infection of a host animal cell by the retro-virus involves the copying of viral RNA into DNA by reverse transcriptase and integration of the viral DNA, including the viral oncogene, into the host cell DNA (Fig. 11.2). The process of gene transfer from the animal genome to viral genome and back to an animal genome may be associated with mutation or rearrangement of the normal gene.

Oncogenes of non-viral origin present in animal tumours are formed from normal genes by somatic mutation or by an event which leads to an abnormal increase in the expression of the gene (Fig. 11.2). These events are described in more detail in the following section. Thus each counterpart of an oncogene can be considered to be a normal gene with the potential to be part of the neoplastic process. One or more specific oncogenes are often associated with a given type of animal tumour.

The expression of the normal counterpart of an oncogene in a given type of cell depends on the state of differentiation of the cell and the stage of the cell cycle that the cell has reached. For example, *fos* and c-*myc* are expressed only at certain times during the cell cycle whereas *ras* is expressed in most cells in G_0 phase as well as during the cell cycle.

The activities of the proteins encoded by the normal counterparts of oncogenes are tightly controlled by either regulation of expression of the gene or regulation of the activity of the protein itself. By contrast, proteins encoded by oncogenes are either synthesized in an uncontrolled manner or are constitutively active and are not constrained by the mechanisms which normally regulate their activity. For example, the *src* protein contains a pseudosubstrate site which is thought to inhibit the activity of this protein–tyrosine kinase. This site is absent in the mutant *src* protein so that the protein–tyrosine kinase catalytic site of this protein is constitutively active.

11.5 Tumour suppressor genes

The fusion of a tumorigenic cell with a normal cell frequently results in hybrid cells which are non-tumorigenic. This observation led to the idea that in each cell one or more genes exist, the product(s) of which suppresses the action of another gene product. These other genes may encode proteins which are expressed during embryogenesis and which stimulate cell growth or the structural transformation of cells during this stage of cell development, but which are not required, and indeed are detrimental to the cells, when the cells enter the differentiated state. A gene which suppresses the actions of one of these growth-stimulating or transforming genes is called a tumour suppressor gene. Tumour suppressor genes are also called growth suppressor genes or anti-oncogenes. Although the tumour suppressor genes may be as important as the oncogenes in the development of animal tumours, much less is known about the nature of tumour suppressor genes.

Although it is suspected that there are a large number of tumour suppressor genes, only a few of these have so far been identified. Three of these are the Rb gene, the p53 gene, and the NF1 gene. The Rb gene encodes a phosphory-lated protein of about 105 kDa molecular weight. The degree of phosphorylation of the Rb protein changes during the cell cycle, although there is no change in the concentration of the protein itself. In the G_0 and G_1 phases the hyposphorylated species predominates whilst in the S and G_2/M phases the hyperphos-phorylated species predominates. It appears that the hypophosphorylated species has the ability to inhibit cell proliferation.

In cells of retinoblastoma and osteosarcoma tumours both alleles of the Rb gene are mutated with loss of the functional Rb protein. At least three viral oncogene proteins, adeno E1A, SB4OLT, and papilloma virus E7, are known to form specific complexes with the normal Rb protein. Since each of these oncogene proteins is a nuclear protein with similarities to the *myc* proteins, the role of the normal Rb protein may be to form a complex with a *myc*-like protein and inhibit its function.

The p53 gene encodes a nuclear protein with a molecular weight of 53 kDa. This protein also forms complexes with certain transforming proteins from DNA tumour viruses. These proteins include the SV40 large T antigen, the E1B protein of adenovirus and the E6 protein of HPV-16 and HPV-18. The p53 protein can be phosphorylated by p34 kinase and by casein kinase II. These or other protein kinases probably play an important role in the regulation of the function of p53. The p53 protein may be a sequence-specific DNA binding protein which inhibits the expression or function of the c-*myc* protein.

The NF-1 protein is a *ras* GTP-ase activating protein (*ras*-GAP) which binds tightly to the *ras* proteins. Since it stimulates the hydrolysis of GTP by the *ras* protein, NF-1 may inhibit the action of the *ras* protein by decreasing the amount of GTP bound to this protein.

11.6   Conversion of normal genes to their oncogenic counterparts

The conversion of a gene its oncogenic counterpart involves either a change in one or more bases in the protein-coding region of the gene or a change in regulation of the expression of the gene. The term 'activation' is broadly used to described these processes.

There are at least five mechanisms by which a gene may be converted to its corresponding oncogene. These are (i) the introduction of one or more point mutations in the protein-coding region of the gene; (ii) the deletion or substitution of sequences of amino acids in the protein-coding region; (iii) rearrangement of the location of the gene in the chromosomes (translocation);

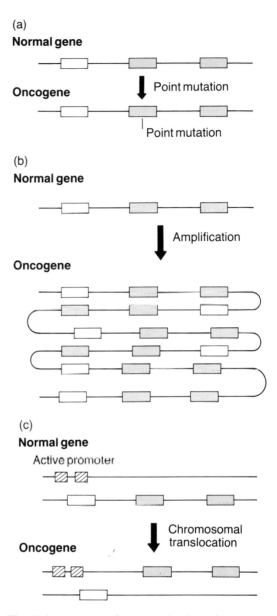

Fig. 11.3 Pathways for the activation of the normal counterpart of an oncogene to an oncogene without the agency of a retrovirus. In the schemes shown, the gene has three exons (rectangular boxes), two of which are transcribed to mRNA (filled rectangles). (a) A point mutation in one of the bases in a region which encodes mRNA. (b) Amplification of the gene. (c) A chromosomal translocation in which the two mRNA coding exons are brought under the control of a more active promoter (hatched rectangles). From Alitalo *et al.* (1987).

(iv) amplification of the gene; or (v) a greatly increased rate of transcription of the gene without a mutation in the base sequences of the gene, such as may occur as a result of the insertion of DNA from a retrovirus. The word 'oncogene' has been used broadly to describe any gene which, when altered in any one of these ways, can induce the transformation of an established cell line, such as NIH-3T3 fibroblasts. An increased rate of transcription of the normal counterpart of an oncogene generally leads to the transformation of an established cell line.

Point mutations are somatic mutations which lead to a change in one of the amino-acid residues in the protein coding region of the gene (Fig. 11.3(a)). For example, generation of the *ras* oncogenes involves point mutations. The amplification of a gene arises from events which lead to the generation of multiple copies of the gene (Fig. 11.3(b)). For example, in neuroblastoma cells, N-*myc* is frequently amplified, and in mouse adrenocortical tumour, K-*ras* is amplified.

A chromosomal rearrangement involves the translocation of DNA from one chromosome to another (Fig. 11.3(c)), or from one region of a chromosome to another region of the same chromosome. This may bring the gene under the control of a different genetic regulatory domain (Fig. 11.3(c)). Two examples of chromosomal rearrangements are activation of c-*myc* in Burkitt's lymphoma and activation of *abl* in Philadelphia chromosome-positive leukaemias.

Several of the oncogenic protein–tyrosine kinases without transmembrane regions and extracellular domains are formed by chromosome translocations. The cells of patients with chronic myeloid leukaemia and those of some patients with acute lymphoblastic leukaemia contain an abnormal chromosome, the Philadelphia chromosome. This is formed by the translocation of DNA between chromosomes 9 and 22 (the t(9;22) (q34;q11) translocation). This trans-

location often results in formation of the *bcr–abl* and *all–abl* fused genes. The products of these genes, p210$^{bcr-abl}$ and p190$^{all-abl}$, both have tyrosine kinase activity. Another example of the formation of an oncogenic protein–tyrosine kinase by chromosome translocation is the v-*fgr* oncogene. This oncogene is formed by fusion of the γ-actin gene with the gene for an unknown protein–tyrosine kinase. An interesting aspect of this gene fusion is the possibility that the γ-actin gene may play a role in oncogenic activity.

The processes just described can account for the conversion of most normal genes to their oncogene counterparts. The properties of the proteins encoded by each group of oncogenes described in Table 11.1 will now be discussed in turn. The first to be considered is the *sis* oncogene which encodes a growth factor.

11.7 The *sis* oncoprotein: a mutated growth factor

The c-*sis* gene encodes the B chain, which is one of two chains comprising platelet-derived growth factor (PDGF). The growth factor is probably an important mitogen in the proliferation of connective tissue cells. Several forms of this growth factor are secreted from a number of types of cell, for example platelets. The forms secreted are an AB heterodimer, designated PDGF, and AA homodimer, and a BB homodimer which is designated PDGF-2. The predominant form of PDGF is PDGF-2. The molecular weights of the A and B chains are 14–18 and 16 kDa, respectively. The two subunits which compose the hetero- and homodimers are linked by disulphide bonds.

The product of the c-*sis* gene undergoes substantial post-translational modification. The primary translation product of c-*sis* has a molecular weight of 26 kDa. This is processed to form a homodimer of molecular weight 56 kDa and in which the two chains are linked by disulphide bonds. This molecule is further processed to yield a dimer of 35 kDa. PDGF and PDGF-2 stimulate cell growth by binding to plasma-membrane receptors on target cells, for example fibroblasts, glial cells, and smooth-muscle cells. Two types of receptors have been identified. These are α (or A)-type receptors which bind AB heterodimers (PDGF), BB (PDGF-2) homo-dimers, and AA homodimers; and β (or B)-type receptors which bind BB homodimers and possibly AB heterodimers.

The v-*sis* oncogene is found in the genome of the simian sarcoma virus. This virus can transform some animal cells. The v-*sis* oncogene encodes a polypeptide chain which contains a region completely homologous with the B chain of normal PDGF flanked by two polypeptide chains which are part of the B chain precursor molecule (Fig. 11.4). One of these flanking poly-peptides is linked to the *env* protein at the amino terminus. The structure of the v-*sis* oncoprotein was first determined in 1983 (Waterfield *et al.* 1983; Doolittle *et al.* 1983; Devare *et al.* 1983).

Cells transfected with the v-*sis* oncogene syn-thesize and secrete a modified form of PDGF-2 (that is a modified form of the BB homodimer). If these cells also possess receptors for PDGF-2, the modified PDGF-2 binds to these receptors, activates the receptor protein–tyrosine kinase, and induces growth (Fig. 11.5). Some exper-iments indicate that, in contrast to the binding of normal PDGF-2 to receptors on the plasma membrane, interaction of the modified form of PDGF-2 with PDGF receptors can also occur at an intracellular site within the cytoplasmic space. In an established cell line such as NIH-3T3 fibroblasts, the presence of the v-*sis* gene induces transformation of the cells. Over-expres-sion of normal c-*sis* gene can also stimulate cell growth and, in an appropriate cell line, transfor-mation of the cell.

The process by which the growth of a cell is stimulated by PDGF or another growth factor synthesized and secreted by that same cell is termed 'autocrine stimulation' (Dulak and Temin 1973). Some evidence that this type of mechanism accounts for the action of modified PDGF-2 in cells transfected with the v-*sis* gene

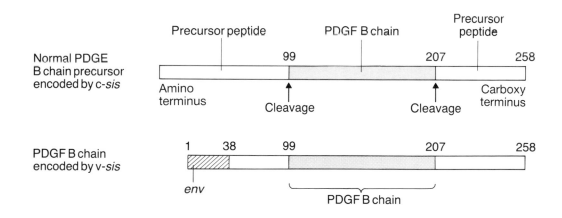

Fig. 11.4 Structures of the precursor of the PDGF B chain encoded by the c-*sis* gene and the protein encoded by the v-*sis* oncogene. The amino terminus of the primary translation product of the v-*sis* oncogene is linked to a polypeptide chain of 38 amino acids derived from the viral *env* gene. The primary translation product of the c-*sis* gene undergoes post-translational modification. This involves cleavage at amino-acid residues 99 and 207. The amino-acid residues from position 99 to position 207 in the v-*sis* polypeptide are identical to those in the PDGF B chain polypeptide.

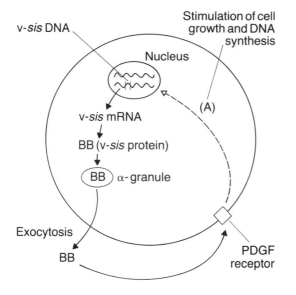

Fig. 11.5 Integration of the v-*sis* oncogene with the DNA of an animal cell can induce the autocrine stimulation of cell growth. Transcription of the v-*sis* oncogene leads to the formation of a dimeric protein composed of two modified platelet-derived growth factor (PDGF) B chains. The modified BB dimer is transferred to α-granules and secreted by exocytosis. In the extracellular space, modified BB dimers bind to receptors for PDGF and stimulate cell growth and division.

has been obtained using antibodies to modified PDGF-2. In some, but not all, experiments these antibodies inhibit cell proliferation induced by v-*sis*. The oncogenic PDGF-2 secreted by a given type of cell may also bind to PDGF receptors on other types of cell which express these receptors. The result of this binding is a stimulation of the growth of these cells.

11.8 The oncogenic protein–tyrosine kinases

11.8.1 *Role of carboxy-terminal tyrosine residue in oncogenic transformation*

As described in Chapter 4 (Section 4.8), the protein–tyrosine kinases encoded by the normal counterparts of oncogenes can be divided into two groups. These are the *erb*-B, *fms*, and a

number of other kinases, which are homologous with plasma-membrane receptors, and the *src*, *abl*, and a number of other kinases, which do not possess a membrane-spanning sequence or an extracellular domain.

The ability of oncogenes which encode protein–tyrosine kinases to transform established cell lines *in vitro* is due to the unusually high intrinsic catalytic activity of the protein–tyrosine kinase domains of these proteins. This high catalytic activity seems to be caused by the absence in the oncogenic protein of a critical tyrosine residue which is present in the carboxy terminus of the protein encoded by the normal gene (Fig. 11.6). This is *tyr* 1173 in the c-*erb*-B kinase, tyr 969 in the c-*fms* kinase and *tyr* 527 in the c-*src* kinase. Autophosphorylation of this critical tyrosine residue in each of these normal cellular proteins inhibits the activity of the protein–tyrosine kinase (Fig. 11.6).

It is thought that the inhibition of protein–tyrosine kinase activity is due to binding of the phosphorylated tyrosine residue to the active site of the kinase in the manner of a product analogue or pseudosubstrate. Interaction of an agonist with a plasma-membrane receptor kinase, or the interaction of an appropriate activator protein with a protein–tyrosine kinase which does not posess a membrane-spanning sequence or an extracellular domain probably alters the conformation of the protein–tyrosine kinase and allows the active site to interact with target proteins. The oncogenic protein–tyrosine kinases, which lack the critical tyrosine residue, are not subject to inhibition and hence are constitutively active, even in the absence of the normal agonist or activator (Fig. 11.6).

Evidence which indicates that *tyr* 527 plays an important role in regulation of the activity of the normal c-*src* protein has been obtained from experiments conducted using site-directed mutagenesis. When *tyr* 527 is replaced by phe, the protein–tyrosine activity of the mutant is 5-

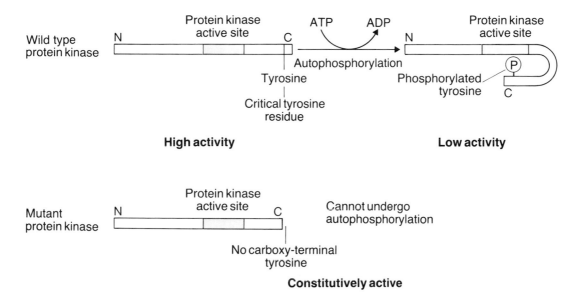

Fig. 11.6 A critical tyrosine residue at the carboxy terminus of a number of protein–tyrosine kinases encoded by the normal counterparts of oncogenes plays an important role in regulation of the activity of these kinases. This tyrosine residue is normally maintained in a phosphorylated form by an autophosphorylation reaction. This results in inhibition of the activity of the kinase. Oncogenic forms of protein–tyrosine kinases lack tyrosine residues in the carboxy terminus. The absence of phosphorylation of the carboxy-terminal tyrosine residue in these mutant forms of the enzyme may be responsible, at least in part, for the high protein–tyrosine kinase activities of these proteins. The amino terminus and carboxy terminus are represented by the symbols 'N' and 'C', respectively.

to 10-fold greater than that of the c src kinase which contains tyrosine at position 527. When introduced into NIH-3T3 fibroblasts, the mutant gene, which contains phe 527, will induce cell transformation.

The substrates for the protein–tyrosine kinases encoded by oncogenes and their normal counterparts were described in Chapter 4 (Section 4.8). The phosphorylation of these substrates leads principally to alterations in the activities of enzymes and proteins which regulate DNA transcription and protein synthesis, and to alterations in the activities of enzymes and proteins which control the structure of the cytoskeleton.

The high intrinsic protein–tyrosine kinase activity of an oncogenic protein–tyrosine kinase protein probably induces the transformation of an established cell line in two ways. One is a

much faster rate of phosphorylation by the oncogenic protein–tyrosine kinase of those substrates normally phosphorylated by the kinase. The second is the phosphorylation of abnormal substrates by the oncogenic protein–tyrosine kinase as a result of an altered substrate specificity and an altered intracellular location of the mutant protein–tyrosine kinase.

11.8.2   *The* erb-B, fms, *and other oncogenic protein–tyrosine kinases: mutated plasma-membrane receptors*

There are at least nine genes which encode protein–tyrosine kinases with homology to plasma-membrane receptors. The normal and oncogenic forms of these genes are listed in Table 11.2. The *erb*-B and *fms* genes encode receptors for the growth factors EGF and CSF-1, respectively. The receptors encoded by the

Table 11.2   *Oncogenes and their normal counterparts which encode protein–tyrosine kinases which share homology with plasma-membrane receptors*

Oncogene	Normal counterpart of oncogene	Polypeptide product of normal gene
v-*erb* B	c-*erb* B	EGF receptor
v-*fms*	c-*fms*	CSF-1 receptor (gp 130/170)
v-*neu*	c-*erb*-B-2	Receptor for unidentified growth factor (P185). Similar, but not identical to, EGF receptor
v-*ros*	c-*ros*	Receptor for unidentified growth factor (homology with insulin receptor)
v-*trk* and *onc* D	c-*trk*	Receptor for unidentified growth factor
trp-met	c-*met*	Hepatocyte growth factor receptor
v-*kit*	c-*kit*	Receptor for mast cell growth factor
sea	c-*sea*	Receptor for unidentified growth factor
ret	c-*ret*	Receptor for unidentified growth factor

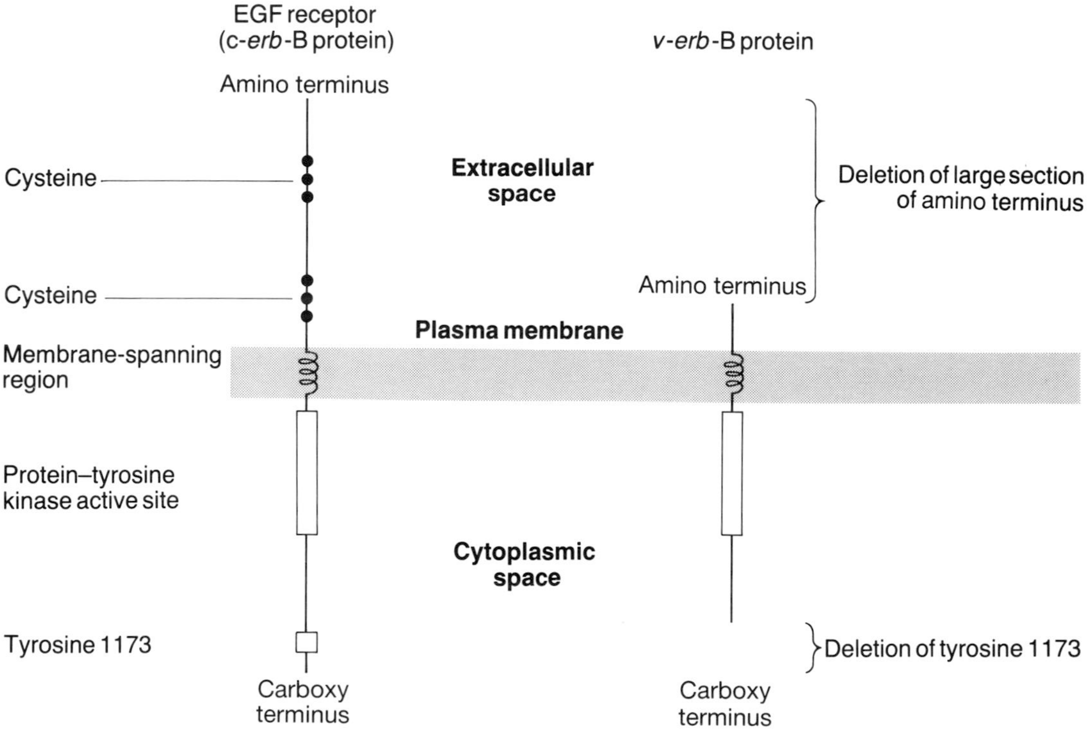

Fig 11.7   Comparison of the primary structures of the EGF receptor, which is encoded by the c-*erb*-B gene, and the protein encoded by the v-*erb*-B oncogene. In formation of the v-*erb*-B oncogene protein, most of the amino-acid residues in the external domain and a small number of amino-acid residues at the carboxy terminus of the EGF receptor have been deleted. The amino-acid sequence of v-*erb*-B protein is identical to the sequence of the corresponding region of the EGF receptor protein. Tyr 1173 represents the major site of autophosphorylation on the EGF receptor protein. Phosphorylation at this site is thought to be essential for regulation of the activity of the EGF receptor protein–tyrosine kinase.

neu, ros, trk, met, sea, and *ret* genes have not yet been fully identified.

The v-*erb*-B oncogene was first identified as one of the genes present in the genome of an avian erythroblastosis retrovirus. The DNA derived from this retrovirus also contains the v-*erb*-A oncogene, the properties of which are described later in Section 11.11. Oncogenic forms of the *erb*-B gene have generally only been found in the genomes of retroviruses: with one exception, none has been detected in animal tumours of non-viral origin.

The protein encoded by the v-*erb*-B oncogene corresponds to the transmembrane domain and most of the cytoplasmic domain of the EGF receptor (Fig. 11.7). This receptor binds TGF-*a* as well as EGF. All the extracellular (amino-terminal) domain, with the exception of the 61 amino-acid residues adjacent to the membrane-spanning sequence, as well as a segment of 32 amino-acid residues at the carboxy terminus, have been deleted in formation of the v-*erb* oncogene. The deleted sequence of the carboxy terminus includes tyr 1173 which, in the EGF receptor protein, is normally phosphorylated and is part of the pseudosubstrate site.

The activity of the v-*erb*-B protein–tyrosine kinase is considerably greater than that of the normal EGF receptor protein–tyrosine kinase in the absence of EGF or TGF-*α* and is independent of the presence of EGF or TGF-*α*. As described earlier, the absence of the pseudosubstrate site composed of tyr 1173 and surrounding residues is thought to explain the

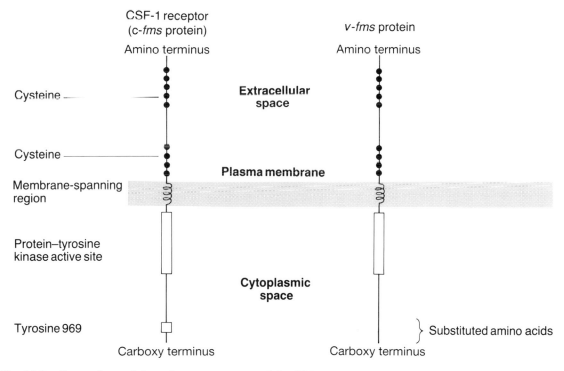

Fig. 11.8 Comparison of the primary structures of the CSF-1 receptor, which is encoded by the c-*fms* gene, and the protein encoded by the v-*fms* oncogene. In the formation of the v-*fms* oncogene the 40 amino acids at the carboxy terminus of the c-*fms* protein have been replaced by 11 unrelated amino acids. With the exception of the 40 amino acids at the carboxy terminus, the amino-acid sequences of the v-*fms* and c-*fms* proteins are identical.

high intrinsic protein–tyrosine kinase activity of the v-*erb*-B protein. However, other components of the v-*erb*-B protein are probably also responsible for the transformation of cultured cells *in vitro*. This is indicated by the observation that the deletion of sections of the carboxy-terminal residues of the v-*erb*-B protein reduces its ability to transform cultured cells.

Like the *erb*-B gene, oncogenic forms of the *fms* gene have generally only been detected in tumours of viral origin. The protein encoded by the v-*fms* oncogene has retained unchanged the complete extracellular and membrane-spanning sequence and a large portion of the cytoplasmic domain of the CSF-1 receptor (Fig. 11.8). However, the 40 amino acids at the carboxy terminus of the c-*fms* protein have been replaced by 11 unrelated amino-acid residues in the v-*fms* protein. This replacement has involved deletion of the critical tyrosine residue, tyr 969 (Fig. 11.8). The loss of *tyr* 969 is probably the cause of the high intrinsic catalytic activity of the v-*fms* protein–tyrosine kinase.

Cells transformed with the v-*fms* oncogene possess an increased number of binding sites for CSF-1. However, the transforming ability of the v-*fms* oncogene seems to be independent of the amount of CSF-1 bound to these sites. It is most likely due to the high intrinsic catalytic activity of the v-*fms* protein–tyrosine kinase which is independent of the binding of CSF-1.

11.8.3   *The* src, abl, *and other oncogenic protein–tyrosine kinases: mutated non-receptor kinases*

A large number of oncogenes and their normal counterparts encode protein kinases that do not possess a membrane-spanning sequence or an extracellular domain. These oncogenes are listed in Table 11.3. Most of these protein–tyrosine kinases are located at the plasma membrane.

The mature c-*src* protein is bound to the cytoplasmic face of the plasma membrane. This protein–tyrosine kinase is probably activated by its combination with an unknown plasma-membrane receptor. The activated c-*src* kinase phosphorylates a variety of substrates, including enzymes and proteins which control the cell cycle. These properties of the c-*src* kinase are described in more detail in Chapter 4, Section 4.8.3.

Several forms of the v-*src* oncogene have been detected. These are derived from the chicken c-*src* gene. An *src* oncogene of non-viral origin has not been detected in animal tumours. Comparison of the amino-acid sequences of the proteins encoded by the c-*src* and v-*src* genes reveals differences in several amino acids within the first

Table 11.3   *Oncogenes and their normal counterparts which encode protein–tyrosine kinases which do not possess a membrane-spanning sequence or an extracellular domain*

Oncogene	Normal counterpart of oncogene	Intracellular location of kinase
v-*src*	c-*src*	Plasma membrane (cytoplasmic side)
v-*yes*	c-*yes*	Plasma membrane (cytoplasmic side)
lck	c-*lck*	Plasma membrane (cytoplasmic side)
v-*abl*	c-*abl*	Plasma membrane (cytoplasmic side)
bcr-*abl*		
all-*abl*		
v-*fps* (v-*fes*)	c-*fps* (c-*fes*)	Cytoplasmic space
v-*fgr*	c-*fgr*	Plasma membrane (cytoplasmic side)

515 residues (Fig. 11.9). However, the major difference between the normal and oncogenic proteins is the deletion of the 19 amino acids at the carboxy terminus of the c-*src* protein and the replacement of this sequence by a variety of unrelated amino acids in the v-*src* proteins. The critical tyrosine residue, tyr 527, which is present in the c-*src* protein, is deleted in each of the v-*src* proteins. As described earlier, this deletion is probably responsible for the high activity of the v-*src* protein–tyrosine kinase.

The specific activity of the protein–tyrosine kinases encoded by the v-*src* genes is up to 20-fold higher than that of the c-*src* protein–tyrosine kinase. This is shown by the observation that cells transformed by the v-*src* oncogene contain concentrations of phosphotyrosine residues which are 5- to 10-fold higher than those of untransformed cells.

11.9 The *ras* oncoproteins: mutated low molecular weight GTP-binding proteins

Three *ras* genes have been detected in mammalian cells. These are c-H-*ras*, c-K-*ras*, and c-N-*ras*. Oncogenes derived from each of these genes are found in many human cancer cells of non-viral origin, as well as in the genomes of certain retroviruses (Table 11.4). The mammalian *ras* genes were first identified in the Harvey and Kirsten strains of rat sarcoma viruses (Harvey 1964; Kirsten and Mayer 1967). As described in Chapter 3 (Section 3.5), there are also a large number of genes, called *ras*-related genes, which encode proteins with considerable homology to the mammalian *ras* proteins. Other genes in this family include the *rap* and *ral* genes.

Each of the mammalian H-*ras*, K-*ras*, and N-*ras* oncogenes differs from its normal counterpart by only one or two point mutations in the protein-coding region. These lead to an amino-acid substitution in one or two of four critical locations in the nucleotide-binding site. These are gly12, gly13, ala59, and gln61 (Fig. 11.10). Activation of the protein is caused by the substitution of gly12 by any amino acid except proline, the substitution of gly13 by val or asp, the substitution of ala59 by threonine, or the substitution of gln61 by lys, leu, or arg. The *ras* oncogenes found in animal tumours of non-viral origin con-

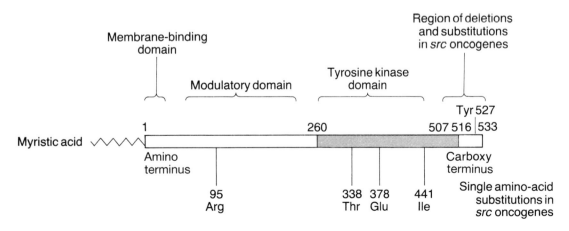

Fig. 11.9 The primary structure of the protein–tyrosine kinase encoded by the c-*src* gene and sites at which mutations occur in formation of v-*src* oncogene proteins. Conversion of the c-*src* gene to v-*src* oncogenes has involved a number of single amino-acid substitutions in the region between amino-acid 1 and amino-acid 507 and considerable alteration in the amino-acid sequence of the carboxy terminus (amino-acids 507 to 533).

Table 11.4 *Origins of the oncogenic* ras *genes found in mammalian cells*

ras oncogenes	Example of origin of oncogene	
	Cell (mammalian tumour)	Retrovirus
H-*ras*	EJ bladder carcinoma	Harvey murine sarcoma virus
K-*ras*-2	Lung carcinoma	Kirsten murine sarcoma virus
N-*ras*	Human neuroblastoma	Not yet detected in viral genome

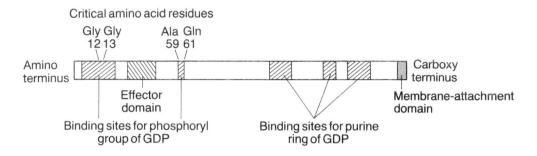

Fig. 11.10 A schematic representation of the primary structure of the normal H-, K-, and N-*ras* proteins showing the location of the amino-acid residues which are mutated in the oncogenic forms of these proteins. These amino-acid residues are located in the guanine nucleotide binding regions. Mutations in the normal *ras* gene which lead to certain amino-acid substitutions at one or more of these sites alter the conformation of the *ras* protein which results in an inhibition of GTP hydrolysis and maintenance of the protein in the GTP-bound conformation.

tain a substitution at only one position whilst the retroviral *ras* oncogenes contain a substitution at two positions. Oncogenic *ras* proteins in which threonine is located at position 59 are autophosphorylated.

As described in Chapter 3, the normal mammalian *ras* proteins link certain extracellular and intracellular signals to reactions involved in cell proliferation and differentiation, although the role of the *ras* proteins in signal transmission is not fully understood. The mechanism of action of these proteins is probably similar to that of the initiation and elongation factors involved in protein synthesis. The normal function of the mammalian *ras* proteins requires the exchange of GTP for GDP and the hydrolysis of GTP.

Analysis of the three-dimensional structures of normal and oncogenic mammalian *ras* proteins by Kim, Nishimura, Ohtsuka, and their colleagues (Tong *et al.* 1989) has indicated that oncogenic mutations in the *ras* gene result in a critical change in the structure of the catalytic site of the *ras* protein. Whilst for most oncogenic *ras* proteins this does not inhibit the binding of GTP, it is responsible for a marked decrease in the rate of GTP hydrolysis (Fig. 11.11). The inability of oncogenic *ras* proteins to hydrolyse GTP probably leads either to a failure to transmit a critical signal which is required to maintain a cell in a differentiated state, or to the constitutive activation of a critical signal which induces cell growth. One of the latter signals is the activa-

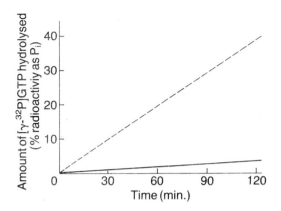

Fig. 11.11 The oncogenic v-H-*ras* protein (full line) hydrolyses GTP at a rate which is considerably slower than the rate of GTP hydrolysis catalysed by the normal c-H-*ras* protein (broken line). From Sweet *et al.* (1984).

tion of protein kinase C although the mechanism by which oncogenic *ras* proteins cause the activation of this protein kinase is not known.

11.10 The sequence-specific DNA-binding proteins encoded by the *myc*, *fos*, and *jun* oncogenes

11.10.1 *Consequences of constitutively high concentrations of the* myc, fos, *and* jun *oncoproteins*

The normal counterparts of the *myc*, *fos*, *jun*, and *myb* genes encode sequence-specific DNA-binding proteins. The properties and some of the probable actions of these proteins are described in Chapter 10. As described in Chapter 10, the cellular concentration of each of the normal *myc*, *fos*, and *jun* proteins increases transiently during the cell cycle in response to the action of a mitogen which switches on the cycle. Each of these proteins binds to a *cis* element in the promoter region of a set of target genes and stimulates the transcription of those genes. The *fos* protein may bind as a heterodimer composed of the *jun* and *fos* proteins.

Cells transformed with oncogenic forms of the *myc*, *fos*, or *jun* genes constitutively express high concentrations of a functional form of the proteins encoded by these genes. This probably leads to a constitutive stimulation of the transcription of the target set of genes for each of these DNA-binding proteins and, consequently, promotes continuous cycles of cell growth and division. In the presence of a complimentary oncogene this can lead to cell transformation. The following sections will describe the nature of the mutations which lead to formation of the *myc*, *fos*, and *jun* oncogenes and how these are thought to result in an increase in the concentration in the nucleus of the oncoproteins encoded by these genes.

11.10.2 *The* myc *oncoproteins*

The principle members of the *myc* gene family are c-*myc*, N-*myc*, and L-*myc*. The c-*myc* gene is found in many types of animal cell. This gene was first detected as an oncogenic form, v-*myc*, in the myelocytomatosis retrovirus. The v-*myc* oncogene is also present in certain other retroviruses which are able to acutely transform infected cells. The N-*myc* and L-*myc* genes were first detected in human neuroblastoma and small lung carcinoma cells, respectively. In each of these cell types the N-*myc* or L-*myc* gene is amplified considerably.

The *myc* genes each contain three exons (Fig. 11.12). The base sequences in exons 2 and 3 are transcribed to mRNA. The three *myc* genes share two highly conserved sequences called the '*myc* boxes'. These are located within the second exon.

Activation of c-*myc* in an animal cell to an environment in which the gene will induce cell transformation involves a rearrangement of the c-*myc* locus. This rearrangement may occur by one of three general mechanisms. The first involves insertion of a viral promoter in a region of the DNA near the c-*myc* gene and a transfer of the control of the transcription of c-*myc* from

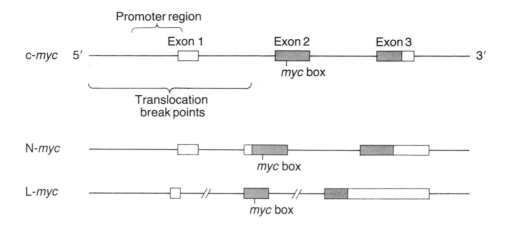

Fig. 11.12 Structures of the c-*myc*, N-*myc*, and L-*myc* genes. Exons are represented by rectangular boxes in which the shaded areas represent translated base sequences. The non-translated exon at the 5' end of the c-*myc* gene is primarily responsible for regulation of the rate of degradation of c-*myc* mRNA. An important promoter region has been identified in the 5' region of this exon. The region of c-*myc* marked 'translocation break points' represents the sequence of DNA in which breaks may occur during chromosome translocations which are found in Burkitt's lymphoma.

the normal cellular promoter to the viral promoter. Insertion of a viral promoter occurs in the induction of B-cell lymphoma in chickens by the avian leukosis virus. The viral DNA integrated with the avian DNA does not, itself, contain a transforming oncogene.

The second mechanism involves formation of the v-*myc* oncogene in the myelocytomatosis virus. The first strain of this virus to be isolated was the MC-29 virus. In people these viruses induce a leukaemic disorder called myelocytomatosis, as well as carcinomas, endotheliomas, and sarcomas. In birds, the viruses induce tumours. In cultured fibroblasts the v-*myc* oncogene also induces transformed but not tumorigenic cells. The genome of the MC-29 virus encodes a single protein of molecular weight 110 kDa. The amino-terminal half of the protein is encoded by the *gag* retroviral gene while the carboxy-terminal half (a 47 kDa peptide) is encoded by exons 2 and 3 of the c-*myc* gene. Exon 1 of the c-*myc* gene is lost in the formation of the v-*myc* oncogene.

A third mechanism by which the c-*myc* locus can be rearranged is chromosomal translocation. The translocation of DNA between human chromosomes 8 and 14 is one of a number of chromosomal translocations which may lead to a greatly enhanced transcription of c-*myc*. This translocation is one of three specific translocations which occur in Burkitt's lymphoma. Each translocation brings c-*myc* under the control of an active promoter. In some 8:14 translocations this is the promoter of the Ig μ-chain gene.

Each of the three mechanisms which cause rearrangement of the c-*myc* locus leads to an increase in the expression of the *myc* gene. The resulting high concentration of *myc* mRNA and protein is responsible for cell transformation. There is generally no mutation in the amino-acid sequences of the c-*myc* protein itself. In the presence of a complimentary oncogene, such as an oncogene encoding one of the protein–tyrosine kinases, or the *mil* or *ras* oncogenes, the presence of a constitutive high concentration of the *myc* protein leads to transformation of the cell.

11.10.3   *The* fos *oncoproteins*

The c-*fos* gene encodes a protein which is designated p55^{c-fos}. Two oncogenic forms of the *fos* gene have been found in the FBJ and FBR osteogenic sarcoma viruses. The protein products of these genes are p55^{v-fos} and p75$^{gag-fos}$, respectively. The p55^{v-fos} protein differs from p55^{c-fos} chiefly in the 49 amino acids in the carboxy-terminal region (Fig. 11.13). This difference is the result of an in-frame deletion which has occurred in the process by which v-*fos* (FBJ) was formed from c-*fos*. The p75$^{gag-fos}$ protein is the product of the fusion of the viral *gag* gene and a mutated form of the c-*fos* gene (Fig. 11.13). A number of amino-acid residues in p55^{c-fos} have been deleted in formation of the *fos* component of the p75$^{gag-fos}$ protein (Fig. 11.13).

The intracellular concentration of c-*fos* mRNA is controlled both by the rate of transcription of the c-*fos* gene and by the rate of degradation of c-*fos* mRNA. Alterations to both of these processes occur following oncogenic activation of c-*fos*. For example, conversion of c-*fos* to the FBR v-*fos* oncogene results in removal of a non-coding base sequence located after the TGA termination site at the 3' region as well as the addition of viral long terminal-repeat sequences. Removal of the non-coding sequence increases the stability of the *fos* mRNA while the long terminal-repeat sequences enhance transcription of the v-*fos* gene.

11.10.4   *The* jun *oncoprotein*

The c-*jun* gene was discovered as an oncogenic form, v-*jun*. The latter is a 0.93 kb insert in the genome of the replication-defective retrovirus, avian sarcoma virus 17 (ASV 17). This virus causes fibrosarcomas in chickens and, when introduced into avian embryonic fibroblasts in culture, induces tumorigenic cells. In the genome of ASV 17, part of the *gag* and *env* genes, and all of the *pol* gene, have been replaced by an altered form of the c-*jun* gene. In the conversion of c-*jun* to v-*jun*, a group of 27 amino-acid resi-

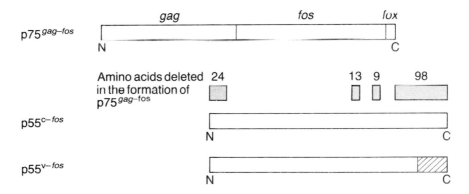

Fig. 11.13   A schematic representation of the primary structures of the protein, p55^{c-fos}, encoded by the c-*fos* gene, the protein p55$^{gag-fos}$, encoded by the v-*fos* oncogene of the FBJ-murine sarcoma virus, and the protein p55^{v-fos}, encoded by the v-*fos* oncogene of the FBR-murine sarcoma virus. 'N' and 'C' represent the amino terminus and carboxy terminus, respectively. The p75$^{gag-fos}$ protein contains a 310 amino-acid polypeptide encoded by the *gag* gene, a 236 amino-acid peptide derived from c-*fos* and a short 8 amino-acid peptide (*fox*). Four regions of the p55^{c-fos} sequence have been deleted in formation of the p75$^{gag-fos}$. The deleted regions and the number of amino acids in each deleted region are indicated by the shaded boxes above p55^{c-fos}. In the p55^{v-fos} polypeptide chain the first 332 amino acids are identical to those of p55^{c-fos}. However, a number of the 49 amino-acid residues at the carboxy terminus of p55^{v-fos} differ from the corresponding residues in p55^{c-fos}. These are shown by the hatched area in p55^{v-fos}.

dues has been deleted from the amino terminal of the molecule and three amino acids in the carboxy terminus have been substituted by non-conservative amino acids.

At least two other genes, *jun*-B and *jun*-D, which are related to c-*jun*, have been detected in animal cells. There is considerable homology between the proteins encoded by the three normal *jun* genes, in the regions of the three major structural domains of the proteins.

The induction of tumours by ASV 17 is probably due to an abnormally high concentration of the *jun* protein rather than to the altered amino-acid sequences which are present in the v-*jun* protein. The over-expression of c-*jun* in a retroviral vector can induce the oncogenic transformation of an established cultured rat cell line.

11.11   The *erb*-A oncoprotein: a mutated DNA-binding receptor protein

The v-*erb*-A oncogene is part of the genome of the avian erythroblastosis virus. This oncogene arose from alteration of the cellular c-*erb*-A gene during transfer from the avian genome to the viral genome (Vennström *et al.* 1982). Infection of chickens with the avian erythroblastosis virus inhibits the differentiation of erythroblasts to erythrocytes and induces a transformed erythroblast phenotype which causes erythroleukaemia.

The genome of the erythroblastosis virus also contains the v-*erb*-B oncogene. As described earlier, this oncogene encodes a truncated version of the EGF receptor. The ability of the avian erythroblastosis virus to induce the transformation of a cell is primarily due to the presence of the v-*erb*-B oncogene. Introduction of the v-*erb*-A gene alone into many established cell lines does not cause cell transformation, although the v-*erb*-A protein is sufficient to transform erythrocyte progenitor cells *in vitro*. However, in established cell lines, v-*erb*-A enhances the transformation induced by the v-*erb*-B oncogene and by other primary oncogenes which induce sarcomas.

The v-*erb*-A oncogene encodes a protein which is a mutant form of a receptor for the thyroid hormones, 3,5,3'-triiodothyronine (T_3) and thyroxine (T_4). Normal receptors for thyroid hormones are encoded by the c-*erb*-A genes. The properties of these were described in Chapter 10 (Section 10.5). The polypeptide encoded by the v-*erb*-A oncogene, $p75^{gag-v-erb-A}$, contains an unchanged DNA-binding domain but an altered hormone-binding domain. This is shown by the observation that $p75^{gag-v-erb-A}$ cannot bind thyroid hormone (Fig. 11.14).

The v-*erb*-A oncoprotein binds to the thyroid hormone response element in the promoter

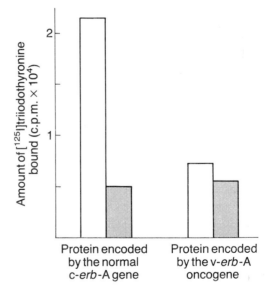

Fig. 11.14   An experiment which shows that the v-*erb*-A protein does not bind triiodothyronine. The ability of the proteins encoded by the normal c-*erb*-A gene and the v-*erb*-A oncogene to bind triiodothyronine was measured using [^{125}I]triiodothyronine. The amount of [^{125}I]triiodothyronine bound was measured in the absence of a competitor (open bars) and in the presence of a 1000-fold excess of unlabelled triiodothyronine (solid bars). From Sap *et al.* (1987).

regions of thyroid hormone-responsive genes. In cells which express thyroid-hormone receptors and which are exposed to thyroid hormone, this results in an inhibition of the normal ability of the thyroid hormone–thyroid-hormone receptor complex to stimulate the transcription of thyroid hormone-responsive genes. Thus the v-*erb*-A oncoprotein acts as a dominant antagonist of the actions of the thyroid hormone–thyroid-hormone receptor complex.

11.12   Summary

The conversion of a normal cell to a tumorigenic cell involves mutations in at least two genes. The mutated genes belong to a small group of genes called oncogenes and to a small group of genes called tumour suppressor genes. The normal counterparts of oncogenes play critical roles in cellular growth and differentiation. Tumour suppressor genes probably encode proteins which inhibit the actions of other proteins which also have critical roles in cell differentiation. Many of these have yet to be defined and only a few tumour suppressor genes have been characterized. Knowledge of the oncogenes has made an important contribution to elucidation of the pathways of intracellular communication by allowing the identification of key proteins in these pathways.

There are over 50 known oncogenes. The normal counterparts of these genes encode growth factors, receptor protein–tyrosine kinases, protein–tyrosine kinases which do not possess a membrane–spanning sequence or an extracellular domain, receptors linked to the generation of intracellular messengers, low molecular weight GTP-binding proteins, sequence-specific DNA-binding proteins, or DNA-binding receptor proteins. An oncogene differs from its normal counterpart by a mutation, base lesion, or a base substitution in the protein-coding region of the gene, or by an alteration in the regulatory region which often leads to an increased expression of the gene. Oncogenes can arise from their normal counterparts as a result of the transfer of a portion of the DNA in an animal cell to the genome of a retrovirus, or by a somatic mutation or chromosomal translocation. The mutant protein encoded by an oncogene is constitutively active or is constitutively expressed. In contrast, the activity and expression of the protein encoded by the normal counterpart of the oncogene is closely regulated.

The v-*sis* oncogene encodes a modified form of the B chain of platelet-derived growth factor (PGDF). A cell transfected with v-*sis* secretes BB dimers of PDGF. If this same cell also possesses PDGF receptors, growth of the transfected cell is stimulated in an autocrine manner.

The v-*erb*-B and v-*fms* genes encode altered forms of the epidermal growth factor (EGF) and colony-stimulating factor (CSF) receptor protein–tyrosine kinases, respectively. A number of oncogenes encode mutated forms of protein–tyrosine kinases which do not possess a membrane-spanning sequence or an extracellular domain. For example, the v-*src* protein–tyrosine kinase contains a number of amino-acid substitutions, the most important of which occurs at tyr 507 near the carboxy terminus. The mutated protein–tyrosine kinases are constitutively active. This is probably due to the lack of a critical tyrosine residue normally present at the carboxy terminus of the proteins. In the normal protein this tyrosine residue is phosphorylated and probably acts as a pseudosubstrate which inhibits protein–tyrosine kinase activity in the absence of a growth factor. The constitutive activity of the oncogenic protein–tyrosine kinases leads to an increased phosphorylation of proteins which are targets for the normal counterparts of these protein–tyrosine kinases and possibly also to the phosphorylation of other proteins.

The oncogenic *ras* proteins differ from the

normal c-*ras* proteins by a change in one or two amino acids at the GTP-binding site. These amino-acid substitutions arise from point mutations in the c-*ras* gene. It is probable that the greatly diminished ability of oncogenic *ras* proteins to hydrolyse GTP leads to constitutive activation or constitutive inhibition of signals normally conveyed by c-*ras* proteins.

The *myc*, *myb*, *fos*, and *jun* oncogenes encode sequence-specific DNA-binding proteins. Generation of the *myc* oncogene leads to a greatly increased rate of transcription of the *myc* gene whilst generation of the *fos* and *jun* oncogenes probably leads to a greatly decreased rate of degradation of the mRNA and proteins encoded by each of these genes. Constitutive expression of high concentrations of the *myc*, *fos*, or *jun* proteins in the absence of mitogens leads to activation of transcription of sets of genes which are targets for the *myc*, *fos*, or *jun* DNA-binding proteins and to a constitutive stimulation of cell growth.

Oncogenic v-*erb*-A encodes a mutant form of the thyroid-hormone receptor. Compared with the c-*erb*-A protein, the normal form of the thyroid-hormone receptor, the v-*erb*-A protein has retained its ability to bind DNA but has lost the binding site for thyroid hormone. In cells which express thyroid-hormone receptors, the v-*erb*-A protein inhibits the stimulation of DNA transcription by the normal thyroid hormone–thyroid-hormone receptor complex.

References

Alitalo, K., Koskinen, P., Makela, T. P., Saksela, K., Sistonen, L., and Winqvist, R. (1987). *myc* oncogenes: activation and amplification. *Biochim. Biophys. Acta*, **907**, 1–32.

Balmain, A. and Pragnell, I. B. (1983). Mouse skin carcinomas induced *in vivo* by chemical carcinogens have a transforming Harvey-*ras* oncogene. *Nature*, **303**, 72–4.

Capon, D. J., Chen, E. Y., Levinson, A. D., Seeburg, P. H., and Goeddel, D. V. (1983). Complete nucleotide sequences of the T24 human bladder carcinoma oncogene and its normal homologue. *Nature*, **302**, 33–7.

Collett, M. S. and Erikson, R. L. (1978). Protein kinase activity associated with the avian sarcoma virus *src* gene product. *Proc. Natl Acad. Sci. USA*, **75**, 2021–4.

Copeland, N. G., Zelenetz, A. D., and Cooper, G. M. (1979). Transformation of NIH-3T3 mouse cells by DNA of Rous sarcoma virus. *Cell*, **17**, 993–1002.

Czernilofsky, A. P., Levinson, A. D., Varmus, H. E., Bishop, J. M., Tischer, E., and Goodman, H. M. (1980). Nucleotide sequence of an avian sarcoma virus oncogene (*src*) and proposed amino acid sequence for the gene product. *Nature*, **287**, 198–203.

Czernilofsky, A. P., Levinson, A. D., Varmus, H. E., Bishop, J. M., Tischer, E., and Goodman, H. M. (1983). Corrections to the Rous sarcoma virus. *Nature*, **301**, 736–8.

Devare, S. G., Reddy, E. P., Law, J. D., Robbins, K. C., and Aaronson, S. A. (1983). Nucleotide sequence of the simian sarcoma virus genome: demonstration that its acquired cellular sequences encode the transforming gene product p28^{sis}. *Proc. Natl Acad. Sci, USA.*, **80**, 731–5.

Doolittle, R. F., Hunkapiller, M. W., Hood, L. E., Devare, S. G., Robbins, K. C., Aaronson, S. A., and Antoniades, H. N. (1983). Simian sarcoma virus *onc* gene, v-*sis*, is derived from the gene (or genes) encoding a platelet-derived growth factor. *Science*, **221**, 275–7.

Dulak, N. C. and Temin, H. M. (1973). Multiplication-stimulating activity for chicken embryo fibroblasts from rat liver cell conditional medium: a family of small polypeptides. *J. Cell. Physiol.*, **81**, 161–70.

Eva, A. and Aaronson, S. A. (1983). Frequent activation of c-*kis* as a transforming gene in fibrosarcomas induced by methylcholanthrene. *Science*, **220**, 955–6.

Fasano, O., Taparowsky, E., Fiddes, J., Wigler, M., and Goldfarb, M. (1983). Sequence and structure of the coding region of the human H-*ras*-1 gene from T24 bladder carcinoma cells. *J. Mol. Appl. Genetics*, **2**, 173–80.

Harvey, J. J. (1964). An unidentified virus which causes the rapid production of tumours in mice. *Nature*, **204**, 1104–5.

Hunter, T. and Sefton, B. M. (1980). Transforming gene product of Rous sarcoma virus phosphorylates tyrosine. *Proc. Natl Acad. Sci. USA*, **77**, 1311–15.

Kirsten, W. H. and Mayer, L. A. (1967). Morphologic responses to murine erythroblastosis virus. *J. Natl Cancer Inst.*, **39**, 311–35.

Krontiris, T. G. and Cooper, G. M. (1981). Transforming activity of human tumour DNAs. *Proc. Natl Acad. Sci. USA*, **78**, 1181–4.

McGrath, J. P., Capon, D. J., Smith, D. H., Chen, E. Y., Seeburg, P. H., Goeddel, D. V., and Levinson, A. D. (1983). Structure and organisation of the human Ki-*ras* protooncogene and a related processed pseudo gene. *Nature*, **304**, 501–6.

Oppermann, H., Levinson, A. D., Levintow, L., Varmus, H. E., and Bishop, J. M. (1979). Uninfected vertebrate cells contain a protein that is closely related to the product of the avian sarcoma virus transforming gene (*src*). *Proc. Natl Acad. Sci. USA*, **76**, 1804–8.

Perucho, M., Goldfarb, M., Shimizu, K., Lama, C., Fogh, J., and Wigler, M. (1981). Human-tumour-derived cell lines contain common and different transforming genes. *Cell*, **27**, 467–76.

Sap, J., Munoz, A., Damm, K., Goldberg, Y., Ghysdael, J., Leutz, A. *et al.* (1986). The c-*erb*-A protein is a high-affinity receptor for thyroid hormone. *Nature*, **324**, 635–40.

Scolnick, E. M., Papageorge, A. G., and Shih, T. Y. (1979). Guanine nucleotide-binding activity as an assay for *src* protein of rat-derived murine sarcoma viruses. *Proc. Natl Acad. Sci. USA*, **76**, 5355–9.

Schwartz, D. E., Tizard, R., and Gilbert, W. (1983). Nucleotide sequence of Rous sarcoma virus. *Cell*, **32**, 853–69.

Shih, C., Shilo, B.-Z., Goldfarb, M. P., Dannenberg, A., and Weinberg, R. A. (1979). Passage of phenotypes of chemically transformed cells via transfection of DNA and chromatin. *Proc. Natl Acad. Sci.*

USA, **76**, 5714–18.

Shih, C., Padhy, L. C., Murray, M., and Weinberg, R. A. (1981). Transforming genes of carcinomas and neuroblastomas introduced into mouse fibroblasts. *Nature*, **290**, 261–4.

Shimizu, K., Birnbaum, D., Ruley, M., Fasano, O., Suard, Y., Edlund, L. *et al.* (1983). The structure of the Ki-*ras* gene of the human lung carcinoma cell line Calu-1. *Nature*, **304**, 497–500.

Stehelin, D., Varmus, H. E., Bishop, J. M., and Vogt, P. K. (1976). DNA-related to the transforming gene(s) of avian sarcoma viruses is present in normal avian DNA. *Nature*, **260**, 170–3.

Sukumar, S., Notario, V., Martin-Zanca, D., and Barbacid, M. (1983). Induction of mammary carcinomas in rats by nitroso-methylurea involves malignant activation of H-*ras*-1 locus by single point mutations. *Nature*, **306**, 658–61.

Sweet, R. W., Yokoyama, S., Kamata, T., Feramisco, J. R., Rosenberg, M., and Gross, M. (1984). The product of *ras* is a GTPase and the T24 oncogenic mutant is deficient in this activity. *Nature*, **311**, 273–5.

Takeya, T., Feldman, R. A., and Hanafusa, H. (1982). DNA sequence of the viral and cellular *src* gene of chicken. The complete nucleotide sequence of an *Eco* RI fragment of recovered avian sarcoma virus which codes for gp37 and pp60^*src*. *J. Virol.*, **44**, 1–11.

Taparowsky, E., Shimizu, K., Goldfarb, M., and Wigler, M. (1983). Structure and activation of human N-*ras* gene. *Cell*, **34**, 581–6.

Tong, L., de Vos., A. M., Milburn, M. V., Jancarik, J., Noguchi, S., Nishimura, S. *et al.* (1989). Structural differences between a *ras* oncogene protein and the normal protein. *Nature*, **337**, 90–3.

Vennström, B. and Bishop, J. M. (1982). Isolation and characterisation of chicken DNA homologous to the two putative oncogenes of avian erythroblastosis virus. *Cell*, **28**, 135–43.

Waterfield, M. D., Scrace, T., Whittle, N., Stroobant, P., Johnsson, A., Wasteson, A. *et al.* (1983). Platelet-derived growth factor is structurally related to the putative transforming protein p28^*sis* of simian sarcoma virus. *Nature*, **304**, 35–9.

Further reading

Barbacid, M. (1987), *ras* Genes. *Ann. Rev. Biochem.*, **56**, 779–827.

Bishop, J. M. (1983). Cellular oncogenes and retroviruses. *Ann. Rev. Biochem.*, **52**, 301–54.

Bishop, J. M. (1991). Molecular themes in oncogenesis. *Cell*, **64**, 235–48.

Bradshaw, R. A. and Prentis, S. (1987). *Oncogenes and growth factors*. Elsevier, Amsterdam.

Cole, M.D. (1986). The *myc* oncogene: its role in transformation and differentiation. *Ann. Rev. Genetics*, **20**, 361–84.

Hunter, T. (1991). Cooperation between oncogenes. *Cell*, **64**, 249–70.

Jove, R. and Hanafusa, H. (1987). Cell transformation by the viral *src* oncogene. *Ann. Rev. Cell Biol.*, **3**, 31–56.

Lewin, B. (1991). Oncogenic conversion by regulatory changes in transcription factors. *Cell*, **64**, 303–12.

Marshall, C. J. (1991). Tumor suppressor genes. *Cell*, **64**, 313–26.

Varmus, H. E. (1984). The molecular genetics of cellular oncogenes. *Ann. Rev. Genetics*, **18**, 553–612.

12 *Interactions between pathways of intracellular communication*

12.1 Parallel pathways and interactions between these pathways

The previous chapters were devoted to a definition of each of the known pathways of communication within the animal cell and have provided a description of the components which constitute these pathways. With some exceptions, each pathway was treated in isolation, or a section of the complete pathway was examined. However, many extracellular signals activate more than one intracellular signalling pathway. This activation is due either to the initiation of a signal along two or more pathways starting at the plasma membrane, or to secondary effects of one signalling pathway on components of another pathway. In addition, most cells are exposed to more than one agonist simultaneously. This results in activation of more than one intracellular signalling pathway.

Table 12.1 *Examples of interactions between pathways of intracellular communication*

Regulation by $[Ca^{2+}]_i$ of cyclic AMP concentration
Regulation by protein kinase C of cyclic AMP concentration
Regulation by cyclic AMP of $[Ca^{2+}]_i$
Synergism between protein kinase C and (Ca^{2+} calmodulin)-dependent protein kinases
Inhibition of the actions of receptors and G proteins by protein kinase C
Control of Ins 1,4,5 P_3 concentration and $[Ca^{2+}]_i$ by protein kinase C
Interactions between sequence-specific DNA-binding proteins

Most pathways of intracellular communication interact with at least one other intracellular pathway. Some examples of these interactions are listed in Table 12.1. Sometimes the interactions are described as 'cross talk' between pathways, although this term is a little imprecise. Interactions between pathways can be complex and the full implications of these are not yet fully understood. One set of interactions about which considerable knowledge has been obtained are those between Ca^{2+} and cyclic AMP. The existence of multiple pathways of intracellular communication and of interactions between these pathways is well illustrated by the actions of mitogens in inducing cell proliferation.

In this chapter, the interactions between cyclic AMP and Ca^{2+} will be examined further, and the stimulation of mitogenesis and the cellular actions of insulin used as examples of systems which employ multiple parallel pathways that interact with each other. These examples will be used to identify some of the general themes which underlie the processes which constitute any pathway of intracellular communication and to indicate likely directions of future research.

12.2 Interactions between the Ca^{2+} and cyclic AMP pathways

In a number of types of cell, for example platelets, β-cells of the pancreas, and smooth-muscle cells, an agonist or the combination of two or more agonists induces increases in the intracellular concentrations of both $[Ca^{2+}]_i$ and cyclic AMP. The changes in the concentrations of these two intracellular messengers often exhibit different time-courses. These changes in $[Ca^{2+}]_i$ and cyclic AMP may arise from the actions of two different agonists at two different plasma-membrane receptors, one of which causes an increase in cyclic AMP concentration and the other an increase in $[Ca^{2+}]_i$. Alternatively, they may arise from the interaction of one type of agonist with one type of receptor which causes an increase in the concentration of one intracellular messenger (Ca^{2+} or cyclic AMP) which, in turn, increases the concentration of the other intracellular messenger. At the molecular level, these interactions are achieved by cyclic AMP-dependent protein kinase, which can modify the movement of Ca^{2+} across intracellular membranes, and by (Ca^{2+} + calmodulin)-dependent protein kinase, which can modify the formation and degradation of cyclic AMP.

Interactions between cyclic AMP and Ca^{2+} have been studied extensively by H. Rasmussen and his colleagues. Although these studies have classified some major types of interaction between these two intracellular messenger pathways, there is still much to be learned before a full description of these interactions can be provided for any given cell type.

Three types of interaction between Ca^{2+} and cyclic AMP have been identified. In the first, an increase in $[Ca^{2+}]_i$ alters the activities of enzymes which synthesize or degrade cyclic AMP. In most cells, Ca^{2+} activates cyclic AMP phosphodiesterase and, depending on the cell type, may activate or inhibit adenylate cyclase. In the second type of interaction, an increase in the concentration of cyclic AMP alters the activities of Ca^{2+} channels and Ca^{2+} transporters. In some excitable cells, for example heart muscle cells, cyclic AMP-dependent protein kinase activates voltage-operated Ca^{2+}

channels. This leads to an increase in the maximum value of $[Ca^{2+}]_i$ achieved each time the channel is opened. In other cell types, for example platelets and smooth-muscle cells, cyclic AMP-dependent protein kinase activates the plasma membrane or endoplasmic (Ca^{2+} + Mg^{2+}) ATPase. This leads to a decrease in $[Ca^{2+}]_i$. Cyclic AMP-dependent protein kinase can also stimulate the plasma-membrane (Na^+ + K^+)ATPase. This may induce a decrease in $[Ca^{2+}]_i$ through alteration of the Na^+ gradient across the plasma membrane and the subsequent activation of Ca^{2+} outflow through the Na^+-Ca^{2+} exchange system.

The third type of interaction between cyclic AMP and Ca^{2+} occurs at the site of phosphorylation of the target proteins. For example, phosphorylation of (Ca^{2+} + calmodulin)-dependent protein kinase or protein kinase C by cyclic AMP-dependent protein kinase alters the sensitivity of these enzymes to Ca^{2+}. There are many examples in which cyclic AMP-dependent protein kinase and (Ca^{2+} + calmodulin)-dependent protein kinase phosphorylate the same or different target enzymes in a particular metabolic pathway. For example, glycogen phosphorylase kinase and glycogen synthetase in the pathways of glycogen metabolism and pyruvate kinase in the glycolytic pathway can each be phosphorylated by both cyclic AMP-dependent protein kinase and (Ca^{2+} + calmodulin)-dependent protein kinase.

12.3 Stimulation of cell proliferation: an example of parallel pathways of intracellular communication

Cultured Swiss 3T3 fibroblasts, which are partially transformed cells, cease to grow and enter the resting state, G_0, when the growth medium becomes depleted of growth factors. These quiescent cells can be induced to enter the G_1 phase of the cell cycle, to grow, re-initiate DNA

Table 12.2   *The relative effectiveness of a number of mitogenic growth factors in stimulating the re-initiation of DNA synthesis in quiescent Swiss 3T3 fibroblasts. The effects of each growth factor added alone (the diagonal) or the effects of the combination of two growth factors are shown. The amount of DNA synthesis is described quantitatively by the symbols (−), no DNA synthesis; (+), lowest amount of synthesis; and (+ + + +), maximal amount of synthesis. The addition of serum in place of growth factors gives maximal stimulation of DNA synthesis. From Rozengurt (1986)*

Mitogen	Mitogen					
	PDGF	Bombesin	Vasopressin	Insulin	EGF	PGE$_1$
PDGF	+ + +	+ + + +	+ + +	+ + + +	+ + + +	+ + +
Bombesin	+ + + +	+ +	+ +	+ + + +	+ + +	+ +
Vasopressin	+ + +	+ +	−	+ + +	+ +	+ +
Insulin	+ + + +	+ + + +	+ + +		+ + +	+ + +
EGF	+ + + +	+ + +	+ +	+ + +	−	+
PGE$_1$	+ + +	+ +	+ +	+ + +	+	−

Table 12.3   *The sequence of cell-cycle events which is initiated by the actions of mitogens*

Interaction of mitogens with plasma-membrane receptors

Formation of intracellular messengers and activation of protein kinases

Transcription of primary response genes (not dependent on protein synthesis)

Transcription of late genes (dependent on protein synthesis)

Increased rate of biosynthetic reactions

Synthesis of DNA and duplication of chromosomes

Separation of the chromosomes to form two daughter nuclei

Cytokinesis (division of the cytoplasm and the cellular membranes)

synthesis, and to divide by the re-addition of growth factors to the growth medium. Platelet-derived growth factor (PDGF) and bombesin can act alone to induce mitogenesis whilst a number of other growth factors act synergistically. The individual growth factors and combinations of two growth factors which induce mitogenesis in Swiss 3T3 fibroblasts, and the relative effectiveness of these growth factors in stimulating DNA synthesis, are listed in Table. 12.2.

Mitogens initiate a complex sequence of events which constitute the steps of the cell cycle (Table 12.3). For Swiss 3T3 fibroblasts, each cycle of cell division takes about 12 h to complete. The process of mitosis occupies 1–2 h. At least four major targets are activated or modified by mitogens. These are sequence-specific DNA-binding proteins, the p34^{cdc2} protein–serine (threonine) kinase which controls the cell cycle, enzymes which catalyse biosynthetic reactions, and enzymes and proteins which induce changes in the shape of the cytoskeleton (Fig. 12.1).

In their natural environment, proliferating cells are often exposed to combinations of external mitogenic signals. Different combinations of pathways of intracellular communication are activated by the main environmental signals which stimulate mitogenesis. Both PDGF and bombesin activate the Ca^{2+} and protein kinase C pathways (Fig. 12.2). In addition, each of these agonists induces the synthesis of PGE$_1$. This metabolite of arachidonic acid is released from the cell, acts on a plasma-membrane receptor, and increases the intracellular concentration of cyclic AMP (Fig. 12.2). While PDGF also activates the PDGF receptor protein–tyrosine kinase, bombesin can stimulate proliferation apparently without activation of a protein–tyrosine kinase (Fig. 12.2).

Insulin, which in Swiss 3T3 fibroblasts acts

at insulin-like growth factor-1 (IGF_1) receptors, plus PGE_1 and insulin plus vasopressin, are examples of environmental signals which induce the activation of one protein–tyrosine kinase pathway and either the cyclic AMP or the Ca^{2+} plus protein kinase C pathways (Fig. 12.3). However, these combinations of pathways do not seem to be essential since mitogenesis can also apparently be induced by the activation of two protein–tyrosine kinase pathways, those initiated by insulin and EGF (Fig. 12.3). Thus it seems that at least two different pathways of intracellular communication must be activated

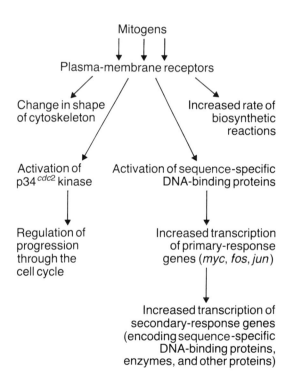

Fig. 12.1 The main categories of intracellular processes that are stimulated by mitogens and which lead to cell proliferation. The single arrows between the plasma-membrane receptors and the individual intracellular processes represent one or more pathways of intracellular communication. Some of these individual pathways are described in Figs 12.2 and 12.3. Each of the processes shown is probably initiated at different times after the binding of mitogens to plasma-membrane receptors.

in order to induce mitogenesis. Of the pathways which can be activated, several possible combinations appear to be equally effective.

Oncogenes can also activate parallel pathways of intracellular communication. Transfection of an established culture of fibroblasts, such as NIH-3T3 fibroblasts, with a single gene, one of the *ras* oncogenes, leads to dramatic changes in cell growth and structure. The cells continue to proliferate in the absence of mitogens and show an altered morphology. The synthesis of relatively large amounts of the oncogenic *ras* protein and the actions of this mutant protein dominate the functions conducted by normal *ras* proteins.

Whilst the precise functions of the low molecular weight GTP-binding proteins encoded by the normal counterparts of the *ras* oncogenes are not known, it is known that the oncogenic *ras* protein hydrolyses GTP at a much slower rate than its normal counterpart and is either constitutively active or is unable to transmit a critical signal. This results in constitutive activation of at least two pathways of intracellular communication. One is the protein kinase C pathway which, in conjunction with at least one other activated pathway, stimulates cell proliferation in a mitogen-independent manner; the other is probably involved in determining the shape of the cytoskeleton and the distribution of cellular membranes. Activation or inhibition of this latter pathway may lead to an alteration in cell morphology.

12.4 Pathways of intracellular communication initiated by insulin

Although insulin was the first hormone discovered, and the insulin receptor was one of the first hormone receptors for which the structure was determined, the mechanism by which insulin exerts it effects on cells is still not well understood. Insulin has diverse effects on cell function including the stimulation of glucose oxidation,

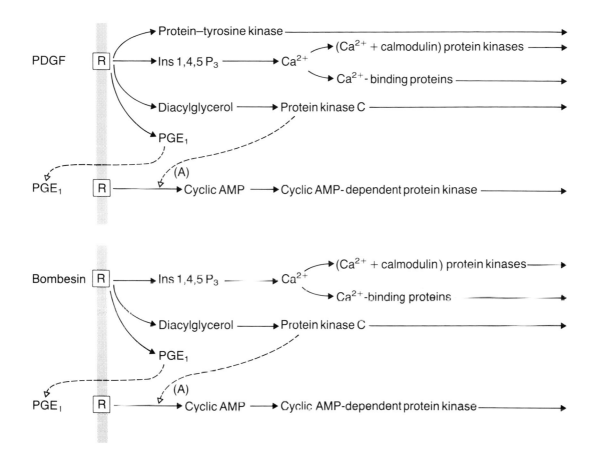

Fig. 12.2   The initial pathways of intracellular communication that are activated when PDGF or bombesin bind to their plasma-membrane receptors (R) and act to induce the proliferation of Swiss 3T3 fibroblasts. One or more of these pathways links plasma-membrane receptors to each of the intracellular processes described in Fig. 12.1. Bombesin and PDGF each induce the synthesis of prostaglandin E_1 (PGE_1) which moves out of the cell to the extracellular fluid and binds to a receptor on the plasma membrane. This, in turn, activates adenylate cyclase and increases the intracellular concentration of cyclic AMP. Adenylate cyclase is also activated (A) by phosphorylation catalysed by protein kinase C.

stimulation of glycogen and triglyceride synthesis, inhibition of lipolysis and proteolysis, and stimulation of the synthesis of a number of proteins. One of the actions of insulin that has received particular attention is the stimulation of glucose uptake in skeletal muscle and adipose tissue. In the cells of these tissues, insulin stimulates the translocation of a distinct insulin-regulatable glucose transporter from an intracellular-membrane pool of transporters, called the low density microsomes, to the plasma membrane. The action of insulin also results in an activation of the transporters.

The combination of insulin with its plasma-membrane receptor leads to the phosphorylation of serine or threonine residues on specific intracellular target proteins and to the dephosphorylation of serine phosphate or threonine phosphate residues on other specific target proteins. Insulin probably exerts most of its effects on the phosphorylation state of these target proteins through a series of protein kinases and

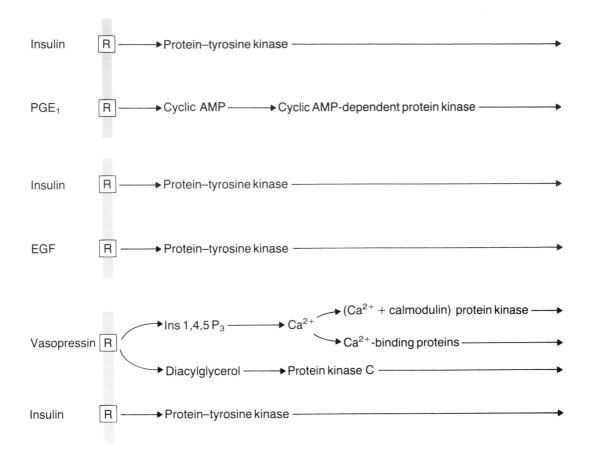

Fig. 12.3 The initial pathways of intracellular communication that are activated when combinations of two growth factors, through interaction with their plasma-membrane receptors (R), act synergistically to induce the proliferation of Swiss 3T3 fibroblasts. One or more of these pathways links plasma-membrane receptors to each of the intracellular processes described in Fig. 12.1. In Swiss 3T3 fibroblasts, insulin exerts its effects by binding to the receptor for insulin-like growth factor-1 (IGF-1).

phosphoprotein phosphatases which, by mechanisms that are not well understood, are probably linked to the insulin receptor protein–tyrosine kinase. A subset of insulin effects, including some of those on regulatory enzymes in the pathways of intermediary metabolism, are mediated by a decrease in the intracellular concentration of cyclic AMP. Other subsets of insulin action may be mediated by the activation of protein kinase C, the activation of phosphatidylinositol kinase, and by an inositol phosphate

glycan mobile messenger. However, the roles of these enzymes and inositol phosphate glycan in the action of insulin are not firmly established.

Many investigators have searched for the existence of a mobile intracellular messenger for insulin. A number of possible candidates have been proposed during the past 20 years. In 1986, Saltiel and Cuatrecasas discovered that insulin stimulates the hydrolysis of glycosyl-phosphatidylinositol to yield inositol phosphate glycan and a species of diacylglycerol. The full structures of glycosyl-phosphatidylinositol and inositol phosphate glycan have not been determined. Inositol phosphate glycan is a complex polysaccharide which contains inositol phosphate glucosamine. Glycosyl-phosphatidylinositol, from which inositol phosphate glycan is derived, is a complex glycosylated phosphatidylinositol.

In cell-free systems, inositol phosphate glycan mimics a number of the actions of insulin, including activation of pyruvate dehydrogenase and cyclic AMP phosphodiesterase. The results of these *in vitro* experiments suggest that inositol phosphate glycan could mediate many of the actions of insulin on intermediary metabolism. However, there is no evidence to indicate that this molecule acts as an intracellular messenger for insulin in intact cells.

12.5   Some general themes which emerge from consideration of the pathways of intracellular communication

A number of general themes emerge from an overview of the present knowledge of pathways of intracellular communication. Some of these themes will be considered briefly in this section, beginning with the idea that many signal pulses are transient. For example, pronounced increases in $[Ca^{2+}]_i$ and Ins 1, 4, 5 P_3 may last for only a minute, and those in cyclic AMP for several minutes. Other examples are the mitogen-induced increases in the concentration of proteins, such as the *fos* and *myc* proteins, encoded by the immediate early genes. These increases occur over a period of about 15 min. The transient nature of all these signals is largely due to strong feedback-control mechanisms. Inhibition by protein kinase C of receptor or G protein function, inhibition by increased $[Ca^{2+}]_i$ and by protein kinase C of Ins 1, 4, 5 P_3 generation, and rapid degradation of immediate early proteins and the mRNA which encodes

these proteins are examples of some of these feedback-control mechanisms.

Many of the components of intracellular signalling pathways might be regarded as switches which direct the flow of information along a particular pathway. One of the best example of these switches are the oligomeric G proteins. These direct a specific extracellular signal, received by a plasma-membrane receptor, to a specific intracellular effector protein. Another example of switches are the monomeric GTP-binding proteins which are required for vesicle secretion. These probably act as a switch which ensures that secretory vesicles are directed to the correct target membrane.

The transmission of intracellular signals is principally dependent on two types of molecular interaction involving proteins and metabolites. These are allosteric interactions, which utilize specific sequences of amino-acid residues in a polypeptide chain, and sequence-independent interactions. Examples of allosteric interactions are the activation of protein–serine (threonine) kinase by mobile intracellular messengers, the inhibition of protein kinase activity by pseudo-substrate regions, and the activation of the monovalent cation channel by cyclic GMP in cells of the retina. Examples of sequence-independent interactions are the binding of calmodulin to calmodulin-binding proteins, the binding of sequence-specific DNA-binding proteins to DNA, and the interaction of proteins containing signal sequences with their receptors, in the process by which these proteins are directed to specific regions of the cell such as the nucleus.

H. R. Bourne (1988) has used the term 'signal transducer protein' to describe the general features of key proteins involved in intracellular communication. This general model proposes that all such proteins possess a detector and a generator component while some may also possess a timing device (timer) and a modulator

(Fig. 12.4). The detector receives the primary input signal, the generator creates the output signal, the timer determines the duration of the signal pulse, and the modulator allows modification of signal transmission by a secondary input signal. While this is probably an over generalization of the functions of a number of signalling proteins, it does help to gain a picture of the role of the proteins within a signalling network.

An example of the structure of a signal transducer protein is the protein complex composed of an agonist receptor, an oligomeric G protein, and an effector protein, such as adenylate cyclase. The input signal for this system is an agonist, the output signal is cyclic AMP, the timer is the oligomeric G protein which hydrolyses GTP at a given rate, and the modulation is achieved by phosphorylation of the receptor or oligomeric G protein by a protein kinase such as protein kinase C.

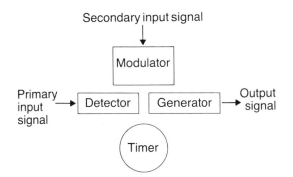

Fig. 12.4 A scheme which shows the general design of a signal transducing protein or protein complex proposed by Bourne (1988). This generalized model can be applied to most proteins involved in the transmission of signals in cells. Examples are plasma-membrane receptor–G protein–effector protein complexes, protein kinases, and sequence-specific DNA-binding proteins. All these proteins contain a signal detector, which recognizes a primary input signal, and a signal generator, which forms the output signal. The protein or protein complex may also contain a modulator which allows a secondary input signal to influence signal transduction by the detector and generator, and a timer, which regulates the duration of the signal pulse transmitted between the detector and generator.

Some multienzyme signal transducer complexes may allow interactions between different signalling pathways. Ullrich and Schlessinger (1990) have proposed that such complexes may be involved in the transmission of signals which originate from the PDGF and epidermal growth factor (EGF) receptors. These complexes probably consist of the receptor protein–tyrosine kinase, phosphatidylinositol 4,5 bisphosphate-specific phospholipase C_γ, the *ras* GTPase activating protein (*ras* GAP), phosphatidylinositol 3-phosphate kinase, and the *raf* protein–serine (threonine) kinase. The existence of such putative enzyme complexes may allow one agonist, such as PDGF, to activate a large number of intracellular signalling pathways.

Specific pathways of intracellular communication are composed of different combinations of a fixed number of signalling elements. For example, a relatively small number of sequence-specific transcription factors can probably regulate the transcription of a large number of different genes. Moreover, different combinations of mobile intracellular messenger systems and protein–tyrosine kinase systems can deliver a specific extracellular signal (which may be composed of a change in the extracellular concentrations of more than one agonist) to induce a specific cellular response.

In some instances an extracellular signal elicits the activation of one or more of several parallel signalling pathways which each appear to convey the same information to a specific intracellular target protein (Fig. 12.5). The existence of these parallel pathways may reflect a redundancy that has evolved in order to prevent a breakdown in signalling, or it may reflect subtle qualitative and quantitative differences in the responses induced by different agonists or by different combinations of agonists.

The last theme to be considered is how the nature of the pathways of intracellular communication reflects the evolution of these path-

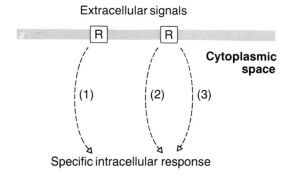

Extracellular signals

Cytoplasmic space

(1)   (2)   (3)

Specific intracellular response

Fig. 12.5 A schematic representation of the idea of redundancy in the transmission of a signal from plasma-membrane receptors to induce a specific response within the cell. Three different parallel signalling pathways (1, 2, and 3), one or more of which may be redundant, are shown linking two plasma-membrane receptors (R) to yield a specific intracellular response.

ways. The target proteins activated by any particular mobile intracellular messenger or protein kinase system do not usually fall into one particular category of structure or function. Thus one particular protein kinase does not regulate only sequence-specific DNA-binding proteins, another does not regulate only rate-limiting enzymes in metabolic pathways, and another, enzymes and proteins which regulate the structure of the cytoskeleton. Moreover, the actions of each of cyclic AMP, cyclic GMP, Ca^{2+}, diacylglycerol, and Ins 1, 4, 5 P_3 are not confined to a particular set of intracellular functions. Rather, a particular protein kinase or mobile intracellular messenger affects a variety of different processes which, at first examination, appear to be haphazard and do not appear to follow a logical sequence.

Achievement of the desired end-response of a cell seems to have remained pre-eminent in evolution of the system of intracellular communication. This means that an evolutionary

need, for example the signal required for stimulation of the release of secretory granules, has been met by the pathway or pathways of intracellular communication most fitted to meet that need.

12.6   Directions of future research

Future research on intracellular communication is likely to reveal new information in two major areas. The first is completion of the knowledge of the steps which compose each individual pathway of intracellular communication. Examples of steps in these pathways that have not yet been fully defined include the nature of all the genes, the transcription of which is increased by mitogens or other agonists, and the nature and function of the proteins encoded by these genes; the nature, location, and function of all the target proteins for the protein–tyrosine kinases and for protein kinase C, and how these kinases interact with these targets within the cytoplasmic space of the cell; the nature and function of all the target proteins for other protein kinases such as cyclic AMP-dependent and $(Ca^{2+} + calmodulin)$-dependent protein kinases; the effects that protein kinases exert on the structure of the cytoskeleton; and details of the signal transmission mediated by a number of proteins encoded by oncogenes such as the *ras* proteins.

The second major area of new information is likely to be a description of how the different intracellular signalling pathways are integrated in space (the physical pathway through the cytoplasmic space) and time. A complete description of the pathways of intracellular communication will only be possible when this integration is achieved. This phase of research is still some way off. It may ultimately require a computer program which can simulate the multiple signalling pathways, the timing of signal pulses, the direction of the signals, and interactions between the different signalling pathways.

12.7 Summary

In most cells, more than one pathway of intracellular communication is activated by signals in the extracellular environment. This can result from either the action of a single agonist or the actions of more than one agonist. An example of the use of multiple parallel pathways of intracellular communication is the stimulation of cell proliferation by mitogens. These agonists activate at least two of the pathways that are mediated by Ca^{2+}, protein kinase C, cyclic AMP, or a receptor protein–tyrosine kinase. In most cells there are interactions between the different pathways of intracellular communication. The most clearly defined interactions are those between Ca^{2+} and cyclic AMP, protein kinase C and plasma membrane receptors and G proteins, protein kinase C and inositol polyphosphates, and between different sequence-specific DNA-binding proteins.

Insulin is another example of an extracellular signal which probably activates more than one pathway of intracellular communication. Elucidation of the intracellular mechanisms of insulin action have proved difficult and the results inconclusive. Most actions of insulin are probably mediated by the insulin receptor protein–tyrosine kinase. Some subsets of the effects of insulin may be mediated by a decrease in the concentration of cyclic AMP, the activation of protein kinase C, the action of an inositol phosphate glycan, a molecule with a complex structure which is derived from glycosyl-phosphatidylinositol, and the activation of phosphatidylinositol kinase. However, with the exception of cyclic AMP, the roles of these pathways in insulin action have not been firmly established.

Several general themes emerge from consideration of the known pathways of intracellular communication. These themes include the transient nature of many intracellular signals, the action of signalling proteins as switches, the role of allosteric interactions, the role of interactions between proteins which are amino-acid sequence independent, the combination of a number of different signalling elements to constitute a particular signalling pathway, and the existence of parallel signalling pathways which apparently deliver the same final signal but which may represent a redundancy in signalling power which protects the cell against a breakdown in signal transduction.

Future research on pathways of intracellular communication is likely to provide new information in two main areas—the completion of elucidation of all the components of each signalling pathway, for example the sequence of events which links the activation of protein–tyrosine kinases and cellular responses, and the development of a description of each signalling pathway in terms of the timing of the signal pulse, its spatial location within the cell, and its integration with other signalling pathways.

References

Bourne, H. R. (1988). Summary: signals past, present and future. *Cold Spring Harbor Symp. Quant. Biol.*, **53**, 1019–31.

Rozengurt, E. (1986). Early signals in the mitogenic response. *Science*, **234**, 161–6.

Saltiel, A. R. and Cuatrecasas, P. (1986). Insulin stimulates the generation from hepatic plasma membranes of modulators derived from an inositol glycolipid. *Proc. Natl Acad. Sci. USA*, **83**, 5793–7.

Ullrich, A. and Schlessinger, J. (1990). Signal transduction by receptors with tyrosine kinase activity. *Cell*, **61**, 203–12.

Further reading

Alkon, D. L. and Rasmussen, H. (1988). A spatial–temporal model of cell activation. *Science* **239**, 998–1005.

325 Interactions between pathways of intracellular communication

Bray, D. and Vasiliev, J. (1989). Networks from mutants. *Nature*, **338**, 203–4.

Cantley, L. C., Auger, K. R., Carpenter, C., Duckworth, B., Graziani, A., Kapeller, R., and Soltoff, S. (1991). Oncogenese and signal transduction. *Cell*, **64**, 281–302.

Hunter, T. (1991). Cooperation between oncogenes. *Cell*, **64**, 249–70.

Low, M. G. and Saltiel, A. R. (1988). Structural and functional roles of glycosyl-phosphatidylinositol in membranes. *Science*, **239**, 268–75.

Rasmussen, H. (1981). *Calcium and cAMP as synarchic messengers*. Wiley, New York.

Rozengurt, E. (1989). Signal transduction pathways in mitogenesis. *Br. Med. Bulletin*, **45**, 515–28.

Index